Fogoros' Electrophysiologic Testing

Fogoros' Electrophysiologic Testing

Seventh Edition

Richard N. Fogoros, MD
Danville
PA, USA

John M. Mandrola, MD
Louisville
KY, USA

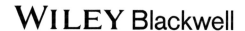

This edition first published 2023
© 2023 John Wiley & Sons Ltd

Edition History
John Wiley & Sons Ltd (6e, 2018)

The right of Richard N. Fogoros and John M. Mandrola to be identified as the authors of this work has been asserted in accordance with law.

Registered Offices
John Wiley & Sons, Inc., 111 River Street, Hoboken, NJ 07030, USA
John Wiley & Sons Ltd, The Atrium, Southern Gate, Chichester, West Sussex, PO19 8SQ, UK

For details of our global editorial offices, customer services, and more information about Wiley products visit us at www.wiley.com.

Wiley also publishes its books in a variety of electronic formats and by print-on-demand. Some content that appears in standard print versions of this book may not be available in other formats.

Library of Congress Cataloging-in-Publication Data applied for

ISBN: 9781119855675 (hardback)

Cover Design: Wiley
Cover Images: © Artem Rudik/Shutterstock; © AlexLMX/Shutterstock

Set in 10/12pt WarnockPro by Straive, Chennai, India
Printed and bound by CPI Group (UK) Ltd, Croydon, CR0 4YY

C9781119855675_270724

Contents

Contents

Preface to the Seventh Edition

Our goal in producing this seventh edition of *Electrophysiologic Testing* is the same as it has been from the beginning – to demystify the field of cardiac electrophysiology for the nonelectrophysiologist. This book is meant for students, residents, cardiology fellows (or even cardiologists!), primary care physicians, physician assistants, nurses, technicians, and anyone else who needs a basic and relatively quick understanding of electrophysiology and cardiac arrhythmias. As always, we have aimed to explain, as clearly and simply as possible, the key concepts of the mechanisms, evaluation, and treatment of cardiac arrhythmias, as elucidated in the electrophysiology laboratory.

In this edition, we have striven to update what needed to be updated without losing sight of that original, motivating goal. To keep things as simple as possible, in this edition we have deemphasized (or eliminated) aspects of electrophysiologic testing that were once important to electrophysiologists, but today are of mainly historical interest. Throughout the book, we have focused on the basic aspects of cardiac electrophysiology that are critical to understanding and treating cardiac arrhythmias. We have most extensively updated the chapters on ablation therapy, the most rapidly evolving aspect of clinical electrophysiology. Additionally, we have added a new chapter on conduction system pacing, which we believe will become very important to clinicians in the near future.

We sincerely hope and trust that this seventh edition of *Electro-physiology Testing* will remain as helpful to a new generation of readers as, we are told, past editions have been to previous generations.

Richard N. Fogoros, MD
Danville, PA

John M. Mandrola, MD
Louisville, KY

Part I

Disorders of the Heart Rhythm: Basic Principles

1

The Cardiac Electrical System

The heart spontaneously generates electrical impulses, and these electrical impulses are vital to all cardiac functions. On a basic level, by controlling the flux of calcium ions across the cardiac cell membrane, these electrical impulses trigger cardiac muscle contraction. On a higher level, the heart's electrical impulses organize the sequence of muscle contractions during each heartbeat, important for optimizing the cardiac stroke volume. Finally, the pattern and timing of these impulses determine the heart rhythm. Derangements in this rhythm often impair the heart's ability to pump enough blood to meet the body's demands.

The heart's electrical system is fundamental to cardiac function. The study of the electrical system of the heart is called cardiac electrophysiology, and the main concern of the field of electrophysiology is the mechanisms and therapy of cardiac arrhythmias. The electrophysiology study (EP study) is the most definitive method of evaluating the cardiac electrical system. It is the subject of this book.

As an introduction to the field of electrophysiology and to the EP study, this chapter reviews the anatomy of the cardiac electrical system and describes how the electrical impulse is generated and propagated.

The anatomy of the heart's electrical system

The heart's electrical impulse originates in the sinoatrial (SA) node, located high in the right atrium near the superior vena cava. The impulse leaves the SA node and spreads radially across both atria. When the impulse reaches the atrioventricular (AV) groove, it encounters the "skeleton of the heart," the fibrous structure to which

Fogoros' Electrophysiologic Testing, Seventh Edition. Richard N. Fogoros and John M. Mandrola.
© 2023 John Wiley & Sons Ltd. Published 2023 by John Wiley & Sons Ltd.

the valve rings are attached, and which separates the atria from the ventricles. This fibrous structure is electrically inert and acts as an insulator – the electrical impulse cannot cross this structure. The electrical impulse would be prevented from crossing over to the ventricular side of the AV groove if not for the specialized AV conducting tissues: the AV node and the bundle of His (Figure 1.1).

As the electrical impulse enters the AV node, its conduction is slowed because of the electrophysiologic properties of the AV nodal tissue. This slowing is reflected in the PR interval on the surface electrocardiogram (ECG). Leaving the AV node, the electrical impulse enters the His bundle, the most proximal part of the rapidly conducting His–Purkinje system. The His bundle penetrates the fibrous skeleton and delivers the impulse to the ventricular side of the AV groove.

Once on the ventricular side, the electrical impulse follows the His bundle as it branches into the right and left bundle branches. Branching of the Purkinje fibers continues distally to the furthermost reaches

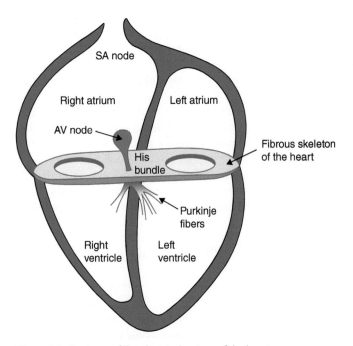

Figure 1.1 Anatomy of the electrical system of the heart.

of the ventricular myocardium. The electrical impulse is thus rapidly distributed throughout the ventricles.

The "job" of the heart's electrical system is to organize the sequence of myocardial contraction with each heartbeat. First, as the electrical impulse spreads over the atria toward the AV groove, the atria contract. The delay provided by the AV node allows for complete atrial emptying before the electrical impulse reaches the ventricles. Once the impulse leaves the AV node, it is distributed rapidly throughout the ventricular muscle by the Purkinje fibers, providing for brisk and orderly ventricular contraction.

We next consider the character of the electrical impulse, its generation, and its propagation.

The cardiac action potential

The cardiac action potential is one of the most misunderstood topics in cardiology. The fact that electrophysiologists claim to understand it is also a leading cause of the mystique that surrounds them and their favorite test, the EP study. Since the purpose of this book is to debunk the mystery of electrophysiology studies, we must gain a basic understanding of the cardiac action potential. Fortunately, it's easier than legend would have it.

Although most of us would like to think of cardiac arrhythmias as an irritation or "itch" of the heart (and of antiarrhythmic drugs as a balm or a salve that soothes the itch), this notion of arrhythmias is wrong and can lead to the faulty management of patients with arrhythmias. In fact, the behavior of the heart's electrical impulse and of the cardiac rhythm is largely determined by the shape of the action potential; the effect of antiarrhythmic drugs is determined by how they change that shape.

The inside of the cardiac cell, like all living cells, has a negative electrical charge compared to the outside of the cell. The resulting voltage difference across the cell membrane is called the *transmembrane potential*. The resting transmembrane potential (which is -80 to -90 mV in cardiac muscle) is the result of an accumulation of negatively charged molecules (called ions) within the cell. Most of the body's cells are happy with this arrangement and live out their lives without considering any other possibilities.

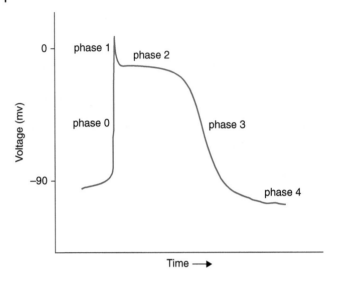

Figure 1.2 The cardiac action potential.

Cardiac cells, however, are different – they are excitable cells. When excitable cells are stimulated appropriately, tiny pores or channels in the cell membrane open and close sequentially in a stereotyped fashion. The opening of these channels allows ions to travel back and forth across the cell membrane (again in a stereotyped fashion), leading to patterned changes in the transmembrane potential. When these stereotypic voltage changes are graphed against time, the result is the cardiac action potential (Figure 1.2). The action potential reflects the electrical activity of a single cardiac cell.

Figure 1.2 shows the five phases of the action potential, which encompass three general periods: depolarization, repolarization, and the resting phase.

Depolarization

The depolarization phase (phase 0) is where the "action" of the action potential is. Depolarization occurs when the rapid sodium channels in the cell membrane are stimulated to open. When this happens, positively charged sodium ions rush into the cell, causing a rapid, positively directed change in the transmembrane potential. The resultant voltage spike is called *depolarization*. When we speak of the heart's electrical impulse, we are speaking of this depolarization.

Depolarization of one cell tends to cause adjacent cardiac cells to depolarize, because the voltage spike of a cell's depolarization causes the sodium channels in the nearby cells to open. Thus, once a cardiac cell is stimulated to depolarize, the wave of depolarization (the electrical impulse) is propagated across the heart, cell by cell.

The speed of depolarization of a cell (reflected by the slope of phase 0 of the action potential) determines how soon the next cell will depolarize, and thus determines the speed at which the electrical impulse is propagated across the heart. If we do something to change the speed at which sodium ions enter the cell (and thus change the slope of phase 0), we therefore change the speed of conduction (the conduction velocity) of cardiac tissue.

Repolarization

Once a cell is depolarized, it cannot be depolarized again until the ionic fluxes that occur during depolarization are reversed. The process of getting the ions back to where they started is called *repolarization*. The repolarization of the cardiac cell roughly corresponds to phases 1 through 3 (i.e., the width) of the action potential. Because a second depolarization cannot take place until repolarization occurs, the time from the end of phase 0 to late in phase 3 is called the *refractory period* of cardiac tissue.

Repolarization of the cardiac cells is complex and incompletely understood. The main ideas behind repolarization, however, are simple.

- Repolarization returns the cardiac action potential to the resting transmembrane potential.
- It takes time to do this.
- The time that it takes to do this, roughly corresponding to the width of the action potential, is the refractory period of cardiac tissue.

There is an additional point of interest regarding repolarization of the cardiac action potential. Phase 2 of the action potential, the so-called plateau phase, can be viewed as interrupting and prolonging the repolarization that begins in phase 1. This plateau phase, which is unique to cardiac cells (e.g., it is not seen in nerve cells), gives duration to the cardiac potential. It is mostly mediated by the slow calcium channels, which allow positively charged calcium ions to slowly enter the cell, thus interrupting repolarization and prolonging the refractory period. The calcium channels have other important effects in electrophysiology, as we will see.

The resting phase

For most cardiac cells, the resting phase (the period of time between action potentials, corresponding to phase 4) is quiescent, and there is no net movement of ions across the cell membrane.

For some cells, however, the so-called resting phase is not quiescent. In these cells, there is leakage of ions back and forth across the cell membrane during phase 4, in such a way as to cause a gradual increase in transmembrane potential (Figure 1.3). When the transmembrane potential is high enough (i.e., when it reaches the threshold voltage), the appropriate channels are activated to cause the cell to depolarize. Because this depolarization, like any depolarization, can stimulate nearby cells to depolarize in turn, the spontaneously generated electrical impulse can be propagated across the heart. This phase 4 activity, which leads to spontaneous depolarization, is called *automaticity*.

Automaticity is the mechanism by which the normal heart rhythm is generated. Cells in the SA node (the pacemaker of the heart) normally have the fastest phase 4 activity within the heart. The spontaneously occurring action potentials in the SA node are propagated as described earlier, resulting in normal sinus rhythm. If, for any reason, the automaticity of the sinus node should fail, there are

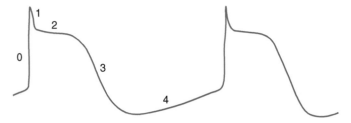

Figure 1.3 Automaticity. In some cardiac cells, there is a leakage of ions across the cell membrane during phase 4, in such a way as to cause a gradual, positively directed change in transmembrane voltage. When the transmembrane voltage becomes sufficiently positive, the appropriate channels are activated to automatically generate another action potential. This spontaneous generation of action potentials due to phase 4 activity is called automaticity.

usually secondary pacemaker cells (often located in the AV junction) to take over the pacemaker function of the heart, but at a slower rate. Thus, the shape of the action potential determines the conduction velocity, refractory period, and automaticity of cardiac tissue. Later, we will see how these three electrophysiologic characteristics directly affect the mechanisms of cardiac rhythms, both normal and abnormal. To a large extent, the purpose of the EP study is to assess the conduction velocities, refractory periods, and automaticity of various portions of the heart's electrical system.

Localized variations in the heart's electrical system

In understanding cardiac arrhythmias, it is important to consider two issues involving localized differences in the heart's electrical system: variations in the action potential and variations in autonomic innervation.

Localized differences in the action potential

Different cardiac cells have differently shaped action potentials. The action potential we have been using as a model (see Figure 1.2) is a

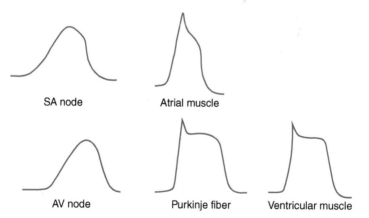

SA node   Atrial muscle

AV node   Purkinje fiber   Ventricular muscle

Figure 1.4 Localized differences in the cardiac action potential. Cardiac action potentials from different locations within the heart have different shapes. These differences account for the differences seen in the electrophysiologic properties of various tissues within the heart.

typical Purkinje fiber action potential. Figure 1.4 shows representative action potentials from several key locations of the heart – note the differences in shape.

The action potentials that differ most radically from the Purkinje fiber model are found in the SA and AV nodes. Note that the action potentials from these tissues have slow instead of rapid depolarization phases (phase 0). This slow depolarization occurs because SA and AV nodal tissues lack the rapid sodium channels responsible for the rapid depolarization phase (phase 0) seen in other cardiac tissues. In fact, the SA and AV nodes are thought to be entirely dependent on the slow calcium channel for depolarization. Because the speed of depolarization determines conduction velocity, the SA and AV nodes

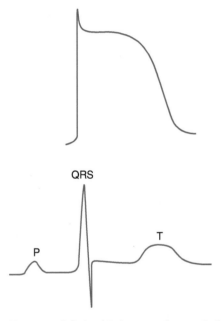

Figure 1.5 Relationship between the ventricular action potential (top) and the surface ECG (bottom). The rapid depolarization phase (phase 0) of the action potential is reflected in the QRS complex on the surface ECG. Because phase 0 is almost instantaneous, the QRS complex yields directional information on ventricular depolarization. In contrast, the repolarization portion of the action potential has significant duration (phases 2 and 3). Consequently, the portion of the surface ECG that reflects repolarization (the ST segment and T wave) yields little directional information. PR interval, beginning of P to beginning of QRS; ST segment, end of QRS to beginning of T; QT interval, beginning of QRS to end of T.

conduct electrical impulses slowly. The slow conduction in the AV node is reflected in the PR interval on the surface ECG (Figure 1.5).

Localized differences in autonomic innervation

In general, an increase in sympathetic tone, for example during exercise, causes enhanced automaticity (pacemaker cells fire more rapidly), increased conduction velocity (electrical impulses are propagated more rapidly), and decreased action potential duration and thus decreased refractory periods (cells become ready for repeated depolarizations more quickly). Parasympathetic tone has the opposite effect (i.e., depressed automaticity, decreased conduction velocity, and increased refractory periods).

Sympathetic and parasympathetic fibers richly innervate both the SA and the AV node. In the remainder of the heart's electrical system, while sympathetic innervation is abundant, parasympathetic innervation is relatively sparse. Thus, changes in parasympathetic tone have a relatively greater effect on the SA and AV nodal tissues than on other tissues of the heart. This fact has implications for the diagnosis and treatment of some heart rhythm disturbances.

Relationship between action potential and surface ECG

The cardiac action potential represents the electrical activity of a single cardiac cell. But the surface ECG reflects the electrical activity of the entire heart – essentially, the sum of all the action potentials of all cardiac cells. Consequently, the information one can glean from the surface ECG derives from the characteristics of the action potential (see Figure 1.5).

For most cardiac cells, the depolarization phase of the action potential is essentially instantaneous (occurring in 1–3 ms) and occurs sequentially, from cell to cell. Thus, the instantaneous wave of depolarization can be followed across the heart by studying the ECG. The P wave represents the depolarization front as it traverses the atria, and the QRS complex tracks the wave of depolarization as it spreads across the ventricles. Changes in the spread of the electrical impulse, such as occur in bundle branch block or transmural myocardial infarction, can be readily diagnosed by inspecting the ECG. Because the depolarization phase of the action potential is relatively instantaneous, the P wave and the QRS complex can yield specific directional information (i.e., information on the sequence of depolarization of cardiac muscle).

In contrast, the repolarization phase of the action potential is not instantaneous – indeed, repolarization has significant duration. While depolarization occurs from cell to cell sequentially, repolarization occurs in many cardiac cells simultaneously. For this reason, the ST segment and T wave (the portions of the surface ECG that reflect ventricular repolarization) give little directional information, and abnormalities in the ST segments and T waves are most often (and quite properly) interpreted as being nonspecific. The QT interval represents the time of repolarization of the ventricular myocardium and reflects the average action potential duration of ventricular muscle.

2

Abnormal Heart Rhythms

Abnormalities in the electrical system of the heart result in two general types of cardiac arrhythmia: heart rhythms that are too slow (brady-arrhythmias) and heart rhythms that are too fast (tachyarrhythmias).

Bradyarrhythmias

There are two broad categories of abnormally slow heart rhythms – the failure of pacemaker cells to generate appropriate electrical impulses (disorders of automaticity) and the failure to propagate electrical impulses appropriately (heart block).

Failure of impulse generation

Failure of sinoatrial (SA) nodal automaticity, resulting in an insufficient number of electrical impulses emanating from the SA node (i.e., sinus bradycardia [Figure 2.1]), is the most common cause of bradyarrhythmias. If the slowed heart rate is insufficient to meet the body's demands, symptoms result. Symptomatic sinus bradycardia is called *sick sinus syndrome*. If sinus slowing is profound, subsidiary pacemakers located near the atrioventricular (AV) junction can take over the pacemaker function of the heart. The electrophysiology study (EP study), as we will see in Chapter 5, can be useful in assessing SA nodal automaticity.

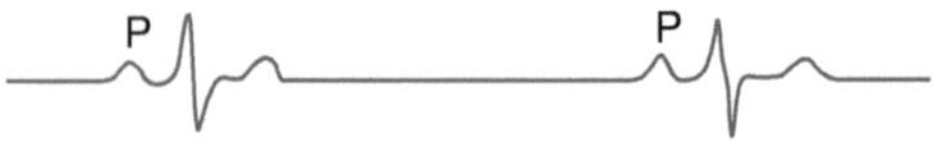

Figure 2.1 Sinus bradycardia.

Failure of impulse propagation

The second major cause of bradyarrhythmias is the failure of the electrical impulses to conduct normally. While conduction block can occur anywhere in the heart, the most common area is the AV junction. This condition, known as *heart block* or *AV block*, implies an abnormality of conduction velocity and/or refractoriness in the conducting system. Because conduction of the electrical impulse to the ventricles depends on the function of the AV node and the His–Purkinje system, heart block is virtually always due to AV nodal or His–Purkinje disease.

Heart block is classified into three categories based on severity (Figure 2.2). First-degree AV block means that, while all atrial impulses are transmitted to the ventricles, intraatrial conduction, conduction through the AV node, and/or conduction through the His bundle is slow (manifested on the electrocardiogram, ECG, by a prolonged PR interval). Second-degree AV block means that conduction to

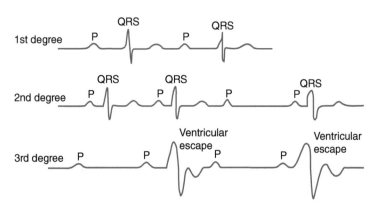

Figure 2.2 Three categories of heart block. In first-degree block (top tracing), all atrial impulses are conducted to the ventricles but conduction is slow (the PR interval is prolonged). In second-degree block (middle tracing), some atrial impulses are conducted and some are not. In third-degree block (bottom tracing), none of the atrial impulses are conducted to the ventricles.

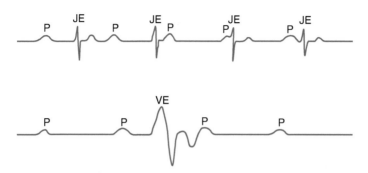

Figure 2.3 Examples of escape pacemakers. When block is localized to the AV node (top tracing), junctional escape pacemakers (JE) are usually stable enough to prevent hemodynamic collapse. When block is located in the distal conducting tissues (bottom tracing), escape pacemakers are usually located in the ventricles (VE) and are slower and much less stable.

the ventricles is intermittent; that is, some impulses are conducted and some are blocked. Third-degree AV block means that block is complete and no atrial impulses are conducted to the ventricles.

If third-degree AV block is present, then sustaining life depends on the function of subsidiary pacemakers distal to the site of block. The competence of these subsidiary pacemakers, and therefore the patient's prognosis, depends largely on the site of block (Figure 2.3). When block is within the AV node, subsidiary pacemakers at the AV junction usually take over the pacemaker function of the heart, resulting in a relatively stable, nonlife-threatening heart rhythm, with a rate that can exceed 50 beats/min. On the other hand, if block is distal to the AV node, the subsidiary pacemakers tend to produce a profoundly slow (usually less than 40 beats/min) and unstable heart rhythm.

If heart block is less than complete (i.e., first or second degree), it is still important to pinpoint the site of block to either the AV node or the His–Purkinje system. First- or second-degree block in the AV node is benign and tends either not to progress or to progress slowly. Permanent pacing is rarely required. First- and especially second-degree block distal to the AV node, on the other hand, tend to progress to a higher degree of block and prophylactic pacing can be indicated if there are symptoms.

Differentiating the site of heart block can usually be done noninvasively by studying the surface ECG and taking advantage of the fact that the AV node has rich autonomic innervation and the His–Purkinje system does not. Sometimes, however, the EP study is useful in locating the site of block. Chapter 5 considers heart block in detail.

Tachyarrhythmias

Cardiac tachyarrhythmias can cause significant mortality and morbidity. It is the ability of the EP study to address the evaluation and treatment of tachyarrhythmias that has brought this procedure into widespread use. We will discuss three mechanisms for tachyarrhythmias: automaticity, reentry, and triggered activity.

Automaticity

Automaticity accounts for normal pacemaker function of the heart. But when abnormal acceleration of phase 4 activity occurs in some location of the heart, an automatic tachyarrhythmia is said to occur (Figure 2.4). Such an abnormal automatic focus can occur anywhere in the heart.

Automaticity accounts for less than 10% of all abnormal tachyarrhythmias. Automatic tachyarrhythmias are usually recognizable by their characteristics and the settings in which they occur.

To understand automatic tachyarrhythmias, it helps to consider the characteristics of sinus tachycardia, which is a *normal* automatic tachycardia. Sinus tachycardia usually occurs as a result of appropriately increased sympathetic tone (for instance, in response to increased metabolic needs during exercise). When sinus tachycardia develops, the heart rate gradually increases from the basic (resting)

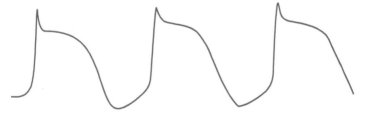

Figure 2.4 Abnormal automaticity causes the rapid generation of action potentials and thus inappropriate tachycardia.

sinus rate; when sinus tachycardia subsides, the rate likewise decreases gradually.

Similarly, automatic tachyarrhythmias often display a warm-up and warm-down in rate when the arrhythmia begins and ends. Analogous to sinus tachycardia, automatic tachyarrhythmias can have metabolic causes, such as acute cardiac ischemia, hypoxemia, hypokalemia, hypomagnesemia, acid–base disorders, high sympathetic tone, and the use of sympathomimetic agents. Therefore, automatic arrhythmias are often seen in acutely ill patients. For example, acute pulmonary disease can lead to multifocal atrial tachycardia, the most common type of automatic atrial tachycardia. Induction of, and recovery from, general anesthesia can cause surges in sympathetic tone, and automatic arrhythmias (both atrial and ventricular) can result. In addition, acute myocardial infarction is often accompanied by early ventricular arrhythmias that are likely automatic in mechanism.

Of all the tachyarrhythmias, automatic arrhythmias most closely resemble an "itch of the heart," and it is tempting to apply the salve of antiarrhythmic drugs. Antiarrhythmic drugs can sometimes decrease automaticity. However, automatic arrhythmias should most often be treated by identifying and reversing the underlying metabolic cause.

Automatic tachyarrhythmias cannot be induced by programmed pacing techniques, so these arrhythmias are generally not amenable to provocative study in the electrophysiology laboratory.

Reentry

Reentry is the most common mechanism for tachyarrhythmias; it is also the most important, because reentrant arrhythmias cause the deaths of hundreds of thousands of people every year. Fortunately, reentrant arrhythmias lend themselves to study in the electrophysiology laboratory. In fact, it was the recognition that most tachyarrhythmias are reentrant in mechanism and that the EP study can help in assessing reentrant arrhythmias that sparked the widespread proliferation of electrophysiology laboratories in the early 1980s.

Unfortunately, the mechanism of reentry is not simple to explain or to understand, and the prerequisites for reentry seem on the surface to be unlikely at best. The failure to understand (and possibly to believe in) reentry has helped the EP study to remain an enigma to most people in the medical profession. The following explanation of reentry therefore errs on the side of simplicity and might offend some electrophysiologists. If the reader can keep an open mind and accept this explanation for now, we hope to show later (in Chapters 6 and 7) that reentry is a compelling explanation for most cardiac tachyarrhythmias.

Reentry requires that the following criteria are met (Figure 2.5). First, two roughly parallel conducting pathways (shown as pathways A and B) must be connected proximally and distally by conducting tissue, thus forming a potential electrical circuit. Second, one of the pathways (pathway B in our example) must have a refractory period that is substantially longer than that of the other pathway. Third, the pathway with the shorter refractory period (pathway A) must conduct electrical impulses more slowly than the other pathway.

If all these prerequisites are met, reentry can be initiated when an appropriately timed premature impulse is introduced to the circuit (Figure 2.6). The premature impulse must enter the circuit at a time when pathway B (the one with the long refractory period) is still refractory from the previous depolarization and at a time when pathway A (the one with the shorter refractory period) has already

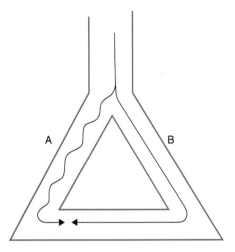

Figure 2.5 Prerequisites for reentry. An anatomic circuit must be present in which two portions of the circuit (pathways A and B in the figure) have electrophysiologic properties that differ from one another in a critical way. In this example, pathway A conducts electrical impulses more slowly than pathway B, while pathway B has a longer refractory period than pathway A.

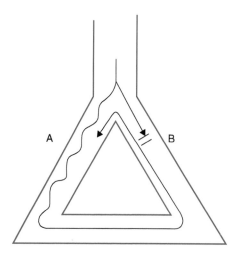

Figure 2.6 Initiation of reentry. If the prerequisites in Figure 2.5 are present, an appropriately timed premature impulse can block in pathway B (which has a relatively long refractory period) while conducting down pathway A. Because conduction down pathway A is slow, pathway B has time to recover, allowing the impulse to conduct retrogradely up pathway B. The impulse can then reenter pathway A. A continuously circulating impulse is thus established.

recovered and is able to accept the premature impulse. While pathway A slowly conducts the premature impulse, pathway B has a chance to recover. By the time the impulse reaches pathway B from the opposite direction, pathway B is no longer refractory and is able to conduct the beat in the retrograde direction (upward in the figure). If this retrograde impulse reenters pathway A and is conducted antegradely (as it is likely to be, given the short refractory period of pathway A), a continuously circulating impulse is established, spinning around and around the reentrant loop. All that remains in order for this reentrant impulse to usurp the rhythm of the heart is for the impulse to exit from the circuit at some point during each lap and thereby depolarize the myocardium outside the loop.

Just as reentry can be initiated by premature beats, it can be terminated by premature beats (Figure 2.7). An appropriately timed impulse can enter the circuit during reentry and collide with the reentrant impulse, thus abolishing the reentrant arrhythmia.

Because reentry depends on critical differences in conduction velocities and refractory periods in the various pathways of the reentrant circuit, and because conduction velocity and refractory periods are

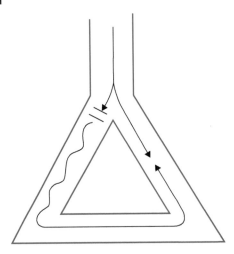

Figure 2.7 Termination of reentry. An appropriately timed premature impulse can enter the circuit during a reentrant tachycardia, collide with the reentrant impulse as shown, and terminate reentry.

determined by the shape of the action potential, it should be obvious that the action potentials in pathway A and pathway B are different from one another. This means that drugs that change the shape of the action potential might be useful in the treatment of reentrant arrhythmias.

Reentrant circuits are common. Some are present at birth, especially those causing supraventricular tachycardias (e.g., reentry associated with AV bypass tracts or with dual SA and AV nodal tracts). More malignant forms of reentrant circuit, however, are usually not congenital but are acquired as cardiac disease develops during life. In reentrant ventricular tachyarrhythmias, the reentrant circuits arise in areas where normal cardiac tissue is interspersed with patches of scar tissue, forming many potential anatomic circuits. Thus, ventricular reentrant circuits usually occur only when scar tissue develops in the ventricles (such as during a myocardial infarction or with cardiomyopathic diseases, such as myocarditis.).

Theoretically, if all the anatomic and electrophysiologic criteria for reentry are present, any impulse that enters the circuit at the appropriate time will induce a reentrant tachycardia. The time from the end of the refractory period of pathway A to the end of the refractory period of pathway B, during which reentry can be induced, is called the *tachycardia zone.* Treating reentrant arrhythmias sometimes involves trying to narrow or abolish the tachycardia zone (by increasing the refractory period of pathway A or decreasing the refractory period of pathway B).

Because reentrant arrhythmias can be reproducibly induced and terminated with appropriately timed impulses, they are ideal for study in the electrophysiology laboratory. In fact, it is mainly the inducibility of reentrant arrhythmias that distinguishes them from automatic arrhythmias in the electrophysiology lab. By inducing reentrant arrhythmias in a controlled setting, the location of the anatomic circuit can be mapped and critical areas ablated.

Triggered activity

Electrophysiologists try to divide the universe of tachyarrhythmias into two parts – automatic arrhythmias (which cannot be induced in the laboratory) and reentrant arrhythmias (which can be induced). This is a useful and practical way of thinking about tachyarrhythmias. Simple and convenient classification systems are usually wrong, however, and this classification system is no exception.

There are other mechanisms for tachyarrhythmias, no doubt including some that have not yet been identified. While most of these other mechanisms can safely be ignored, at least one appears commonly in the clinical setting – triggered activity.

Triggered activity has some features of both automaticity and reentry and can be difficult to distinguish in the electrophysiology laboratory. Like automaticity, triggered activity involves the leakage of positive ions into the cardiac cell, leading to a bump on the action potential (Figure 2.8a) in late phase 3 or early phase 4. This bump is called an *afterdepolarization*. If these afterdepolarizations are of sufficient magnitude to engage the rapid sodium channels (i.e., if they reach the threshold voltage), another action potential can be generated (Figure 2.8b). Thus, triggered activity resembles automaticity in that new action potentials can be generated by leakage of positive ions into the cell. Many electrophysiologists classify triggered activity as a subgroup of automaticity.

Unlike automaticity (and like reentry), however, triggered activity is not always spontaneous (and therefore not truly automatic). Triggered activity can be provoked by premature beats. Thus, triggered activity, like reentry, can be induced with programmed pacing techniques.

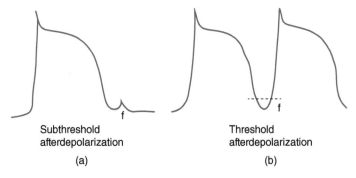

Subthreshold
afterdepolarization

(a)

Threshold
afterdepolarization

(b)

Figure 2.8 Triggered activity. (a) In some circumstances, premature cardiac action potentials will display a late bump (called an afterdepolarization). (b) If the afterdepolarization is of sufficient magnitude, the rapid sodium channels are engaged and a second action potential is generated.

Theoretically, because it can be induced during electrophysiologic testing, triggered activity poses a potential threat to the use of the inducibility of an arrhythmia as the major criterion for diagnosing a reentrant mechanism. If an arrhythmia is induced, the following have been proposed as ways of differentiating between reentry and triggered activity: triggered activity resembles automaticity in displaying warm-up and warm-down; triggered activity is felt to depend on calcium channels and thus may respond to calcium channel blockers; in distinction to most reentrant arrhythmias, inducing arrhythmias due to triggered activity may require introducing a pause into the sequence of paced beats used for induction (such arrhythmias, called "pause-dependent" arrhythmias, will be discussed in Chapter 7); reentry is the more likely mechanism in the presence of underlying structural cardiac disease.

The clinical significance of triggered activity has become more clear in recent years. Triggered activity is most likely the mechanism for digitalis-toxic supraventricular and ventricular arrhythmias, as well as some of the rare cases of ventricular tachycardia that respond to calcium-blocking agents. More importantly, triggered activity is now thought to be the mechanism of torsades de pointes – the polymorphic, pause-dependent ventricular arrhythmias often associated with the use of certain drugs, most notably certain antiarrhythmic drugs.

Triggered activity as a cause of ventricular arrhythmias will be discussed more fully in Chapter 7.

3

Treatment of Arrhythmias

Pharmacologic therapy

Antiarrhythmic drugs are not arrhythmia suppressants in the same way that menthol is a cough suppressant. They do not work by soothing irritable areas. In fact, most antiarrhythmic drugs work merely by changing the shape of the cardiac action potential. By changing the action potential, these drugs alter the conductivity and refractoriness of cardiac tissue – and make reentry less likely to occur.

Channels and gates

Antiarrhythmic drugs change the shape of the action potential by altering the channels that control ionic fluxes across the cardiac cell membrane. The class I antiarrhythmic drugs, which affect the rapid sodium channel, provide the clearest example (Figure 3.1).

The rapid sodium channel is controlled by two gates: the m gate and the h gate. In the resting state (a), the m gate is closed and the h gate is open. When an appropriate stimulus occurs, the m gate opens (b) and positively charged sodium ions enter the cell rapidly, causing the cell to depolarize (phase 0 of the action potential). After a few milliseconds, the h gate slams shut (c), closing the sodium channel and ending phase 0.

Class I antiarrhythmic drugs work by binding to the h gate, making it behave as if it is partially closed (d). In this case, when the m gate is stimulated to open, the opening through which sodium ions enter the cell is narrower (e). Consequently, it takes longer to depolarize the

Fogoros' Electrophysiologic Testing, Seventh Edition. Richard N. Fogoros and John M. Mandrola.
© 2023 John Wiley & Sons Ltd. Published 2023 by John Wiley & Sons Ltd.

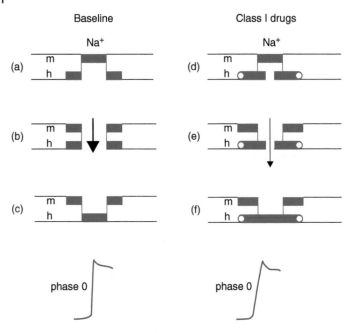

Figure 3.1 The effect of class I drugs on the rapid sodium channel. Images (a) through (c) display the baseline (drug-free) state. In (a), the resting state, the m gate is closed and the h gate is open. The cell is stimulated in (b), causing the m gate to open, thus allowing positively charged sodium ions to enter the cell rapidly (large arrow). In (c), the h gate shuts and sodium transport stops (i.e., phase 0 ends). Images (d) and (e) display the effect of adding a class I antiarrhythmic drug (open circles). (d) shows the class I drug binding to the h gate, making it behave as if it is partially closed. When the cell is stimulated in (e), the m gate still opens normally but the channel through which sodium ions enter the cell is narrower and sodium transport is slower. It subsequently takes longer to reach the end of phase 0 (f), and the slope of phase 0 is decreased.

cell (i.e., the slope of phase 0 is decreased). Because the speed of depolarization determines how quickly adjacent cells will depolarize (and therefore the speed of impulse propagation), class I drugs as a group tend to decrease the conduction velocity of cardiac tissue.

Although their precise sites of action have not all been worked out, most antiarrhythmic drugs act in a similar fashion: that is, by altering the function of the various channels that control transport of ions across cardiac cell membranes. The resultant changes in the cardiac action potential (Figure 3.2) cause changes in the conduction velocity,

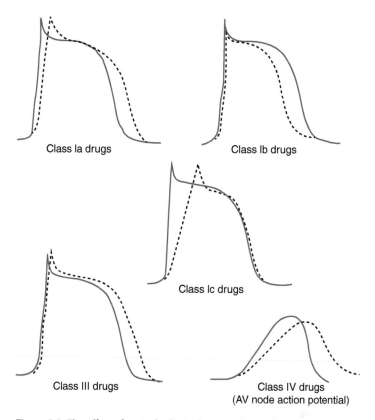

Figure 3.2 The effect of antiarrhythmic drugs on the cardiac action potential. The solid lines represent the baseline action potential and the dotted lines represent the changes that result in the action potential when various classes of antiarrhythmic drug are given. The Purkinje fiber action potential is shown, except in the case of class IV drugs, for which the AV nodal action potential is depicted.

refractoriness, and automaticity of cardiac tissue, and also provide the basis for the classification of antiarrhythmic drugs.

Classification of antiarrhythmic drugs

Table 3.1 lists the most frequently used classification system for antiarrhythmic drugs.

Class I is reserved for drugs that block the rapid sodium channel (as shown in Figure 3.1). Because drugs assigned to class I

Table 3.1 Classification of antiarrhythmic drugs.

Class I	Bind to sodium channel, decrease speed of depolarization	
Class II	β-blocking drugs, decrease sympathetic tone	
	Atenolol	Nadolol
	Bisoprolol	Carvedilol
	Labetolol	Propranolol
	Metoprolol	Timolol
		Nebivolol
	Affect mainly SA and AV nodes (indirectly by blocking P receptors)	
Class III	Increase action potential duration	
	Amiodarone	N-acetylprocainamide
	Dronedarone	Sotalol
	Ibutilide	Dofetilide
Class IV	Calcium channel blockers	
	Diltiazem	Verapamil
	Affect mainly SA and AV nodes (direct membrane effect, see Figure 3.2)	
Class V	Digitalis agents	
	Digitoxin	Digoxin
	Affect mainly SA and AV nodes (indirectly by increasing vagal tone)	

AV, atrioventricular; SA, sinoatrial.

block the sodium channel in varying degrees and also have varying effects on action potential duration, class I is currently broken down into three subgroups (Table 3.2). Class Ia drugs (quinidine, procainamide, disopyramide) slow conduction velocity and increase refractory periods. Class Ib drugs (lidocaine, tocainide, mexiletine, phenytoin) actually have little effect on depolarization when used in systemic doses (although in high concentrations these drugs too can block sodium transport – this is why lidocaine is an excellent local anesthetic agent). In systemic doses, class Ib drugs decrease action potential duration and shorten refractory periods but have little effect on conduction velocity. Class Ic drugs (flecainide and propafenone) have a pronounced depressant effect on conduction velocity, with relatively little effect on refractory periods.

Table 3.2 Subclassification of class I antiarrhythmic agents.

Class Ia	**Quinidine, procainamide, and disopyramide**
	Slow upstroke of action potential ++
	Prolong duration of action potential ++
	Decrease conductivity, increase refractoriness
Class Ib	**Lidocaine, phenytoin, tocainide, and mexiletine**
	Minimal effect on upstroke of action potential
	Shorten duration of action potential
	Decrease refractoriness
Class Ic	**Flecainide, propafenone, and moricizine***[a]*
	Marked slowing of upstroke of action potential ++++
	Minimal effect on action potential duration +
	Marked decrease in conductivity, little effect on refractoriness

[a] The classification of moricizine is controversial, and some place it in class Ib. It is placed in class Ic here to emphasize its class Ic-like proarrhythmic potential.

β-blocking agents are assigned to class II. These drugs have little direct effect on the action potential and work mainly by decreasing the sympathetic tone.

Class III drugs (amiodarone, dofetilide, dronedarone, ibutilide, N-acetylprocainamide, sotalol) increase the action potential duration and therefore refractory periods, and have relatively little effect on the conduction velocity.

Class IV includes the calcium channel blockers. They mainly affect the sinoatrial (SA) and atrioventricular (AV) nodes, because these structures are almost exclusively depolarized by the slow calcium channels.

Class V includes digitalis agents, whose antiarrhythmic effects are related to the increase in parasympathetic activity caused by these drugs.

Effects of antiarrhythmic drugs

Most antiarrhythmic drugs are felt to ameliorate automatic tachyarrhythmias to some extent, although it must again be stressed that the primary treatment for automatic arrhythmias is to remove the underlying cause. Many antiarrhythmic drugs slow the phase 4 ionic fluxes that are responsible for automaticity.

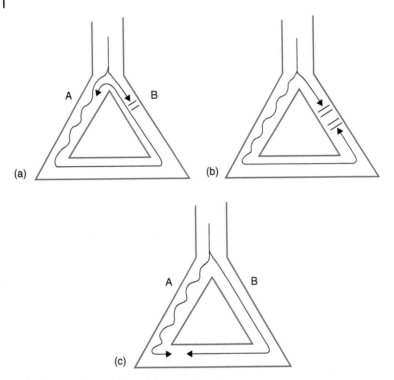

Figure 3.3 Effect of antiarrhythmic drugs on a reentrant circuit. (a) A prototype reentrant circuit (the same as that described in Figures 2.5 and 2.6). (b) Changes that may occur with administration of a class Ia drug. The refractory period of pathway B may be sufficiently prolonged by the drug to prevent reentry from occurring. (c) Changes that may occur with administration of a class Ib drug. The refractory period of pathway B may be shortened, so that the refractory periods of pathways A and B are nearly equal. A premature impulse would then be more likely to either conduct or block down both pathways, thus preventing the initiation of reentry.

Figure 3.3 shows two examples of how antiarrhythmic drugs may affect reentrant circuits. Figure 3.3a shows a reentrant circuit with the same characteristics as described in Chapter 2. Figure 3.3b illustrates the changes that can occur if a class Ia drug is administered. These drugs increase refractory periods. By further lengthening the already long refractory period of pathway B, the class Ia drugs can convert unidirectional block to bidirectional block, thus chemically amputating one pathway of the reentrant circuit. Figure 3.3c shows what happens if a class Ib drug is given. These drugs shorten the duration of the action potential, thus decreasing the refractory period. In this example, a class Ib drug shortens the refractory period of pathway B, thus rendering the refractory periods in pathways A and B relatively equal. (In other words, the *tachycardia zone* is significantly narrowed.) Without a difference in refractory periods between the two pathways of the anatomic circuit, reentry cannot be initiated.

The drug effects illustrated in Figure 3.3 should not be taken literally. The key point in understanding how drugs affect reentry is this: because reentry requires a critical relationship between the refractory periods and the conduction velocities of the two pathways of the reentrant circuit, and because antiarrhythmic drugs alter the refractory periods and conduction velocities, these drugs can make reentry less likely to occur.

Proarrhythmia

Unfortunately, there is another side to that coin. Consider the following scenario: a patient with a previous myocardial infarction and complex ventricular ectopy (but no sustained tachyarrhythmias) has an anatomic circuit whose electrophysiologic characteristics are like those shown in Figure 3.3b. In other words, while the anatomic circuit is present, the electrophysiologic characteristics necessary to activate the circuit are not present. If this patient is placed on a class Ib drug, it is possible to selectively decrease the refractory period of pathway B, giving this circuit the characteristics shown in Figure 3.3a. In other words, the antiarrhythmic drug may make a sustained tachycardia more likely to occur. A similar scenario may develop if a class Ia drug is used in a patient with a circuit resembling the one shown in Figure 3.3c. By increasing the refractory period of pathway B, the benign circuit may be converted to a potentially malignant one. To put it another way, when we administer an antiarrhythmic drug, we may be just as likely to increase as to decrease the tachycardia zone within a potential reentrant circuit – and thus make a sustained arrhythmia more likely instead of less likely.

The phenomenon just described is *proarrhythmia*. Although proarrhythmia is a common occurrence, for many years it was poorly recognized by many physicians who used antiarrhythmic drugs. Failure to recognize that drug therapy is actually worsening arrhythmias can lead to inappropriate therapy (such as increasing or adding to the offending drug) and sometimes to death. Herein lies the problem with considering antiarrhythmic drugs to be simply arrhythmia suppressants. Proarrhythmia is an inherent property of antiarrhythmic drugs: the mechanism that controls reentrant arrhythmias is the same mechanism that can worsen arrhythmias. Unfortunately, whether a drug will improve or worsen an arrhythmia is difficult to predict before actually administering it. Proarrhythmia, therefore, is a possibility for which one must be vigilant whenever using antiarrhythmic drug therapy.

Drug toxicity

Proarrhythmia is probably the most important, and is certainly the most universal, type of toxicity seen with antiarrhythmic drugs. The form of proarrhythmia just mentioned – that is, the worsening of reentrant arrhythmias – can be seen with any class of antiarrhythmic drug.

In addition, antiarrhythmic drugs that prolong the action potential duration can produce a second type of proarrhythmia called *torsades de pointes*. Torsades de pointes (discussed in more detail in Chapter 7) is a polymorphic, pause-dependent ventricular tachycardia that is associated with prolongation of the QT interval and the subsequent development of triggered activity. (Triggered activity was described briefly in Chapter 2.) Torsades commonly causes syncope and can result in sudden death. It can be seen in a subset of otherwise normal individuals – probably 3–4% of the population at large – who are prone to develop triggered activity whenever something acts to prolong their cardiac action potentials. Thus, antiarrhythmic drugs in classes Ia and III tend to cause torsades in such individuals. Table 3.3 lists the relative risk of drug-induced proarrhythmia of both types for the various antiarrhythmic drugs.

Besides proarrhythmia, antiarrhythmic drugs as a group are often poorly tolerated due to side-effects. Table 3.4 lists some of the more common side-effects of antiarrhythmic drugs.

Amiodarone, a class III agent, deserves special recognition. It alters all four classes of ion channels, has a long half-life (up to 100 days), and complex metabolism. Adverse effects of amiodarone are best thought

Table 3.3 Relative risk of drug-induced proarrhythmia.

Drug	Risk of exacerbation of reentry	Risk of torsades de pointes
Class Ia		
Quinidine	++	++
Procainamide	++	++
Disopyramide	++	++
Class Ib		
Lidocaine	+	0
Mexiletine	+	0
Phenytoin	+	0
Class Ic		
Flecainide	+++	0
Propafenone	+++	0
Moricizine	+++	+
Class III		
Amiodarone	+	+
Dronedarone	+	+
Sotalol	+	+++
Ibutilide	+	+++
Dofetilide	+	+++

of in two categories: side-effects and organ toxicity. Side-effects are quickly reversible and most often gastrointestinal (nausea and anorexia) and neurologic (tremor, insomnia). The three most common organ toxicities are thyroid (both low and high activity), liver, and pulmonary. While amiodarone is – on average – the most effective arrhythmia suppressant, its adverse effects limit usage. In selected patients, and with proper surveillance, amiodarone can be quite useful.

The general rule with antiarrhythmic drugs is that, due to these complexities, they should be used only when arrhythmias are significantly symptomatic or life-threatening.

Table 3.4 Common side-effects of antiarrhythmic drugs.

Hypotension	Negative inotropy	Bradycardia
IV procainamide	β-blockers	β-blockers
IV quinidine	Flecainide	Calcium blockers
IV phenytoin	Disopyramide	Amiodarone
IV bretylium		
CNS effects	**GI effects**	**Hepatic effects**
All class Ib	All drugs, especially quinidine, procainamide and class Ib	Amiodarone
Amiodarone		Phenytoin
P-blockers		Dronedarone
Flecainide		
Pneumonitis	**Blood dyscrasias**	**Autonomic effects**
Amiodarone	Quinidine	Disopyramide
Tocainide	Tocainide	Quinidine
	Phenytoin	β-blockers
		Digitalis
		Sotalol

Other notable toxicities

Procainamide – drug-induced lupus

Amiodarone – peripheral neuropathy, proximal myopathy, skin discoloration, skin photosensitivity, **hypothyroidism, hyperthyroidism**

Disopyramide – urinary hesitancy

Dronedarone – increases mortality with heart failure

CNS, central nervous system; GI, gastrointestinal; IV, intravenous.

Nonpharmacologic therapy

Reversing the underlying cause for arrhythmias

The treatment of cardiac arrhythmias should always begin with an attempt to identify and treat reversible etiologies for the arrhythmias. To those etiologies already listed (including electrolyte and acid–base disturbances, ischemia, and cardiometabolic disorders), we must now add antiarrhythmic drugs. A patient with recurrent arrhythmias who is on antiarrhythmic drug therapy should be regarded in the same way as a patient with fever of unknown origin who is on antibiotic therapy – strong consideration should be given to stopping the drug and reassessing the baseline state. Stopping antiarrhythmic drugs will often improve the frequently recurring arrhythmias.

Surgical and ablation therapy

Surgical procedures can be helpful in the treatment of arrhythmias. Arrhythmias due to cardiac ischemia can respond to revascularization procedures such as coronary artery bypass surgery or percutaneous coronary intervention. The location of reentrant circuits can be mapped (especially those due to AV bypass tracts and to ventricular tachycardias associated with a discrete ventricular aneurysm) and the reentrant circuit can be disrupted surgically. Transcatheter ablation in the electrophysiology laboratory has largely supplanted most types of arrhythmia surgery and is useful for nearly all arrhythmias. (Transcatheter ablation will be discussed in detail in Chapters 8 through 12.) All these procedures carry at least some risk of complications.

Device therapy

Permanent artificial pacemakers are the mainstay of treatment for bradyarrhythmias. Permanent pacemakers consist of a source of electrical current that is attached to cardiac muscle by a wire (lead) and is under the control of an integrated circuit (a small computer). If the heart is not generating intrinsic electrical impulses often enough, the pacemaker sends an electrical current down the lead to stimulate it. (There are now leadless pacemakers – see Chapter 5). The current depolarizes the cardiac cells at the tip of the lead (i.e., an action potential is generated) and that depolarization propagates across the myocardium in the normal fashion.

Pacemakers today are sophisticated and highly programmable. Pacemakers are available that guarantee the normal sequence of AV contraction with each heartbeat. Other pacemakers can use some physiologic variable (such as the patient's level of exercise) to judge the optimal heart rate from moment to moment and vary the rate of pacing accordingly. Selecting the appropriate pacemaker for a patient requires extensive knowledge of the technology available.

Devices are also useful for patients with tachyarrhythmias. Many patients with malignant ventricular tachyarrhythmias are now being offered the implantable cardioverter-defibrillator (ICD). This device monitors the heart rhythm constantly and, if a potentially lethal tachyarrhythmia occurs, can automatically deliver either a painless attempt at overdrive pacing or a large defibrillating current (shock) to the heart to terminate the arrhythmia. The implantable defibrillator has prevented sudden death in thousands of patients who have lethal ventricular arrhythmias, but there are downsides. The use of this device is discussed in detail in Chapter 7.

Part II

The Electrophysiology Study in the Evaluation and Therapy of Cardiac Arrhythmias

4

Principles of the Electrophysiology Study

The electrophysiology study (EP study) can be helpful in evaluating a broad spectrum of cardiac arrhythmias. It can help with assessing the function of the sinoatrial (SA) node, the atrioventricular (AV) node, and the His–Purkinje system; with determining the characteristics of reentrant arrhythmias; with mapping the location of arrhythmogenic foci for potential ablation; and with evaluating the efficacy of devices.

One might expect a test that can accomplish all of this to be extraordinarily complex. On the contrary (although electrophysiologists may not like to admit it), the EP study is performed by doing two simple things: recording the heart's electrical signals and pacing from localized areas within the heart. Using the information obtained from these relatively simple tasks and keeping in mind the concepts outlined in Part I, one can assess and decide on treatment for a wide array of heart rhythm disturbances.

In this chapter, we introduce the principles used in performing the EP study.

Recording and pacing

To discuss intracardiac recording and pacing, we need to introduce two terms that are used by electrophysiologists relating to time measurements. Time measurements are reported in milliseconds (ms, one thousandth of a second), the basic unit of time in electrophysiology.

Fogoros' Electrophysiologic Testing, Seventh Edition. Richard N. Fogoros and John M. Mandrola.
© 2023 John Wiley & Sons Ltd. Published 2023 by John Wiley & Sons Ltd.

Cycle length

When electrophysiologists talk about heart rate, they typically speak in terms of cycle length – the length of time between each heartbeat (Figure 4.1a). Thus, the faster the heart rate, the shorter the cycle length: an arrhythmia with a rate of 100 beats/min has a cycle length of 600 ms, while an arrhythmia with a rate of 300 beats/min has a cycle length of 200 ms. Nonelectrophysiologists must pay close attention when discussing heart rate with electrophysiologists, to avoid some amusing miscommunications.

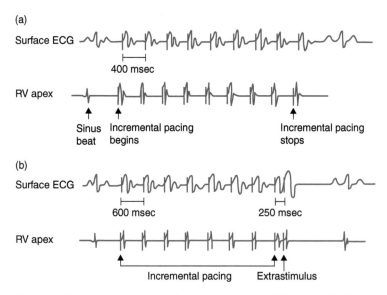

Figure 4.1 Time measurements in the electrophysiology laboratory. This figure depicts pacing from the right ventricular apex. (a) *Cycle length* is the interval of time between heartbeats during either incremental pacing (as in this figure) or a spontaneous rhythm. The cycle length of the incrementally paced beats in (a) is 400 ms. (b) *Coupling interval* is the interval of time between the last normal beat and a premature impulse. In this figure, the normal beats are represented by eight incrementally paced beats at a cycle length of 600 ms. Following the last incrementally paced beat, a single premature stimulus is delivered with a coupling interval of 250 ms.

Coupling interval

When using a pacemaker to introduce a premature impulse, the coupling interval is the time between the last normal impulse and the premature impulse (Figure 4.1b). With earlier premature impulses, the coupling interval is shorter; with later premature impulses, the coupling interval is longer.

The electrode catheter

The EP study is performed by inserting electrode catheters into blood vessels and positioning these catheters in strategic locations within the heart. Once in position, the catheters can be used to perform the two essential tasks of the EP study: recording the heart's electrical signals and pacing.

Electrode catheters consist of insulated wires; at the distal tip of the catheter (the end inserted into the heart [Figure 4.2]), each wire is attached to an electrode, which is exposed to the intracardiac surface. At the proximal end of the catheter (the part not inserted into the body [Figure 4.3]), each wire is attached to a plug, which can be connected to an external device (such as a recording device or an external pacemaker). Apart from the fact that they usually have more than two electrodes, these catheters are similar to many temporary pacemaker catheters used in emergency rooms and coronary care units. The catheter shown in Figures 4.2 and 4.3 is a quadripolar electrode catheter, the type most commonly used in electrophysiology studies. In recent years, electrophysiologists often use recording electrodes with 10–20 electrodes – often in different geometric shapes, such as circular, grid or pent-array formats (Figure 4.4).

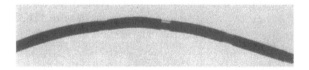

Figure 4.2 The tip of a quadripolar electrode catheter. The electrodes are numbered 1 through 4, the distal (tip) electrode being number 1. The spacing between electrodes is 1 cm.

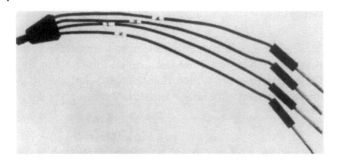

Figure 4.3 The proximal end of a quadripolar electrode catheter. The number on each plug corresponds to the appropriate electrode at the tip of the catheter.

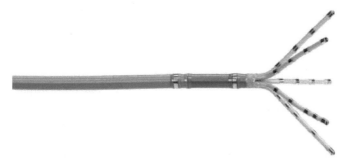

Figure 4.4 PentaRay® mapping catheter, consisting of five flexible branches, each with four electrodes. This is one of several modern electrode catheters which are designed to facilitate electrical mapping from multiple intracardiac locations simultaneously.

Recording intracardiac electrograms

The recording made of the cardiac electrical activity from an electrode catheter placed in the heart is called an *intracardiac electrogram*. The intracardiac electrogram is essentially an electrocardiogram (ECG) recorded from within the heart. The major difference between a body surface ECG and an intracardiac electrogram is that the surface ECG gives a summation of the electrical activity of the entire heart, whereas the intracardiac electrogram records only the electrical activity of a localized area of the heart – the cardiac tissue located near the electrodes of the electrode catheter. Most typically, the intracardiac electrogram records the electrical activity between two

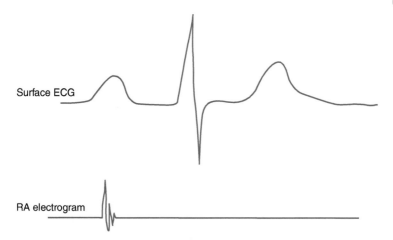

Figure 4.5 Surface ECG and intracardiac electrogram recorded from the high right atrium (RA) during sinus rhythm. The deflection recorded on the RA electrogram reflects the precise moment at which the portion of the right atrium at the tip of the electrode catheter is being depolarized.

of the electrodes (i.e., an electrode pair) at the tip of the catheter. This is called a *bipolar recording configuration.*

The intracardiac electrogram is filtered electronically, so that in general only the rapid depolarization phase of the cardiac tissue (corresponding to phase 0 of the action potential) is recorded. Figure 4.5 shows an intracardiac electrogram recorded from a catheter in the right atrium during normal sinus rhythm. As the wave of depolarization spreading outward from the SA node passes by the catheter, a discrete high-frequency, high-amplitude signal is recorded. This signal indicates the precise moment at which myocardial depolarization occurs at the electrode pair which is being used for recording. By having catheters positioned in several different intracardiac locations, one can accurately measure the conduction time from one location to another. Further, if enough catheter positions are used, one can map the sequence of myocardial depolarization as an electrical impulse traverses the heart.

In summary, the deflection recorded from the electrode catheter represents depolarization of the cardiac tissue in the immediate vicinity of the catheter's electrodes. The intracardiac electrogram plus the pattern of the 12 surface ECG leads allow for precise, localized data on the heart's electrical impulse.

Pacing

The electrode catheter is also used for pacing. To pace, a pulse of electrical current is carried by the electrode catheter from an external pacemaker to the intracardiac surface, where it causes cardiac cells near the catheter's electrodes to depolarize. The depolarization of these cardiac cells is then propagated across the heart, just as an electrical impulse arising in the SA node is propagated. To pace is to artificially generate a cardiac impulse. By careful positioning of the electrode catheter, one can initiate electrical impulses from almost any desired intracardiac location.

During the EP study, pacing is used to introduce premature electrical impulses, delivered in predetermined patterns and at precisely timed intervals. Such pacing is called *programmed stimulation.*

There are several reasons for performing programmed stimulation. Precisely timed premature impulses allow us to measure the refractory periods of cardiac tissue. By introducing premature impulses in one location and recording electrograms in other locations, one can assess the conduction properties of the intervening cardiac tissue and the pattern of myocardial activation. Programmed stimulation can also help to assess the automaticity of an automatic focus and to study the presence and characteristics of reentrant circuits.

Programmed stimulation consists of two general types of pacing: incremental and extrastimulus (Figure 4.6).

Incremental pacing (or burst pacing) consists of introducing a train of paced impulses at a fixed cycle length. The incremental train may last for a few beats or for several minutes.

The *extrastimulus* technique consists of introducing one or more premature impulses (called extrastimuli), each at its own specific coupling interval. The first extrastimulus is introduced at a coupling interval timed, either from an intrinsic cardiac impulse or from the last of a short train of incrementally paced impulses. (This train is usually eight beats in duration, owing to tradition rather than to scientific reasons.) The generally accepted nomenclature for the extrastimulus technique is illustrated in Figure 4.6. The term "S1" (stimulus 1) is used for the incrementally paced impulses or the intrinsic beat from which the first extrastimulus is timed; "S2" is used for the first programmed extrastimulus; "S3" stands for the second programmed extrastimulus; and so on. This nomenclature (in which, for example, the number 2

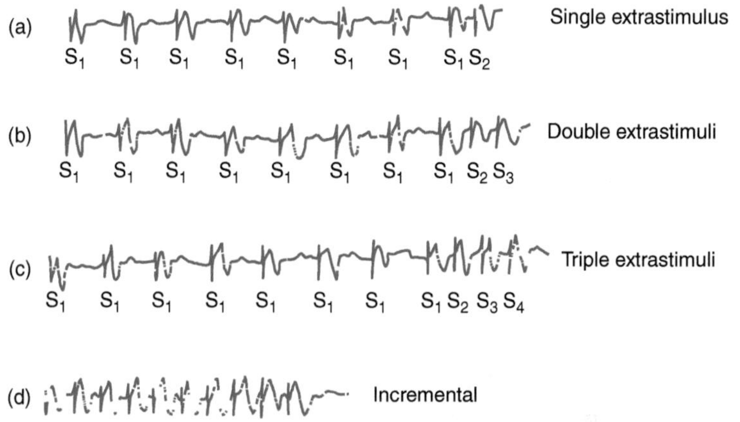

(a) S_1 S_1 S_1 S_1 S_1 S_1 S_1 $S_1 S_2$ Single extrastimulus

(b) S_1 S_1 S_1 S_1 S_1 S_1 S_1 $S_1 S_2 S_3$ Double extrastimuli

(c) S_1 S_1 S_1 S_1 S_1 S_1 S_1 $S_1 S_2 S_3 S_4$ Triple extrastimuli

(d)   Incremental

Figure 4.6 Extrastimulus and incremental pacing. Right ventricular pacing is depicted. (a) Extrastimulus pacing involves introducing one or more extrastimuli, either during the patient's spontaneous rhythm or (as depicted here) following a train of impulses delivered at a fixed cycle length. This panel shows a single extrastimulus. The fixed-cycle-length impulses from which the extrastimuli are timed are referred to as the S1 beats. The first extrastimulus is labeled S2. (b) Same as in (a), except that a second extrastimulus is delivered (labeled S3). (c) Same as in (a) and (b), except that a third extrastimulus is delivered (labeled S4). (d) Incremental pacing consists of a train of paced impulses at a fixed cycle length. The S1 beats in (a) through (c) are incrementally paced impulses.

is attached to the first extrastimulus) causes a lot of confusion among the uninitiated.

Performance of the electrophysiology study

The physical setup of the electrophysiology laboratory

The EP study is a type of heart catheterization, and much of the equipment necessary for electrophysiologic testing can be found in a general cardiac catheterization laboratory. This includes a fluoroscopic unit, a radiographic table, a physiologic recorder, oscilloscopes, instrumentation for gaining vascular access, and emergency equipment. Equipment required specifically for electrophysiologic testing includes a programmable stimulator, a multichannel lead switching box (a junction box), and electrode catheters. An arrangement for a typical electrophysiology laboratory is shown in Figure 4.7.

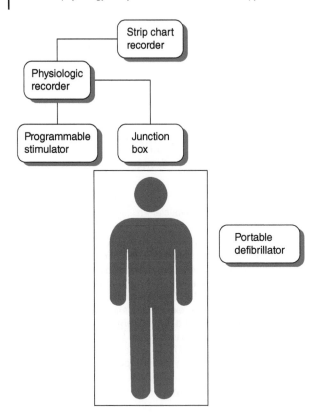

Figure 4.7 Schematic for the layout of a typical electrophysiology laboratory.

The programmable stimulator is a specialized pacing unit built especially for electrophysiology studies. It has the capability to introduce complex sequences of paced beats with an accuracy of within 1 ms. It can also synchronize pacing to the intrinsic heart rhythm and can pace multiple intracardiac sites simultaneously.

The junction box allows the laboratory personnel to control the connections from the electrode catheters to the various recording and pacing devices. With a series of switches, multiple electrode pairs from multiple catheters can be sorted out for recording and pacing.

The physiologic recorder should have enough channels to process three or four surface ECG leads and multiple intracardiac leads (often up to 12). Most electrophysiology laboratories today are equipped with specialized physiologic recorders designed specifically for electrophysiology studies. Such recorders are computer based and provide features such as color-coded intracardiac leads, electronic calipers for precise measurements, and hard disk storage of the entire study. Also integral to most labs is a three-dimensional mapping system for anatomic and electrical characterization of cardiac signals.

Equipment to deal with emergencies is essential, especially because many electrophysiology studies include the intentional induction of arrhythmias, which can cause hemodynamic collapse. This includes a defibrillator, a full complement of cardiac medications, and equipment for maintaining airway support. Likewise, enough trained personnel should always be present to deal with any cardiac emergency. As a minimum, this should include the electrophysiologist, two cardiac nurses who are trained in electrophysiologic procedures (or one nurse and a second physician), and a technician.

Preparation of the patient

Although preparation of the patient will vary somewhat depending on the nature of the study to be performed, all patients having electrophysiology studies should be given a clear understanding of the purpose and nature of the procedure and its potential benefits and harms. As with any procedure in medicine, the patient should sign a statement of informed consent prior to the study.

Ideally, the electrophysiologic evaluation should be performed while the patient is in a baseline state – nonessential drugs should be withdrawn (especially antiarrhythmic agents), any cardiac ischemia or heart failure maximally treated, electrolytes controlled, and every effort made to prevent excessive anxiety, which can cause excessive sympathetic tone. While sedative drugs are often used, anxiety is most easily controlled by adequately preparing the patient for what to expect in the electrophysiology laboratory.

Any cardiac catheterization procedure can cause potentially dangerous arrhythmias, but patients having electrophysiology studies need to be especially aware of this possibility. In particular, patients who are having studies for known or suspected ventricular tachyarrhythmias should be psychologically prepared for the possibility that induction of an arrhythmia might produce loss of consciousness and require defibrillation. Fortunately, the efficacy of electrophysiologic testing and the remarkable safety record achieved in most laboratories go a long way toward allaying the fears of most patients and their families. Detailed discussions with the patient serve not only to guarantee truly informed consent but also to alleviate the patient's anxiety and build his or her confidence in the electrophysiologist.

Insertion and positioning of electrode catheters

The patient is brought to the catheterization laboratory in the fasting state, and the catheterization sites are prepared and draped. The majority of electrophysiology studies can be performed from the venous side of the vascular system, thus precluding the necessity of catheterizing the arterial tree. Under sterile conditions and after local anesthesia is given, catheters are inserted in most instances percutaneously by the modified Seldinger technique (a needle-stick technique that does not require a cutdown). Many operators use ultrasound guidance for access as this helps reduce inadvertent arterial puncture when attempting venous catheterization. When arterial access is needed, ultrasound can reduce "low" sticks in the superficial femoral artery.

Most often, catheters are inserted into the femoral veins (two catheters can safely be inserted into the same femoral vein). Catheters may be inserted from the upper extremities for one of several reasons: for more complicated studies, which require multiple catheters; when there is a contraindication to use of the femoral veins; when a catheter will be left in place at the end of the procedure; or when positioning of the catheter is easier from the upper extremities (such as in coronary sinus catheterization). In these cases, the internal or external jugular veins, subclavian veins, or brachial veins may be used. In those instances where access to the left ventricle is required, the femoral-arterial approach may be used. During complex procedures, a small catheter may be inserted into an artery for continuous monitoring of blood pressure (BP), although there are now reliable noninvasive BP monitors attached to a finger.

Under fluoroscopic or three-dimensional map guidance, the catheters are placed into the proper intracardiac positions. For a simple diagnostic study, generally one catheter is positioned in the high right atrium and the second catheter is placed in the His position (described later). One of these catheters can later be moved to the right ventricle if ventricular pacing is required. For studies of supraventricular tachycardias, additional catheters are commonly placed in the right ventricle and the coronary sinus (thus allowing recordings from all four major cardiac chambers and from the His position).

In the right atrium, catheters are most commonly positioned in the high lateral wall, near the junction of the superior vena cava. This position approximates the location of the SA node and is the region of the atrium that is depolarized earliest during normal sinus rhythm. Pacing from this area results in P-wave configurations that are similar to normal sinus beats.

Pacing and recording from the left atrium are usually accomplished by inserting an electrode catheter into the coronary sinus (Figure 4.8). The os of the coronary sinus lies posterior and slightly inferior to the tricuspid valve. With the advent of deflectable catheters, the coronary sinus os is easily entered from an inferior approach.

Coronary sinus recordings are especially useful because the coronary sinus lies in the AV groove – that is, between the left atrium and the left ventricle. One catheter, therefore, records both left atrial and left ventricular activation. A coronary sinus catheter can easily be used to pace the left atrium, and with a little maneuvering, it can also be used to pace the left ventricle.

Electrode catheters in the right ventricle can be positioned in the apex, septum, or outflow tract for pacing and recording. Placing electrode catheters in the left ventricle is not part of the standard EP study. When it is necessary to do so (e.g., when ablation procedures require access to the left ventricle or left atrium), access can be achieved via either a transseptal approach or retrograde aortic valve approach from the arterial system. The advent of left atrial ablation for atrial fibrillation has led to increased comfort with transseptal access.

The *His bundle electrogram* yields the most information about AV conduction. To record this electrogram, an electrode catheter is passed across the posterior aspect of the tricuspid valve (near the penetration of the His bundle into the fibrous skeleton [Figure 4.9]). The catheter is maneuvered while continuously recording electrograms from several electrode pairs (so that the best pair for recording can be selected), until an electrogram similar to the one shown in Figure 4.9 is seen. The electrode pair that records the His electrogram is thus placed in a strategic location. It straddles the important structures of the AV conduction system and allows one to record the electrical activity of the low right atrium, the AV node, the His bundle, and a portion of the right ventricle – all from one electrode pair.

Once the catheters are in position, the various electrode pairs are set up for recording and pacing. The leads recorded include various surface ECG leads and intracardiac electrograms from each electrode

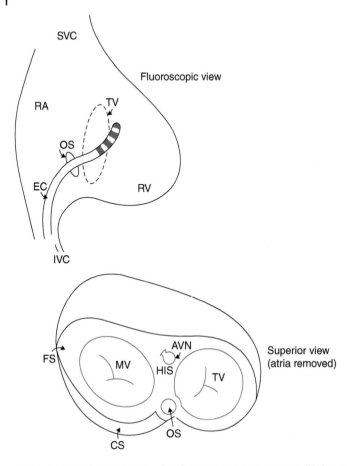

Figure 4.8 A catheter positioned in the coronary sinus can record left atrial and left ventricular electrograms, because the coronary sinus lies in the AV groove between the left atrium and the left ventricle. AVN, AV node; CS, coronary sinus; EC, electrode catheter; FS, fibrous skeleton of the heart; HIS, His bundle; IVC, inferior vena cava; MV, mitral valve; OS, os of the coronary sinus; RA, right atrium; RV, right ventricle; SVC, superior vena cava; TV, tricuspid valve.

catheter. Figure 4.10 shows a typical baseline recording for a typical baseline EP study, displaying surface ECG leads I, II, and V_1 (thus providing a lateral, an inferior, and an anterior lead from which to assess the QRS axis), as well as leads from two intracardiac catheters (high right atrium and His positions). For ventricular recording and

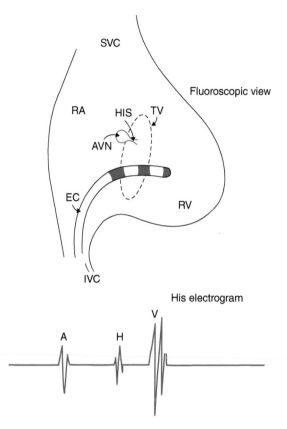

Figure 4.9 Positioning of the His bundle catheter. The His bundle electrogram is recorded from a catheter that lies across the posterior aspect of the tricuspid valve. Abbreviations are the same as in Figure 4.7. See Chapter 5 for a description of "A," "H," and "V" spikes on the His electrogram.

pacing, the right atrial catheter is moved to the right ventricle after atrial pacing is completed.

The basic electrophysiology protocol

The protocol used in electrophysiology studies varies according to the specific type of procedure being performed, but most electrophysiologic procedures follow the same general outline.

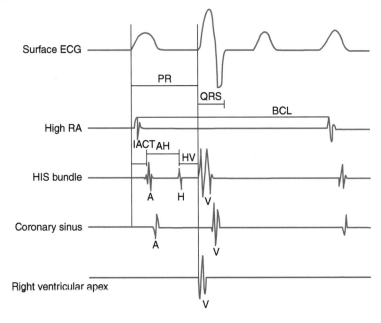

Figure 4.10 Typical baseline recording of intracardiac electrograms. In this figure, one surface ECG lead is shown, as well as intracardiac electrograms from the high right atrium (RA), His bundle, coronary sinus, and right ventricular apex. Conduction intervals are as follows: BCL (basic cycle length) is the interval between successive A waves (measured from the RA catheter); PR interval is the time from the beginning of the P wave to the beginning of the QRS complex (measured from the surface ECG); QRS duration is the width of the QRS complex on the surface ECG; IACT (intraatrial conduction time) is the interval from the SA node to the AV node and is measured from the beginning of the P wave on the surface ECG to the A deflection on the His bundle electrogram. The AH and HV intervals are discussed in detail in Chapter 5.

1. Measurement of baseline conduction intervals.
2. Atrial pacing.
   - Assessment of SA nodal automaticity and conductivity
   - Assessment of AV nodal conductivity and refractoriness
   - Assessment of His–Purkinje system conductivity and refractoriness
   - Induction of atrial arrhythmias
3. Ventricular pacing.
   - Assessment of retrograde conduction
   - Induction of ventricular arrhythmias

Chapters 5, 6, and 7 discuss the individual steps of the EP study in detail. Before proceeding to specifics, however, we need to review the principles of how one can evaluate the electrophysiologic properties of the heart and assess and treat reentrant arrhythmias through the simple expediency of recording and pacing from intracardiac electrodes.

Evaluation of the electrophysiologic properties of the heart

By recording and pacing from electrode catheters, one can evaluate the fundamental electrophysiologic properties of the heart – namely, automaticity, conduction velocity, and refractory periods.

Automaticity

The EP study can be used to assess the normal automaticity of the SA node, thanks to the phenomenon known as *overdrive suppression.* An automatic focus such as the SA node can be overdriven by a more rapidly firing pacemaker. This means that the more rapid pacemaker depolarizes the SA node faster than it can be depolarized by its intrinsic automaticity. When the overdriving pacemaker stops, there is often a relatively long pause before the SA node recovers and begins depolarizing spontaneously again. The pause induced in an automatic focus by a temporarily overdriving pacemaker is called overdrive suppression.

Overdrive suppression of the SA node is accomplished in the electrophysiology laboratory by pacing the atrium rapidly (thus overdriving the SA node), then suddenly turning off the pacemaker and measuring how long it takes for the SA node to recover. A diseased SA node tends to have a grossly prolonged recovery time after overdrive pacing. The evaluation of SA nodal dysfunction is covered in detail in Chapter 5.

Overdrive suppression of automatic foci is also clinically relevant when patients are dependent on subsidiary escape pacemakers to sustain life (e.g., patients with complete heart block and ventricular escape rhythms). These subsidiary pacemakers are automatic foci like the SA node and are thus subject to overdrive suppression. If such a patient receives a temporary pacemaker and after a time the temporary pacemaker suddenly loses capture (as temporary pacemakers sometimes do), the patient may be left with a prolonged, possibly fatal asystolic episode due to overdrive suppression of the escape pacemaker. In such patients, careful positioning of the temporary pacemaker to guarantee excellent pacing thresholds in a very stable location is essential, and every precaution must be taken to keep the temporary lead stable (such as enforced bed rest) until a permanent pacemaker can be inserted.

Tachyarrhythmias due to abnormal automaticity (such as automatic ventricular tachycardia due to ischemia) do not lend themselves well to study in the electrophysiology laboratory. Overdrive suppression of such abnormal automatic foci is not a prominent feature and usually cannot be demonstrated. Also, as we have already discussed, automatic arrhythmias cannot be induced during electrophysiologic testing. Thus, the evaluation of automatic tachyarrhythmias is not an indication for an EP study.

Conduction velocity

Conduction velocity refers to the speed of conduction of an electrical impulse across the heart and, as we have noted, is related to the rate of rise (i.e., the slope) of the depolarization phase (phase 0) of the action potential. By measuring the time it takes for an electrical impulse to travel from one intracardiac location to another (referred to as a *conduction interval*), one can use electrode catheters to assess the conduction velocities of various portions of the cardiac electrical system.

The best example of measuring conduction velocity from intracardiac electrograms is given by the His bundle electrogram. As noted previously, this electrogram contains signals from all the critical structures of the AV conducting system. Figure 4.9 represents the His bundle electrogram of a patient in normal sinus rhythm. As shown, the His electrogram contains three major deflections. The first deflection is the A spike. This represents depolarization of the tissue in the low right atrium, just as the electrical impulse enters the AV node. Once in the AV node, the impulse encounters tissue that depolarizes slowly. (As discussed in Chapter 1, the slow depolarization of the AV nodal tissue is a result of the lack of rapid sodium channels in AV nodal cells.) Because the depolarization of the AV node is slow, no high-frequency signal is generated, and the passage of the impulse through the AV node does not produce a deflection on the His bundle electrogram.

When the impulse exits the AV node and zips down the His bundle (again encountering rapidly depolarizing cells), the His bundle deflection (i.e., the H spike) is produced on the electrogram.

As the impulse passes distally through the bundle branches and on to the farther reaches of the Purkinje system, it moves away from the recording electrode pair. Because of their distance from the recording electrodes, the Purkinje fiber depolarizations are not recorded on the His electrogram (although the right bundle branch depolarization is sometimes seen). Finally, as the impulse is spread to the ventricular myocardium, the depolarization of the ventricular muscle near the His catheter produces the V deflection on the His electrogram.

By analyzing the deflections on the His bundle electrogram, the conduction properties of the major structures of the AV conduction system can be deduced. The conduction interval from the beginning of the A deflection to the beginning of the H deflection (the *AH interval*) represents the conduction time through the AV node (normally 50–120 ms). The interval from the beginning of the H deflection to the beginning of the V deflection (the *HV interval*) represents the conduction time through the His–Purkinje system (normally 35–55 ms). Disease in the AV node will often produce a prolongation in the AH interval, whereas disease in the distal conducting system produces a prolongation in the HV interval.

The AH and HV intervals are two of the basic conduction intervals measured at the beginning of the EP study. Other basic conduction intervals (shown in Figure 4.10) include the basic cardiac cycle length, the QRS duration, the PR interval, and the intraatrial conduction interval. The basic cycle length is the interval between successive atrial impulses as measured in the right atrial catheter (in order to approximate the basic rate of depolarization of the SA node). The PR interval is measured from the surface ECG leads and is defined as the interval from the beginning of the P wave to the beginning of the QRS complex. The QRS duration, the interval from the beginning of the QRS complex to the end of the QRS complex, is also measured from the surface ECG leads. The intraatrial conduction interval approximates the conduction time from the sinus node to the AV node and is measured from the beginning of the P wave on the surface ECG to the beginning of the A spike on the His bundle electrogram. Note that the intraatrial conduction interval, the AH interval, and the HV interval are the three basic components of the PR interval.

Depending on the type of EP study being performed and the type of information needed, other conduction intervals may be measured, such as retrograde conduction intervals (from the ventricle to the atrium).

Refractory periods

Thus far, we have defined the refractory period as the period of time after depolarization during which a cell cannot be depolarized again, and we have related the refractory period of a cell to the duration of the action potential. Because we cannot measure a cell's action potential duration in the electrophysiology laboratory, the refractory period must be redefined in such a way as to make it meaningful in the laboratory setting. Thus, the refractory period of cardiac tissue is defined in terms of the tissue's response to premature paced impulses. Here, electrophysiologists have outdone themselves by defining three different kinds of refractory period: the effective refractory period (ERP), the relative refractory period (RRP), and the functional refractory period (FRP).

The *ERP* (Figure 4.11) is the definition that most closely coincides with our original definition of the refractory period. When introducing

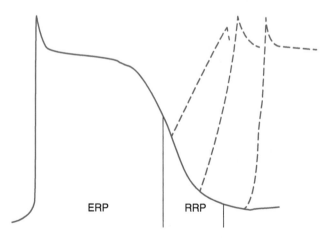

Figure 4.11 Effective and relative refractory periods. During the effective refractory period (ERP), the cell cannot be depolarized. During the relative refractory period (RRP), the cell can be depolarized, but the resultant action potential displays slower phase 0 activity (dotted lines).

a premature impulse, that impulse will fail to propagate through tissue that is refractory. The ERP of a tissue is the longest coupling interval for which a premature impulse fails to propagate through that tissue. In other words, the ERP refers to the latest early impulse that is blocked – if the premature impulse were any later, the tissue would be recovered and would propagate the impulse. In general, the end of ERP occurs sometime during the last third of phase 3 of the action potential.

The *RRP* (Figure 4.11) requires the introduction of a new concept. Recovery from refractoriness turns out to be a gradual process instead of an instantaneous one. As shown, the end of the ERP occurs during phase 3, before a cell is fully repolarized (that is, before phase 4 begins). If a cardiac cell is stimulated after the end of the ERP but before the cell is fully repolarized, the resulting action potential has a slower upstroke (phase 0) and therefore propagates at a slower conduction velocity. The period of time from the end of the ERP to the beginning of phase 4 is called the RRP. Formally, the RRP of a tissue is the longest coupling interval for which a premature impulse results in slowed conduction through that tissue. At the end of the RRP, the tissue is fully recovered.

At least the ERP and RRP can be related in some way to the duration of the action potential. The *FRP* loses even that relationship to our original notion of "refractory period." The FRP of a tissue is the smallest possible time interval between two impulses that can be conducted through that tissue. It is a measure of the output of a tissue. Think of a tiny electrophysiologist standing on the His bundle with a stopwatch, determined to measure the FRP of the AV node. A larger electrophysiologist is pacing the atrium with progressively earlier (i.e., more premature) impulses. The only thing our miniature friend can detect, however, is each electrical impulse exiting the AV node and zipping down the His bundle (do not worry – he is wearing rubber-soled shoes). Each time an impulse exits the AV node and stimulates the His bundle, the tiny electrophysiologist records the time interval since the previous impulse. Eventually, premature impulses stimulating the AV node are so premature that the ERP of the AV node is reached (i.e., the impulse is blocked when it reaches the AV node), and therefore no more impulses are transmitted to the His bundle. The FRP of the AV node is the shortest interval between successive impulses observed by our tiny timer.

What possessed electrophysiologists to invent such a thing as the FRP? First, since the FRP of a tissue is determined by transmission of impulses through that tissue, FRP is a measurement of both the refractoriness and the conduction velocity of a tissue. As shown in the discussion of RRP, refractoriness and conduction velocity are intimately related at narrower coupling intervals. The FRP is a way of quantifying this relationship. Second, the FRP may be clinically relevant more often than the more straightforward types of refractory periods. The best example is in atrial fibrillation, in which much effort is often spent in slowing the ventricular response. The drugs used for this purpose tend both to increase refractoriness and to slow conduction in the AV conducting system. One of the best measures of effective therapy, then, is the narrowest interval between successive QRS complexes (i.e., the FRP of the AV conducting system). Third, when inventing a list of anything (such as types of refractory period), it is best to have at least three items on the list.

The effect of cycle length and autonomic tone on refractory periods and conduction velocity

The refractory period of cardiac tissue is affected by the cycle length. For most tissue, shorter cycle lengths (i.e., faster heart rates) decrease refractory periods. The glaring exception to this general rule is the AV node, in which shorter cycle lengths increase refractory periods.

Autonomic tone affects both refractory periods and conduction velocity. An increase in sympathetic tone increases the conduction velocity and decreases the refractory periods throughout the heart. An increase in parasympathetic tone decreases the conduction velocity and increases the refractory periods. Here, again, there is a differential effect on the AV node, which is far more richly supplied by parasympathetic fibers than is most of the heart. Thus, parasympathetic tone has a disproportionate effect on the AV node.

Evaluation of reentrant arrhythmias

The ability to induce and terminate reentrant arrhythmias renders them amenable to detailed study. Consequently, the EP study has become vitally important in the evaluation and treatment of reentrant tachyarrhythmias. Although the techniques used to study different types of reentrant arrhythmia vary (this will be discussed in detail in Chapters 6 and 7), the principles behind the electrophysiologic evaluation of all types of reentry are the same.

Programmed stimulation in reentrant arrhythmias

The hallmark of the reentrant mechanism is the ability to induce and terminate the arrhythmia with programmed pacing techniques. Figure 2.6 shows the basic principle behind inducing a reentrant arrhythmia. A paced premature impulse enters the reentrant loop at a critical coupling interval, when pathway B is still refractory from the previous impulse (i.e., the premature impulse arrives during the ERP of pathway B) but after the ERP of pathway A, which accepts the early impulse. Note that, if the impulse enters pathway A during its RRP, the requirement for slow conduction down pathway A may be met automatically (since by definition conduction is slow during the RRP). Because of the slow conduction down pathway A, pathway B has time to recover and accepts the premature impulse in the retrograde direction. Reentry is established.

Once a reentrant arrhythmia is established, premature paced impulses encountering the loop can do one of three things (Figure 4.12). First, the early impulse may encounter refractory tissue, which will prevent it from entering the circuit (Figure 4.12a). In this case, the premature beat will not affect the reentrant rhythm. Second, the early paced impulse may enter the loop and conduct down the slow pathway (pathway A) but collide with the reentrant impulse in the fast pathway (Figure 4.12b). In this case, the paced impulse resets the reentrant rhythm. Finally, the early impulse may enter the loop at just the right moment to encounter refractory tissue in pathway A and collide with the circulating wavefront in pathway B (Figure 4.12c). In this case, the reentrant rhythm is terminated.

A paced impulse must reach a reentrant circuit at a critical moment to start or stop an arrhythmia. The ability to arrive at such a critical moment is dependent on several factors, including the distance of the pacing electrode from the reentrant circuit and the refractoriness and conduction velocity of the tissue lying between the catheter and the circuit. If the catheter is far away from the reentrant circuit and if the intervening tissue has long refractory periods and slow conduction,

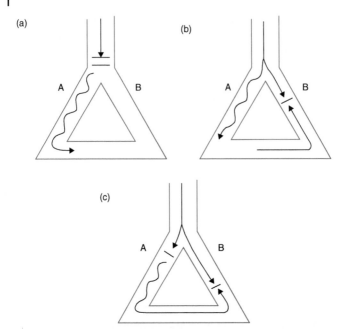

Figure 4.12 Effect of premature impulses on a reentrant arrhythmia. (a) A relatively late premature impulse may encounter refractory tissue that prevents penetration into the reentrant circuit. In this case, reentry is not affected. (b) An earlier premature impulse than that depicted in (a) may enter the reentrant circuit and abolish the reentrant impulse in one pathway (pathway B in this figure) but reestablish reentry by conducting down the opposite pathway (pathway A). In this case, the reentrant rhythm is reset. (c) A very early premature impulse may abolish the reentrant arrhythmia in pathway B while encountering refractory tissue in pathway A. In this case, reentry is terminated.

it is less likely that a paced impulse will reach the reentrant circuit early enough to either induce or terminate an arrhythmia. For this reason, stimulation protocols usually call for pacing from more than one location, to improve the chances of finding a location near the reentrant circuit. In addition, most stimulation protocols call for coupling up to four premature impulses together. The resulting short cycle lengths reduce refractory periods and increase conduction velocity in the intervening tissue, giving subsequent impulses a better chance of reaching the reentrant circuit.

Pacing from various locations during supraventricular tachycardia can help to determine whether certain intracardiac locations are part of the reentrant loop. For instance, pacing from a right ventricular site which does not affect a narrow complex tachyarrhythmia is evidence against a macroreentrant tachycardia that includes both atrial and ventricular tissue in the reentrant loop. Chapter 6 discusses this concept in more detail.

Recording electrograms during reentrant arrhythmias

By recording intracardiac electrograms during reentrant tachycardias, it is possible to characterize the pathways of large reentrant circuits (present in many supraventricular arrhythmias) or to map the general location of small reentrant circuits (present in most ventricular tachycardias). Especially helpful in the evaluation of supraventricular arrhythmias is the pattern of atrial activation during tachycardia. As will be discussed in Chapter 6, some types of reentrant supraventricular arrhythmia show characteristic patterns of atrial activation. A diagnosis can often be made by analyzing the intracardiac atrial electrograms. By recording multiple ventricular electrograms during induced ventricular tachycardia and looking for the earliest ventricular activation site, the general location of the reentrant circuit can be deduced. This mapping helps locate important sites for ablation in the ventricle.

Effect of autonomic maneuvers, antiarrhythmic drugs, and devices on reentry

The EP study can help to determine the effect of autonomic maneuvers on reentrant arrhythmias. By manipulating autonomic tone and reassessing the inducibility of arrhythmias, one can determine whether reentrant arrhythmias are dependent on autonomic tone. In supraventricular arrhythmias, reentry which depends on autonomic tone is strong evidence that the AV node is involved in the reentrant loop. Stimulating the ventricle during the infusion of sympathomimetic agents can help to diagnose catecholamine-dependent ventricular tachycardia. Diagnosing this relatively infrequent type of ventricular tachycardia is important, because this arrhythmia almost always responds to b-blockers.

By studying the characteristics of an induced arrhythmia, one can assess important factors before considering implantable devices. How many different types of arrhythmia are inducible? What are their cycle lengths? What pacing sequences reliably terminate the induced arrhythmias? Does pacing ever degenerate a hemodynamically stable arrhythmia to an unstable one? Are there benign tachyarrhythmias (such as sinus tachycardia) that might fool a device into delivering inappropriate therapy? All these questions can be addressed through careful study in the electrophysiology laboratory.

Complications of electrophysiologic testing

On first learning about the EP study – especially when the purpose of that study is to induce lethal ventricular arrhythmias – many physicians assume that a test that sounds so barbaric must be dangerous. On the contrary, the EP study is remarkably safe, often much safer than the standard cardiac catheterization.

The EP study is a form of heart catheterization, and it necessarily carries the qualitative risks of a heart catheterization. These include cardiac perforation, hemorrhage, thromboembolism, phlebitis, and infection. Because the most common complications of a general heart catheterization involve damage to the arterial tree, and because most electrophysiology studies do not require arterial puncture, the statistical risk of serious vascular damage is actually substantially less with the EP study than with a standard cardiac catheterization. In most laboratories, the cumulative risk of thromboembolism or phlebitis, bacteremia, or hemorrhage requiring transfusion is well below 1%.

One might think that a procedure that sometimes intentionally induces lethal arrhythmias would entail significant mortality. In fact, the risk of death during an EP study approaches zero. Reentrant ventricular arrhythmias are induced in the electrophysiology laboratory under controlled circumstances. Immediate efforts are made to terminate hemodynamically unstable arrhythmias, and it turns out that these arrhythmias are readily terminable if they are treated quickly. In most laboratories, the average length of time for which the patient remains in an induced ventricular tachycardia is less than 30 seconds. Only a small minority of patients with inducible ventricular tachyarrhythmias require DC shocks for termination, and the need to initiate cardiopulmonary resuscitation procedures is exceedingly rare.

5

The Electrophysiology Study in the Evaluation of Bradycardia: The SA Node, AV Node, and His–Purkinje System

As we saw in Chapter 2, the sinoatrial (SA) node, atrioventricular (AV) node, and His–Purkinje system are responsible for generating, propagating, and distributing the heart's electrical impulse, and thus for determining the cardiac rhythm and rate, and optimizing the hemodynamic performance of the heart. Specifically, the SA node continuously regulates the heart rate according to the body's fluctuating needs; the AV node and His bundle transmit electrical impulses from the atria to the ventricles; and the Purkinje system coordinates the contraction of the left and right ventricles.

In this chapter, we will discuss the electrophysiologic problems that produce bradycardia: disorders of the SA node, AV node, and His–Purkinje system, emphasizing how (and when) the electrophysiology (EP) study can help in their evaluation. We will also briefly review pacemaker therapy.

As we do so, the reader will note a recurring theme: while the EP study has provided us with detailed knowledge of how the SA node, AV node, and His–Purkinje system work, now that we have acquired this knowledge we can usually evaluate patients with disorders of these cardiac structures without actually having to perform an EP study. Indeed, the original electrophysiologists were so successful in achieving their prime directive (understanding how the cardiac impulse is formed and propagated) that they nearly put themselves out of business. Fortunately, a second generation of electrophysiologists quickly figured out how to apply electrophysiologic testing to the tachyarrhythmias, thus rescuing the profession – but that is a story for later chapters.

Fogoros' Electrophysiologic Testing, Seventh Edition. Richard N. Fogoros and John M. Mandrola.
© 2023 John Wiley & Sons Ltd. Published 2023 by John Wiley & Sons Ltd.

Evaluation of SA nodal abnormalities

Anatomy of the SA node

The SA node can be thought of as a subendocardial, comma-shaped structure, approximately 3 mm in width and 10 mm in length, the head of which is located laterally to the right atrial appendage, near the junction of the atrium and the superior vena cava, on the crista terminalis. (The crista terminalis is an endocardial ridge extending like a narrow mountain chain from the superior to the inferior vena cava along the lateral right atrium). The tail of the SA nodal "comma" extends downward along the crista terminalis, toward the inferior vena cava.

The SA node receives rich innervation from both sympathetic and parasympathetic fibers; accordingly, its function is strongly influenced by the autonomic nervous system. There is some evidence that autonomic tone helps to determine which portion of the SA node (i.e., the head or the tail) is "firing" at a given time (elevated sympathetic tone tends to trigger the head of the SA node while elevated parasympathetic tone tends to trigger the tail), leading to different appearances of the p-wave on the surface electrocardiogram (ECG).

SA nodal dysfunction

Disease of the SA node is the most common cause of bradycardia. The bradyarrhythmias that accompany SA nodal disease can manifest as intermittent or sustained sinus bradycardia, as sudden episodes of SA nodal arrest or exit block, or as sinus bradycardia alternating with paroxysms of atrial tachyarrhythmias (a condition referred to as "brady-tachy syndrome"). When sinus bradyarrhythmias are sufficient to produce symptoms, *sick sinus syndrome* is said to be present.

(Note that the "official" definition of sinus bradycardia can be misleading. While most textbooks define normal sinus rhythm as having a rate between 60 and 100 beats/min, this range is probably incorrect. Normal, healthy individuals often have resting sinus rates as low as 35 while resting heart rates in the upper 80s or 90s often indicate the presence of occult medical problems, such as anemia or cardiopulmonary or thyroid disorders.)

Bradycardia caused by SA nodal disease is usually benign. That is, people do not commonly die from sinus bradycardia itself. On the other hand, the presence of SA nodal disease is associated with increased mortality – but that excess mortality is often due to non-cardiac causes.

Because sinus bradycardia is usually not lethal, the level of aggressiveness that ought to be used in evaluating and treating suspected SA nodal disease is solely dependent on whether any associated symptoms are thought to be present. If SA nodal disease is causing symptoms (i.e., if sick sinus syndrome is present), permanent pacing is indicated. If there are no symptoms, in general there is no indication for pacing.

By far the most common cause of SA nodal disease is simple fibrosis of the SA node, a condition that is associated with aging and that often is accompanied by diffuse fibrosis within the atria and the AV conducting system. Accordingly, most patients with SA nodal dysfunction are elderly. Other causes of SA nodal dysfunction include atherosclerotic disease involving the SA nodal artery; cardiac trauma (often due to either surgery or catheter ablation), cardiac infiltrative or inflammatory disorders; and thyroid disorders.

Brady-tachy syndrome deserves special mention. This syndrome occurs because the diffuse atrial fibrosis that often accompanies SA nodal dysfunction can produce a propensity for atrial fibrillation or flutter. Individuals with brady-tachy syndrome thus will have intermittent episodes of atrial tachyarrhythmias, with intervening periods of sinus bradycardia. Importantly, because their diseased SA nodes often display exaggerated overdrive suppression (see Chapter 4 and later in this chapter), these patients tend to have very prolonged asystolic pauses when their tachyarrhythmias abruptly terminate. Often, then, their presenting symptoms have little to do directly with either the tachycardia or the sinus bradycardia – instead, they are frequently caused by this posttachycardia asystole. Thus, patients with brady-tachy syndrome can have sudden and relatively severe episodes of lightheadedness, or even frank syncope. Furthermore, because the atrial fibrosis also commonly involves the AV conduction system, during their atrial tachyarrhythmias these patients may have surprisingly well-controlled (or even slow) ventricular responses. Seeing an unexpectedly slow ventricular response in a patient with atrial fibrillation should thus immediately raise the question of a generalized disorder of the conducting system – and the physician should be prepared to administer immediate pacing therapy if cardioversion is contemplated.

Patients with brady-tachy syndrome often end up with chronic atrial fibrillation accompanied by a reasonably well-controlled ventricular response. Indeed, one might be tempted to view this chronic atrial fibrillation as "God's way" of guaranteeing an adequate heart rate in the face of diffuse conducting system disease. While this may be so, in the intervening years patients are often very symptomatic, not to mention at risk for syncope-induced trauma, so sitting on one's hands and waiting for this final, relatively stable rhythm to occur does not constitute adequate therapy.

Although the EP study can help to document the presence of SA nodal dysfunction, it generally cannot help to assess whether such dysfunction is causing symptoms or, therefore, whether pacing therapy is indicated. However, patients sometimes present who have symptoms suggesting significant bradycardia (such as lightheadedness or syncope), without clearly documented bradycardia. In such patients, the EP study can be helpful in determining whether or not the SA node is intrinsically normal.

Evaluating SA nodal function in the electrophysiology laboratory

Sinus node recovery time (SNRT)

A primary manifestation of SA nodal dysfunction is disordered automaticity, where the slope of phase 4 automaticity is reduced in the SA node, resulting in bradycardia.

The test designed to assess SA nodal automaticity in the electrophysiology laboratory is the "sinus node recovery time" (SNRT; Figures 5.1 and 5.2). Measurement of the SNRT is based on the phenomenon of overdrive suppression. Overdrive suppression is the temporary slowing of automaticity seen when an automatic focus is exposed to rapid, extrinsic electrical stimuli. When this overdriving stimulation stops, it takes the automatic focus a few cycles to recover its normal rate of discharge. Until it recovers, it fires more slowly than its original baseline rate; thus, the automatic focus has been transiently "suppressed" by overdrive stimulation. Overdrive suppression is a normal behavior of automatic foci; in SA nodal disease, however, overdrive suppression tends to be exaggerated.

In nature, as we have seen, overdrive suppression of the SA node is caused by atrial tachyarrhythmias. In the electrophysiology laboratory, we provoke it with a temporary pacemaker.

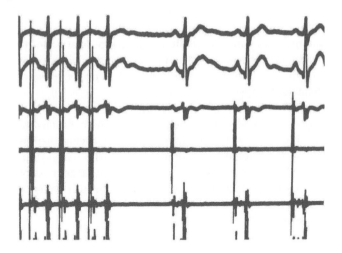

Figure 5.1 A normal sinus node recovery time (SNRT). This figure shows three surface electrocardiogram (ECG) leads (top three tracings), a right atrial (RA) electrogram (fourth tracing), and a His bundle electrogram (fifth tracing). In measuring the SNRT, only the RA electrogram needs to be examined. The first three impulses on the RA electrogram represent the final three paced beats during 30 seconds of incremental pacing. Pacing is stopped, and the interval from the last paced atrial complex to the first spontaneous atrial complex on the RA electrogram is measured. In this instance, the basic cycle length is 800 ms and the SNRT equals 1260 ms. This is a normal value.

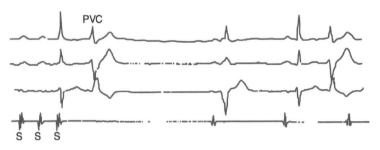

Figure 5.2 An abnormal sinus node recovery time (SNRT). This figure shows three surface ECG leads and the right atrial (RA) electrogram. The last three paced impulses are shown. The interval following termination of pacing (from the RA electrogram) is 2200 ms, an abnormally long SNRT. Note that during the recovery interval, a premature ventricular complex (PVC) is seen. Because this PVC does not conduct retrogradely (this is obvious because no corresponding atrial activity is present on the RA electrogram), the PVC does not affect the sinus node and therefore does not affect measurement of the SNRT.

Measuring SNRT

Measuring the SNRT is simple in concept and in practice, although interpreting the results can be more challenging. An electrode catheter is placed in the high right atrium near the SA node and pacing is initiated to overdrive the SA node. After a while, pacing is terminated and the ensuing "recovery" time from the last paced beat to the next spontaneous sinus beat is measured.

In the formal measurement of SNRT, several pacing sequences are tested, beginning with a pacing rate just slightly faster than the basic sinus rate, and generally ending with a cycle length of 300 ms (200 beats/min). Each pacing sequence is maintained for at least 30 seconds to maximize overdrive suppression and is then abruptly stopped. The first recovery interval (the interval from the last paced atrial complex to the first spontaneous SA nodal depolarization) is normally longer than the prepacing baseline sinus interval, reflecting the degree of overdrive suppression induced by pacing. After pacing is stopped, the SA node gradually returns to its baseline rate over 5–6 beats. In SA nodal disease, two observations are commonly seen. First, the initial recovery interval can be longer than normal. Second, the gradual return to the baseline sinus rate can be interrupted during subsequent recovery intervals by marked "secondary pauses."

By the end of the study, several initial recovery intervals will have been measured, one at each pacing rate. In addition, one or more secondary pauses may have been observed. The official SNRT is deemed to be the longest recovery interval observed during the entire test, whether it is one of the initial recovery intervals or a secondary pause.

An interesting but not surprising observation

One might think that the longest postpacing recovery times would always be seen after the more rapid pacing rates, but this is often not the case. Recovery times measured after slower pacing rates are frequently longer than those measured after faster pacing rates. This phenomenon – longer recovery times after slower overdrive suppression – is attributed to the conduction properties of the SA node itself. If conduction within the perinodal cells (cells that surround the pacemaker cells) is abnormal then SA nodal "entrance block" can occur, wherein some of the paced impulses are blocked from reaching the pacemaker cells. Faster pacing rates can thus actually result in fewer impulses reaching the SA nodal pacemaker cells themselves, and hence in less effective overdrive suppression, than slower pacing rates. This is why a wide range of pacing rates is used when measuring SNRT, instead of just the more rapid pacing rates.

In any case, determining the SNRT is easy enough; deciding whether that SNRT is normal or abnormal is a little more problematic. One difficulty is that overdrive suppression of the SA node, being a normal phenomenon, occurs in everybody. Unfortunately, there is wide variation in SNRTs among apparently normal individuals as well as considerable overlap in measured SNRTs between patients with apparently normal and clearly abnormal SA nodes.

Deciding on the upper normal values for the SNRT, then, is not dictated by nature but by electrophysiologists. "Normal" values vary from laboratory to laboratory, depending on whether electrophysiologists want their measurements to err on the side of sensitivity (in which case a lower value would be used) or specificity (in which case a higher value would be used). A conservative upper limit of "normal" for the SNRT, above which most experts would agree that SA nodal dysfunction is present, is 1500 ms.

Another difficulty in interpreting SNRTs is the fact that the SNRT is related to the underlying heart rate (or the basic cycle length, BCL), such that at slower underlying heart rates, a longer recovery time is normally seen. An SNRT that is abnormal at a shorter BCL could be normal at a longer BCL.

To account for this relationship between SNRT and BCL, electrophysiologists have created two indices, one or both of which are now measured routinely during electrophysiology studies. The first is the corrected sinus node recovery time (CSNRT), which is calculated simply by subtracting the patient's BCL from the SNRT. Thus:

$$CSNRT = SNRT - BCL$$

By convention, the upper limit of "normal" for the CSNRT is 525 ms. In other words, the SNRT should be no more than 525 ms longer than the BCL. The second index commonly used is the ratio of the SNRT to the BCL (SNRT/BCL × 100%). A ratio greater than 160% is usually considered abnormal.

Figure 5.1 demonstrates a normal SNRT. Here, the patient's BCL is 800 ms and the initial recovery interval is 1260 ms. Thus, the SNRT is 1260 ms, the CSNRT (SNRT − BCL) is 460 ms, and the ratio of the SNRT to the BCL is 158%. These values are all within normal limits.

An abnormal SNRT is demonstrated in Figure 5.2. The BCL in this example is also 800 ms. The longest recovery interval (and thus the SNRT) is 2200 ms. The CSNRT is 1400 ms, and the ratio of the SNRT to the BCL is 275%. All of these values are abnormal.

These two examples are straightforward in that all the SNRT measures – the SNRT itself, the CSNRT, and the ratio – are either normal (Figure 5.1) or abnormal (Figure 5.2). Not uncommonly, there will be divergence among these three measures. In such cases, the electrophysiologist must use their clinical judgment in interpreting the test. Given the relatively arbitrary nature of determining normal from abnormal SNRT values in the first place, this circumstance should not add appreciably to one's level of discomfort. Indeed, once you resort to the EP study for determining whether a patient's SA node is normal or not, you are signing up for a certain amount of arbitrariness.

Intrinsic heart rate (IHR)

As previously mentioned, the SA node is richly innervated by both sympathetic and parasympathetic fibers. Occasionally, it can therefore be difficult to determine whether suspected SA nodal dysfunction is actually intrinsic to the SA node or whether it might be due to abnormal autonomic tone. In such cases, it can be helpful to measure the intrinsic heart rate (IHR).

The IHR is assessed by administering drugs to block both branches of the autonomic nervous system and then measuring the resultant heart rate. Classically, autonomic blockade is accomplished by giving both propranolol (0.2 mg/kg) and atropine (0.04 mg/kg). According to the formula devised by Jose, after autonomic blockade the normal IHR $= 118 - (0.57 \times age)$.

Patients presenting with sinus bradycardia but who turn out to have normal IHRs are considered to have normal intrinsic SA nodal function; their bradycardia is apparently due to autonomic influences. Patients with bradycardia and depressed IHRs are considered to have intrinsic SA nodal dysfunction. Alternately, patients with inappropriate sinus tachycardia often have substantially elevated IHRs.

In clinical practice, it is rarely necessary to measure IHR in order to document intrinsic SA nodal disease. An exercise test, for instance, is a much simpler way to accomplish parasympathetic withdrawal in a patient presenting with sinus bradycardia, and a blunted heart rate response to exercise (in the absence of drugs that cause bradycardia, such as β-blockers and calcium blockers) usually clinches the diagnosis of intrinsic SA nodal dysfunction.

Interpreting SA nodal tests: when to carry out electrophysiologic testing

When assessing patients for SA nodal dysfunction, several simple points should be borne in mind. First, SA nodal dysfunction is generally not a lethal condition, and therapy is necessary only to the extent that it produces symptoms. Second, the best way to diagnose SA nodal dysfunction is to see it occurring spontaneously, because the specificity of such an observation is 100%. Thus, ambulatory cardiac monitoring (and not electrophysiologic testing) is the study of choice in assessing SA nodal dysfunction. Third, since the EP study can help to determine only whether SA nodal dysfunction is present (and not whether it causes symptoms), once unexplained sinus bradyarrhythmias are already known to occur, there is generally no reason to consider electrophysiologic testing. Fourth, while the EP study offers methods for evaluating the electrophysiologic properties of the SA node, the specificities and sensitivities of these tests as usually applied are estimated to be only approximately 70%.

With these points in mind, we can confidently state the following guidelines in assessing SA nodal disease.

- Asymptomatic sinus bradyarrhythmias need no evaluation or treatment.
- Asymptomatic abnormal SNRTs or IHRs need no treatment.
- Symptomatic sinus bradyarrhythmias should be treated with pacing, unless they are due to medications or to some other reversible cause.
- The only inarguable indication for performing electrophysiology studies to assess SA nodal function is in the evaluation of patients who present with episodic symptoms suggestive of bradyarrhythmias (especially syncope), and for whom no significant bradycardia is documented during cardiac monitoring.

Evaluation of AV conduction disorders

Atrioventricular conduction disorders are the second major cause of bradyarrhythmias. As with SA nodal disease, the clinician's chief concern with AV conduction disease is deciding whether the affected patient should receive a pacemaker. This decision is based on three essential pieces of data: whether the conduction disorder is producing *symptoms*; the *site* of the conduction disorder; and the *degree* of conduction block. Once again, thanks to what has been learned in the electrophysiology laboratory, we usually do not need to perform invasive testing to make this decision.

Symptoms of AV conduction disorders

The symptoms that occur with AV conduction disease are the same as those that occur with any bradyarrhythmia: lightheadedness, dizziness, presyncope, profound dyspnea on exertion, and syncope. Whatever the site or degree of block, AV block that produces any of these symptoms needs to be treated. Often, however, especially with first- or second-degree block, AV conduction disturbances are totally asymptomatic.

The site of the conduction disorder

Determining the site of the conduction disturbance is important for a simple reason: block that occurs in the AV node (proximal block) is usually benign, whereas block that occurs in the His–Purkinje system (distal block) is potentially lethal.

AV nodal block

Similar to sinus node dysfunction, AV nodal block is often due to aging. However, there can also be reversible causes. Ischemia or infarction involving the right coronary artery (which gives off the AV nodal artery in 90% of patients) can cause AV nodal block. Thus, heart block following an inferior myocardial infarction is usually localized to the AV node, and normal AV conduction almost always recovers (though block can persist for days or even weeks). While drugs that affect AV nodal function – mainly digoxin, β-blockers, and calcium blockers – may produce first-degree and second-degree (Wenckebach-type) AV block, drugs should not be implicated in complete AV block.

Complete heart block localized to the AV node is usually accompanied by the emergence of a relatively reliable escape pacemaker, located just distally to the AV node. This "high junctional" escape rhythm often yields a baseline heart rate of 40–55 beats/min, and responds at least moderately well to increases in sympathetic tone. Congenital complete heart block, which is usually localized to the AV node, illustrates the typical, relatively benign character of AV nodal block.

Since AV nodal block is usually reversible, it can frequently be managed simply by dealing with the underlying cause, although sometimes temporary pacing support is required in the meantime.

His–Purkinje block

In stark contrast to AV nodal block, block occurring distally to the AV node is potentially life-threatening. The potential lethal effect of distal heart block can largely be attributed to the unreliable, unstable, and slow escape pacemakers that tend to accompany this condition. These distal escape pacemakers usually discharge irregularly, 20–40 times per minute, and are prone to fail altogether. Thus, syncope, hemodynamic collapse, and death are much more likely to occur when AV block is located in the His–Purkinje system. Further, distal AV block tends to be chronic and progressive in nature, instead of transient and reversible.

Distal AV block following myocardial infarction is almost always associated with occlusion of the left anterior descending artery, and thus with anterior myocardial infarctions. His–Purkinje block can also be seen with inflammatory and infiltrative cardiac disease, with myocardial fibrosis, and in association with aortic valve and mitral valve calcification.

The degree of AV block

First-degree AV block

In first-degree AV block, all atrial impulses are transmitted to the ventricles, but with prolonged conduction times (Figure 5.3). First-degree block is diagnosed from the ECG; all P waves are conducted but the PR interval is prolonged (usually to between 0.20 and 0.40 seconds but sometimes much longer). In most patients with first-degree AV block, slow conduction is localized to the AV node; slow conduction in the His–Purkinje system can, however, occasionally cause first-degree block. First-degree AV block usually causes no symptoms.

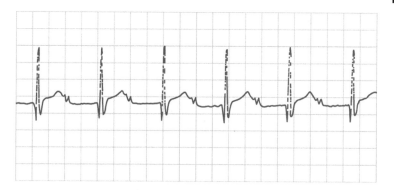

Figure 5.3 First-degree AV block. The PR interval in this figure is approximately 380 ms.

Second-degree AV block: Mobitz classification

In second-degree AV block, intermittent AV block is seen; on the ECG, some P waves are followed by QRS complexes and others are not. Symptoms depend largely on the resultant ventricular rate.

When second-degree AV block is observed, one should attempt to classify the block as either Mobitz type I (also called Wenckebach block) or Mobitz type II. The Mobitz classification helps to localize the site of the second-degree AV block.

In Mobitz type I block, there is a gradual prolongation of the PR interval in the conducted beats immediately preceding a blocked beat (Figure 5.4). The site of Mobitz type I block is usually (but not always) localized to the AV node. (Note that Figure 5.4 shows the unusual case in which Mobitz type I block is due to distal conducting disease.) In Mobitz type II block, the blocked beat occurs suddenly, without any lengthening of the PR intervals in the conducted beats preceding the dropped beat (Figure 5.5). *Mobitz type II block always indicates distal block.*

When differentiating Mobitz I from Mobitz II block, a common mistake is to only compare the PR intervals of successive conducted beats. Sometimes the prolongation in the PR interval from one beat to the next is so subtle that it can be easily missed, in which case Mobitz II block may be mistakenly declared. The best way to tell that the Mobitz I pattern of PR interval prolongation is occurring is to compare the PR interval of the last conducted beat prior to the dropped beat with the PR interval of the first conducted beat after the dropped beat. That is, compare the "longest" conducted PR interval to the "shortest"

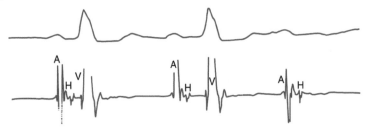

Figure 5.4 Mobitz I AV block. A surface ECG and a His bundle electrogram from a patient with Mobitz I AV block are shown. On the surface ECG, progressive prolongation of the PR interval is seen prior to the nonconducted P wave. Although most instances of Mobitz I AV block are located in the AV node, this example illustrates that Mobitz I block occasionally can be seen with disease in the more distal conducting tissue. As seen in the His bundle electrogram, PR prolongation occurs as a result of gradually slowing conduction beyond the His bundle (i.e., prolonging HV interval), and when block finally occurs, it occurs below the His bundle.

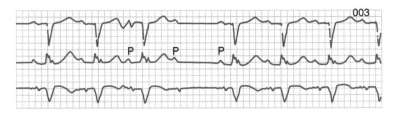

Figure 5.5 Mobitz II AV block. This figure shows three simultaneous surface ECG leads. The nonconducted P wave occurs suddenly, without progressive prolongation in the PR interval. Mobitz II block always indicates distal conducting system disease.

conducted PR interval – a difference between these two PR intervals is almost always easily detectable with Mobitz I block.

It is important to realize that the Mobitz classification can only be used when you can find at least one instance in which two consecutively conducted beats immediately precede a blocked beat. The reason for this limitation is simple – in order for there to be progressive prolongation in the PR interval prior to the dropped beat, at least two consecutively conducted beats must occur. Stating it another way: you cannot use the Mobitz classification with 2 : 1 AV block; by definition, it does not apply (Figure 5.6). Many clinicians make the mistake of automatically classifying 2 : 1 block as Mobitz II, thus misdiagnosing many cases of 2 : 1 AV nodal block as distal block. When 2 : 1 block is

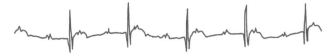

Figure 5.6 2 : 1 AV block. Every other P wave in this figure is nonconducted. The Mobitz classification system cannot be applied here.

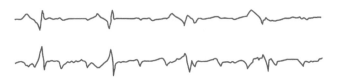

Figure 5.7 Complete heart block with a slow ventricular escape mechanism. Distal heart block is likely in this example.

present, some means other than Mobitz classification must be used to deduce the site of block.

Third-degree AV block

In third-degree AV block, no atrial impulses are conducted to the ventricles – complete AV block is present (Figure 5.7). Maintaining a ventricular rhythm in the presence of third-degree AV block is totally dependent on subsidiary escape pacemakers. As noted earlier, the reliability of those escape pacemakers is related to the site of block. With AV nodal block, the escape pacemakers tend to be relatively reliable; with distal block, they tend to be unreliable and slow. Distal third-degree AV block is much more likely to produce symptoms than third-degree block located in the AV node.

AV dissociation

The presence of AV dissociation can lead to confusion when attempting to discern whether third-degree AV block is present. AV dissociation simply means that the atria and ventricles are each being controlled by their own independent pacemakers. While AV dissociation is present in all cases of complete heart block, complete heart block is *not* present in all cases of AV dissociation. Complete heart block is merely one variety of AV dissociation.

Figure 5.8 illustrates AV dissociation without complete heart block. Here, normal sinus rhythm is present at a rate of 65 beats/min but

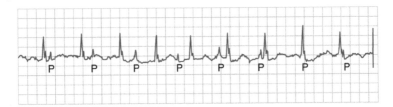

Figure 5.8 AV dissociation without complete heart block. In this tracing, the sinus rate is simply slower than the junctional escape rate. The fourth P wave conducts to the ventricles (since the following QRS complex occurs at a coupling interval that is shorter than the escape interval of the junctional escape).Thus, not all AV dissociation is complete heart block.

an accelerated junctional pacemaker is also present with a rate of 78 beats/min. Thus, the atrial and ventricular rhythms are functioning independently – that is, they are dissociated. Note the fourth P wave in Figure 5.11. This P wave happens to occur at a time when the AV conducting system is no longer refractory from the previous junctional impulse, and it is conducted to the ventricles. Since an appropriately timed atrial complex is conducted, there is no heart block. As a general rule, when the atrial rate is faster than the ventricular rate and no atrial impulses are conducted, complete heart block is present. If the ventricular rate is higher than the atrial rate, AV dissociation without heart block should be suspected.

Treatment of AV block

Table 5.1 summarizes the treatment of AV block based on symptoms, the degree of block, and the site of block. In general, determining the presence or absence of symptoms and the degree of AV block is simple. If there is a problem in deciding on therapy, it almost always lies in localizing the site of AV block.

Localizing the site of AV block
In most cases, localizing the site of block can be done noninvasively, by evaluating the ECG and performing selected autonomic maneuvers.

The ECG can be helpful in several ways. A wide QRS complex indicates the presence of distal conducting system disease and should raise suspicions of infranodal block. In cases of complete heart block, a wide-complex, slow (20–40 beats/min) escape pacemaker is a strong indicator of distal AV block; a narrow-complex and more

Table 5.1 Indications for pacing based on the site and degree of AV block.

	Should a permanent pacemaker be implanted?	
	AV nodal block	Distal block
First-degree AV block	No	No[a]
Second-degree AV block	No[b]	Yes
Third-degree AV block	No[b]	Yes

[a]Unless the HV interval is >100 ms.
[b]Unless symptomatic bradycardia is present.

rapid (40–55 beats/min) escape rhythm suggests AV nodal block (see Figure 2.3). If second-degree AV block is present, the Mobitz classification should be applied (unless the only conduction ratio seen is 2 : 1). Mobitz I block suggests AV nodal disease, whereas Mobitz II block always indicates distal block.

Autonomic maneuvers are useful because the AV node has rich autonomic innervation and the distal conducting system does not. Maneuvers that decrease vagal tone or increase sympathetic tone can be expected to improve AV nodal block but not distal block. Maneuvers that increase vagal tone or decrease sympathetic tone will worsen AV nodal block but not distal block.

Autonomic maneuvers are especially helpful when either Mobitz type I block or 2 : 1 second-degree AV block is present. In AV nodal block, exercise or atropine administration will improve or resolve the block. In distal block, these same maneuvers will not improve the AV block; in fact, the conduction ratio often worsens (e.g. 2 : 1 block may shift to 3 : 1 block; see Figure 5.9). Table 5.2 summarizes noninvasive techniques for localizing the site of AV block.

Occasionally, the site of block remains unclear, even after a careful noninvasive evaluation. In these instances, the EP study virtually always resolves the issue.

The electrophysiology study in the evaluation of AV conduction disorders

The key to localizing AV conduction disorders in the electrophysiology laboratory is the His bundle electrogram. The recording and interpretation of this electrogram are described in detail in Chapter 4.

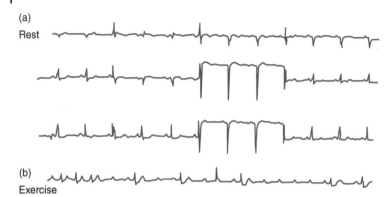

(a)
Rest

(b)
Exercise

Figure 5.9 Exercise-induced worsening of AV conduction. (a) The resting 12-lead ECG of a patient who had intermittent 2 : 1 AV conduction. (b) With exercise, the conduction ratio is markedly worsened, strongly implying distal conducting system disease.

Table 5.2 Noninvasive differentiation of AV nodal and infranodal block.

	AV nodal	Infranodal
Exercise/isoproterenol	Improves	Conduction ratio may worsen
Atropine	Improves	Conduction ratio may worsen
Vagal maneuvers	Worsens	No change
P-blockers	Worsens	No change

In review, the His bundle electrogram consists of three major deflections (Figure 5.10). The A deflection represents depolarization of atrial tissue proximate to the AV node. The H spike represents the depolarization of the His bundle itself. The V spike represents the depolarization of the ventricular myocardium. The AH interval is therefore an approximation of the conduction time through the AV node (normally 50–120 ms) and the HV interval is an approximation of the conduction time through the His–Purkinje system (normally 35–55 ms). Thus, the His bundle electrogram reveals the function of all the major components of AV conduction.

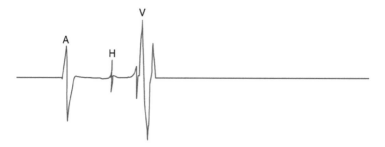

Figure 5.10 Atypical His bundle electrogram.

(a)

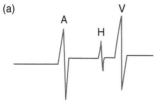

(b)

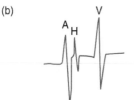

Figure 5.11 His bundle electrogram patterns seen with first-degree AV block. (a) Prolonged conduction in the AV node (the AH interval is prolonged). (b) Prolonged conduction below the AV node (the HV interval is prolonged).

Overt AV conduction disturbances

In the patient with overt AV conduction disturbances, the His bundle electrogram immediately reveals the site of block.

When first-degree AV block is localized to the AV node, a prolonged AH interval will be seen (Figure 5.11a), while first-degree block below the AV node will produce a prolonged HV interval (Figures 5.11b and 5.12). It should be noted that significantly slowed conduction through the His–Purkinje structures can occur without overt first-degree AV block. For instance, a lengthening of the HV interval from 50 to 100 ms

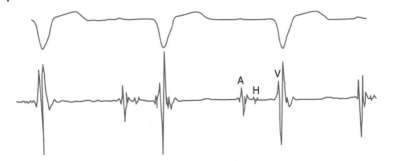

Figure 5.12 Distal first-degree AV block. A surface ECG lead and the His bundle electrogram of a patient with first-degree AV block are shown. The conduction delay can be seen to occur in the distal structures, because the AH interval is normal and the HV interval is prolonged.

(a markedly abnormal value) may prolong the PR interval only from 140 to 190 ms (still within the normal range).

Occasionally, slowed conduction within the His bundle itself can be observed. The normal conduction time through the His bundle (measured by the duration of the H spike on the His–bundle electrogram) is less than 25 ms – a longer H spike duration reflects His–bundle conduction delay. Sometimes, a His–bundle conduction delay is sufficiently severe to produce an actual splitting of the His deflection (Figure 5.13).

While there is no general agreement on whether to treat patients with asymptomatic prolongations in the HV interval, most physicians

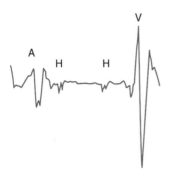

Figure 5.13 Split His. Conduction disease within the His bundle itself is present, because the His bundle is split into two discrete components. A split His potential indicates significant distal conducting system disease.

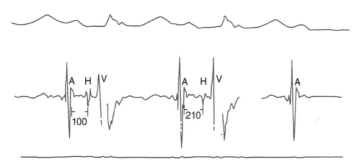

Figure 5.14 Typical Mobitz I AV block. A surface ECG lead and the His bundle electrogram are shown. Note the progressive prolongation of the AH interval (and the PR interval) prior to the nonconducted P wave. The blocked beat occurs when the impulse fails to exit the AV node (the A complex is not followed by an H spike in the blocked beat). This is much more typical for Mobitz I AV block than the example shown in Figure 5.7.

agree that a permanent pacemaker is indicated if the HV interval is very prolonged (i.e., greater than 100 ms) or if a split His is present.

With second-degree AV block of Mobitz type I (Figure 5.14), the intracardiac electrogram usually shows a progressive prolongation of the AH interval in the beats immediately prior to the dropped atrial impulse (indicating a gradual slowing in conduction through the AV node before the dropped beat). With the dropped beat itself, the A deflection is not followed by an H spike, indicating block within the AV node. Again, while Mobitz type I block usually indicates AV nodal block, a Mobitz I pattern is occasionally seen with block in the His–Purkinje system (Figure 5.4).

Mobitz type II block (Figure 5.15) is always located in the His–Purkinje system. Thus, the His bundle electrogram shows a normal AH interval and a stable HV interval in all the conducted beats,

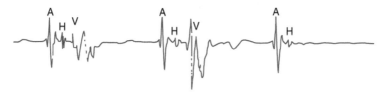

Figure 5.15 Mobitz II AV block. The His bundle electrogram is shown. The beat is dropped after the H spike and has no prior prolongation in either the AH or the HV interval.

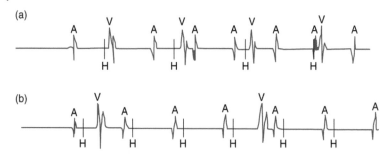

Figure 5.16 His bundle electrograms in complete heart block. (a) With block in the AV node, H spikes are seen prior to the escape V complexes, indicating a high junctional escape pacemaker. No H spikes are seen after the blocked A complexes, indicating block in the AV node. (b) With distal AV block, an H spike follows each nonconducted A complex. The distal ventricular escape complexes are not preceded by H spikes.

but in the dropped beat there is suddenly no ventricular depolarization after the H spike.

With third-degree block within the AV node, the A spikes are not followed by H spikes. Further, since the escape pacemaker is usually proximal to the His bundle, escape pacemaker complexes are usually preceded by His potentials (Figure 5.16a). With third-degree block occurring in the His–Purkinje system, the A spike is followed by an H spike but there is no V spike after the H. The escape ventricular electrogram is not preceded by a His potential, since these escape pacemakers are distal to the His bundle (Figure 5.16b).

Inapparent AV conduction disturbances

Patients may present with symptoms compatible with AV conduction disease but show no conduction abnormalities on either ECG or monitoring. In such cases the EP study can be helpful.

The goal in electrophysiologic testing is to stress AV conduction by pacing the right atrium, while recording the His electrogram to observe what happens. Two primary pacing methods are used, as described in Chapter 4: the extrastimulus technique (in which a single atrial premature stimulus is introduced, after a drive train of stimuli at a fixed cycle length) and incremental pacing.

The extrastimulus technique

This technique is illustrated in Figure 5.17. Following a drive train of several (usually eight) incrementally paced beats (the S1 beats) at a

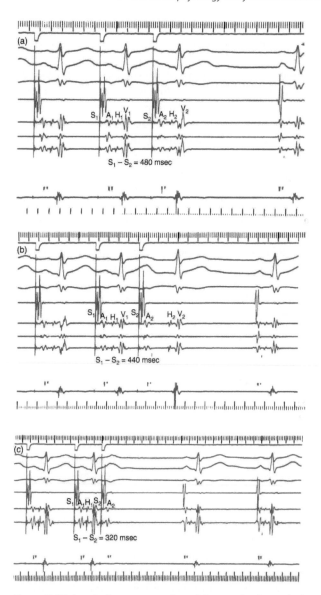

Figure 5.17 A typical response to the atrial extrastimulus technique. Three surface ECG leads, one right atrial electrogram, three His bundle electrograms, and one right ventricular electrogram are shown. (a) The S1–S2 coupling interval of 480 ms is followed by a minimal prolongation of the AH interval. (b) With further shortening of the S1–S2 coupling interval (to 440 ms), progressive prolongation in the AH interval is seen (compare this A2–H2 interval to that in (a)). (c) With an S1–S2 coupling interval of 320 ms, the S2 stimulus is blocked in the AV node (the A2 complex is not followed by an H spike).

fixed cycle length (usually 600 ms), a single premature atrial stimulus is introduced (the S2 beat). The coupling interval between the last S1 beat and the S2 beat is initially relatively long (usually 500 ms), but with each subsequent pacing sequence it is progressively shortened. The goal is to determine *when* AV block first occurs and *where* it first occurs (i.e., in or distal to the AV node) in response to the S2 impulses.

The normal sequence of events is shown in Figure 5.17. The AH interval and HV interval measured during the S1 drive train are considered to represent the baseline AV node and His–Purkinje conduction times. Any prolongations in AH and HV intervals observed with the S2 beat then reflect slowed conduction in response to premature impulses. Initially, the S2 beat is conducted normally, with little or no delay in either the AH or HV intervals (Figure 5.17a). As the S1–S2 coupling interval becomes gradually shorter, the relative refractory period (RRP) of the AV node is reached (i.e., at this point conduction through the AV node becomes prolonged – see Chapter 4 for a review of the definitions of relative, effective, and functional refractory periods [FRPs]). Thus, the AH interval becomes longer (Figure 5.17b). With progressively shorter S1–S2 intervals, the resultant AH interval becomes even longer, until finally the S2 beat is so early that block occurs in the AV node (Figure 5.17c). The coupling interval that produces block in the AV node is the effective refractory period (ERP) of the AV node. By measuring the H1–H2 intervals that result with each pacing sequence, the FRP of the AV node can be determined (the FRP of the AV node is the shortest H1–H2 interval attained). The His–Purkinje ERP is usually significantly shorter than the AV nodal FRP, so that the His–Purkinje structures are usually "protected" by the conduction delays in the AV node. Thus, block in the His–Purkinje system is seldom seen during the extrastimulus technique in normal patients.

Figure 5.18 shows an abnormally prolonged AV nodal ERP. At a coupling interval of 480 ms, the S2 impulse is blocked in the AV node. The significance of this finding would depend largely on whether the patient showed evidence of symptomatic bradyarrhythmias. If so, and if the AV nodal dysfunction were intrinsic (i.e., not reversible), pacing might be considered. Note that in this example, it would be difficult to diagnose concomitant His–Purkinje disease because the long ERP (and thus the long FRP) of the AV node prevents us from evaluating the effect of early impulses on the more distal structures. To evaluate the His–Purkinje system in such a patient, it would be necessary to

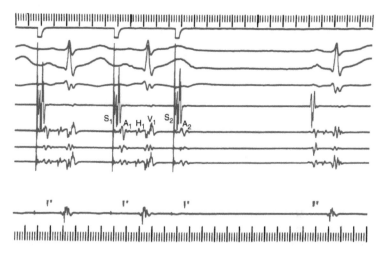

Figure 5.18 Abnormal AV nodal function brought out by the extrastimulus technique. The same leads are depicted as in Figure 5.20. With an S1–S2 coupling interval of 480 ms, block occurs in the AV node.

attempt to improve AV nodal function by administering atropine or isoproterenol.

An example of abnormal His–Purkinje function is shown in Figure 5.19. At an S1–S2 interval of 460 ms, the impulse is conducted normally to the His bundle through the AV node (we know this from the normal AH interval), but infranodal block is present because the impulse is not conducted to the ventricles (i.e., the H spike is not followed by a V spike). Block in the His–Purkinje system at an H1–H2 interval of greater than 400 ms indicates significant distal conducting system disease.

Incremental pacing

With this technique (illustrated in Figure 5.20), long sequences of right atrial pacing are introduced while observing the behavior of the AV node and the His–Purkinje system. A pacing rate slightly faster than the underlying sinus rate is used initially. The pacing rate is gradually increased with each subsequent pacing sequence.

The normal response to incremental pacing is shown in Figure 5.20. At progressively faster atrial pacing rates, the AH interval gradually increases until the refractory period of the AV node is reached, at which time second-degree AV block occurs, typically in a Mobitz I

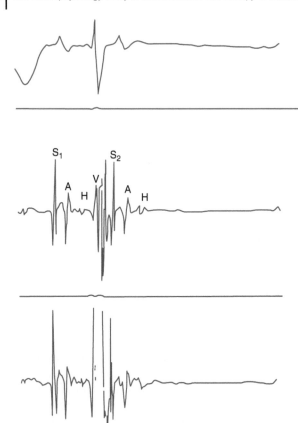

Figure 5.19 Abnormal His–Purkinje function brought out by the extrastimulus technique. With an S1–S2 coupling interval of 460 ms, block occurs below the His bundle (the H spike is not followed by a V complex). A surface ECG lead and two His bundle electrograms are shown.

pattern. In this case, the AH interval gradually prolongs from 110 ms at a paced cycle length of 600 ms (Figure 5.20a) to 160 ms at a cycle length of 450 ms (Figure 5.20b). Finally, in Figure 5.20c, at a cycle length of 400 ms, Mobitz I second-degree AV block is seen (note the gradually increasing AH intervals prior to the dropped beat). The atrial pacing rate at which Mobitz type I block occurs is called the *Wenckebach cycle length*. Normally, this length is less than or equal to 450 ms.

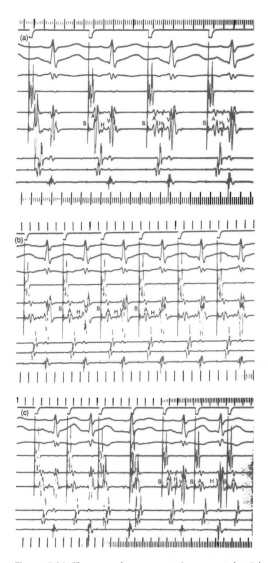

Figure 5.20 The normal response to incremental atrial pacing. Three surface ECG leads followed by one right atrial electrogram, two His bundle electrograms, two coronary sinus electrograms, and one right ventricular electrogram are shown.
(a) Incremental pacing from the high right atrium at a cycle length of 600 ms results in normal AV conduction (as shown in the labeled His bundle electrogram).
(b) At a faster incrementally paced cycle length (450 ms), prolongation in the AH interval (compared to (a)) is apparent. All atrial impulses, however, are conducted.
(c) At a paced cycle length of 400 ms, Mobitz I conduction occurs. Note the progressive prolongation in the AH intervals in the beats preceding the non-conducted P wave. Thus, the Wenckebach cycle length is 400 ms (abnormal value).

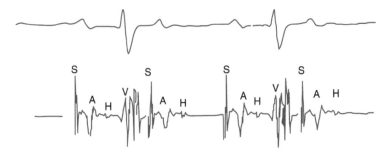

Figure 5.21 Distal AV block during incremental atrial pacing. In this figure, during incremental atrial pacing, 2 : 1 AV block occurs. The His bundle electrogram shows that the block is in the distal conducting system – the AH interval is constant, and there is an H spike in the nonconducted beats.

During incremental atrial pacing, the Wenckebach cycle length is normally encountered before any prolongation of the HV interval is seen. Lengthening of the HV interval, or block in the His bundle, occurring at a paced cycle length of greater than or equal to 400 ms indicates an abnormal distal conducting system. An example of distal block is shown in Figure 5.21. At a cycle length of 460 ms, intermittent second-degree AV block is seen. The His electrogram reveals a constant AH interval, with intermittent block occurring in the His–Purkinje system (in dropped beats, H spikes are not followed by V spikes). Once again, if distal conducting system disease is suspected but the AV nodal refractory periods are too long to allow the His–Purkinje system to be fully evaluated, autonomic maneuvers should be considered to reduce the refractoriness of the AV node and permit further testing of the infranodal conducting system.

Bundle branch block

As we saw in Chapter 1, the His bundle divides into two main branches – the right and left bundle branches. Electrical impulses exiting the AV conduction system are rapidly transmitted through the right and left bundle branches, then through successive branches of Purkinje fibers, and finally to the right and left ventricular myocardium. The bundle branches and Purkinje system distribute the electrical impulse across the ventricular myocardium in such a way as to optimally coordinate the contraction of both ventricles.

The bundle branches and Purkinje fibers are subject to the same sorts of disorders as the rest of the cardiac conducting system. When there is a general slowing of conduction in or distal to the bundle branches, the distribution of the electrical impulse to the ventricular myocardium is delayed, and an intraventricular conduction delay (IVCD) is said to be present. An IVCD is manifested on a surface ECG by a wide QRS complex.

Delayed or blocked conduction is commonly limited specifically to either the right or the left bundle branch, conditions referred to as right bundle branch block (RBBB) or left bundle branch block (LBBB). Thus, RBBB and LBBB are specific varieties of IVCD.

Right bundle branch block (RBBB)

RBBB is a relatively common ECG finding that generally carries little prognostic significance. The incidence of RBBB gradually increases with age, from less than 1% in 50 year olds to approximately 10% in octogenarians. Most younger patients with RBBB have no underlying heart disease.

The right bundle branch remains a relatively discrete structure for a few centimeters after splitting off from the His bundle, and for most of its course it is located just beneath the endocardial surface, where it is subject to stretch and trauma from conditions affecting the right ventricle. Thus, RBBB is common in conditions causing pulmonary hypertension or right ventricular hypertrophy, inflammation, or infarction. RBBB can appear quite abruptly with sudden elevations in right-sided cardiac pressures, as in pulmonary embolism. RBBB can also occur during right heart catheter insertions due to localized trauma to the right bundle branch – this latter form of RBBB, which is seen in roughly 5% of right heart catheterizations, is usually transient.

The prognosis of patients with RBBB is dictated not by the RBBB itself but almost entirely by the type and severity of any underlying heart disease. If there is no underlying heart disease – that is, if RBBB is an isolated finding in an otherwise normal patient – the long-term prognosis appears virtually normal.

As long as the left bundle branch functions normally, patients with RBBB do not appear to suffer from clinically significant ventricular dyssynchrony; that is, left ventricular contractions remain coordinated and efficient.

The presence of RBBB alone is never an indication for a permanent pacemaker.

Left bundle branch block (LBBB)

LBBB, while not uncommon, is seen less frequently than RBBB. The incidence of LBBB is less than 0.5% in 50 year olds, but increases to 5–6% by age 80 (the age-related increase in frequency seen with both varieties of bundle branch block suggests a degenerative disorder of the conducting system, similar to the process that causes SA nodal and AV conduction abnormalities in the same age group).

Younger patients with LBBB usually have no underlying heart disease, in which case the prognosis is thought to be excellent. In older patients, for whom the new onset of LBBB most often indicates the presence of progressive heart disease (most commonly coronary artery disease, cardiomyopathy, or valvular heart disease), LBBB is an independent predictor of mortality.

There are at least two reasons why LBBB may indicate a worse prognosis in patients with underlying heart disease. The first is related to the fact that the left bundle branch almost immediately divides into three major fascicles after splitting off from the His bundle, and thus quickly becomes a relatively diffuse system. For this reason, the presence of LBBB (in contrast to RBBB) both suggests a diffuse pathological process instead of a localized one and frequently indicates that advanced heart disease is present. The second reason is that the LBBB itself produces disordered left ventricular contraction and, in patients with underlying systolic dysfunction, can directly worsen cardiac performance (see Chapter 14, especially Figure 14.1, for an explanation of how LBBB produces ventricular dyssynchrony). In many cases, patients with LBBB and heart failure can be helped with cardiac resynchronization therapy (CRT) – specialized pacemakers that pace both ventricles simultaneously, thus recoordinating ventricular contraction. (See Chapter 14 for a more detailed discussion of CRT.)

The presence of LBBB alone does not constitute an indication for a standard, antibradycardia permanent pacemaker. As noted, however, in some clinical circumstances patients will have an indication for CRT pacemakers by virtue of their LBBB. Further, when performing a right heart catheterization in patients with LBBB, provisions for immediate temporary pacing support should be available, since there is roughly a 5% chance of causing transient RBBB (and thus complete heart block) during the procedure. In addition, some patients experiencing block in one of the fascicles of the left bundle branch in combination with RBBB (a condition known as bilateral fascicular block) and a myocardial infarction have an increased risk of complete heart block and should receive permanent pacemakers.

A brief overview of permanent pacemakers

Major indications for pacemakers

In the preceding discussion, we have touched upon the major indications for permanent pacemakers. The following list makes these indications more explicit.

1. Symptomatic sinus bradycardia.
   - Symptomatic sinus bradycardia at rest.
   - Inability to increase the sinus rate appropriately with exercise (i.e., chronotropic incompetence), thus limiting exercise capacity.
   - Syncope of unknown origin in patients who are shown to have significant SA nodal abnormalities on electrophysiologic testing.
2. AV conduction disease.
   - Acquired third-degree AV block.
   - Second-degree AV block below the AV node.
   - Second-degree AV nodal block if persistent and symptomatic.
   - New bilateral fascicular block following an acute myocardial infarction.
   - Congenital complete heart block with severe bradycardia, significant symptoms, or wide-QRS escape rhythm.
   - Markedly prolonged HV interval (>100 ms) or split His.
3. Other indications for pacing.
   - Cardioneurogenic syncope (also known as vasodepressor syncope; see Chapter 15), in which there is a severe or persistent component of bradycardia, in patients in whom more conservative therapeutic attempts have failed.
   - Syncope of unknown origin in the presence of bilateral fascicular block, where no other cause of syncope can be identified.
   - Bradycardia-induced ventricular tachyarrhythmias

- CRT is indicated for many patients with significant left ventricle (LV) dysfunction (ejection fraction less than 0.35) and wide QRS complex (QRS duration more than 120 ms). CRT is discussed in detail in Chapter 14.

Pacemaker nomenclature

While in practical terms, most pacemakers can be separated into one of two categories – single-chambered or dual-chambered – any pacemaker can be programmed to a potentially bewildering array of "modes." If we view a pacemaker as a tiny computer enclosed within an implantable metal can, the pacing mode can be thought of as the set of instructions – or the software program – that tells the pacemaker how to function under various circumstances.

By convention, pacing modes are described by a *three-letter code.*

The *first letter* indicates the chamber or chambers that are paced. "A" indicates the atrium; "V" indicates the ventricle; and "D" (which stands for "dual chamber") indicates both atrium and ventricle.

The *second letter* indicates the chamber or chambers in which sensing occurs. Again, "A" indicates the atrium; "V" indicates the ventricle; "D" indicates both atrium and ventricle; and "O" means no sensing is occurring.

The *third letter* indicates how the pacemaker responds to a sensed event. "I" means that a sensed event causes inhibition of the pacing impulse (and resets the timing intervals). "T" means a sensed event triggers a pacing impulse. "D," which is only used in dual-chambered devices, means there is a "dual" (or two kinds of) response – a sensed event can either inhibit or trigger a pacing impulse, depending on circumstances. "O" means that a sensed event neither inhibits nor triggers a pacing impulse – it is "ignored."

In addition, *a fourth letter* is often employed to indicate that rate-responsive pacing is being used. Rate-responsive pacing incorporates a sensor into the pacing system that continually monitors the physiologic needs of the patient. The rate of pacing is thereby adjusted to the physiologic requirements of the patient from moment to moment. The sensors used most commonly in today's pacemakers monitor either activity or respiratory rate – the more active the patient or the more rapidly they are breathing, the higher the rate of pacing (within a programmed limit). The fourth letter "R" is added to the three-letter code if rate-responsive pacing is active.

Common modes of pacing

For practical purposes, only two modes are used with any frequency: the VVI (or AAI) mode for single-chambered pacemakers and the DDD mode for dual-chambered pacemakers.

VVI or AAI pacing

Single-chambered pacemakers function in the VVI mode when the pacing lead is positioned in the ventricle and in the AAI mode when the lead is in the atrium. These pacemakers simply maintain a minimum programmable heart rate. Each timing sequence is initiated by either a paced impulse or a sensed (i.e., intrinsic) impulse. If an intrinsic beat does not occur (i.e., is not sensed) by the end of this timing sequence, a paced impulse is delivered and a new timing sequence is begun (thus a VVI pacemaker paces in the ventricle [V] and senses intrinsic beats occurring in the ventricle [V], and a sensed event causes it to inhibit pacing and resets the timing sequence [I]). Essentially, then, the doctor programs a minimum heart rate, and whenever the patient's IHR falls below that value, pacing occurs at the programmed rate; if the IHR is above the programmed rate, pacing is inhibited. An electrogram from a VVI pacemaker is illustrated in Figure 5.22.

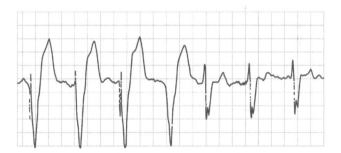

Figure 5.22 This surface ECG tracing is from a patient with a VVI pacemaker. A VVI pacemaker paces the ventricle at a fixed rate, unless intrinsic ventricular activity is sensed during the pacemaker escape interval (the length of time after a QRS complex during which the pacemaker waits for an intrinsic QRS complex before firing). The first four beats show ventricular pacing. After the fourth paced beat, an intrinsic QRS complex occurs during the pacemaker escape interval. This inhibits the pacemaker from firing and resets the pacemaker escape interval. Two more intrinsic QRS complexes occur, and the pacemaker remains appropriately inhibited.

AAI pacemakers work in exactly the same way, except that the pacing lead is located in the atrium instead of the ventricle. AAI pacing is used exclusively in patients with isolated SA nodal dysfunction; that is, patients who show no evidence of AV conduction disease. For such patients, AAI pacing provides both rate support and AV synchrony and is an excellent choice. AAI pacing is not used commonly in the United States (apparently, American doctors are afraid of either occult AV conduction disease or American lawyers) but is employed quite frequently in many other countries.

VVI pacemakers offer perfectly acceptable protection from brad-yarrhythmias but do not restore AV synchrony. In general, VVI pacemakers are used in patients who are felt to need only rare to occasional ventricular pacing support.

Practically speaking, almost all single-chambered pacemakers in use today are programmed to rate-responsive modes (i.e., either AAIR or VVIR pacing modes), so the rate of pacing is not fixed but adjusts from minute to minute according to the needs of the patient. Since AAI pacing is used exclusively in patients with SA nodal disease, and thus in patients who are likely to have a blunted heart rate response to exercise, it is difficult to imagine a circumstance in which AAI pacing would be chosen over AAIR pacing. VVIR pacemakers are a good choice for patients with chronic atrial fibrillation.

DDD pacing

Modern dual-chambered pacemakers almost always function in the DDD mode. In DDD pacing, pacing occurs in both the right atrium and the right ventricle (D), sensing in both the atrium and the ventricle (D), and a sensed event can either trigger or inhibit a pacing output (D) (see Figure 5.23).

DDD pacemakers are designed to preserve the normal sequence of AV contraction under a wide range of circumstances and, if the SA node is functioning normally, to allow tracking of the intrinsic sinus rate. Atrial pacing occurs if the intrinsic atrial rate falls below the minimum programmed heart rate. After a paced or sensed atrial event, the pacemaker will wait a certain length of time (i.e., the programmed AV interval) for the ventricle to depolarize. If no intrinsic ventricular activity is detected during that interval, the ventricle is then paced.

Most dual-chambered pacemakers used today offer a rate-responsive mode (i.e., the DDDR mode) to allow higher heart rates in response to physiologic needs, even if the SA nodal dysfunction is present.

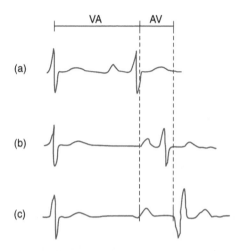

Figure 5.23 DDD pacing is designed to maintain AV coordination under most circumstances. DDD pacing can be described largely by considering two escape intervals: the VA interval and the AV interval (both of which are programmable with DDD pacemakers). When a QRS complex occurs (either intrinsic or paced), the VA interval is reset. If no intrinsic atrial or ventricular activity is sensed by the end of the VA interval, an atrial pacing spike is delivered. Once an atrial event occurs (either a paced or an intrinsic atrial event), the AV interval is initiated. If no intrinsic ventricular activity occurs during the AV interval, a ventricular pacing spike is delivered at the end of that interval. (a) An intrinsic P-QRS complex occurs during the VA interval, and all pacing is inhibited. (b) No atrial or ventricular activity is sensed during the VA interval, and atrial pacing occurs. During the ensuing AV interval, normal conduction occurs to the ventricle, so ventricular pacing is inhibited. (c) Same as in (b), except that this time conduction to the ventricles does not occur during the AV interval, so the ventricle is also paced.

DDDR pacing is ideal for patients with both SA nodal and AV conduction disorders.

CRT pacing

CRT – also known as *biventricular pacing* – is done not to provide bradycardia support but instead to improve left ventricular hemo- dynamic function in patients with both systolic heart failure and significant IVCDs. CRT therapy is discussed in detail in Chapter 14.

Complications intrinsic to pacemaker therapy

While pacemakers have saved countless lives, and have improved the quality of life in countless others, these medical devices are not without their complications. Indeed, at least four potential problems are related to pacemaker therapy itself: pacemaker syndrome, pacemaker tachycardia, inappropriate rate tracking, and ventricular dyssynchrony.

Pacemaker syndrome

The major clinical problem inherent in VVI/R pacing is pacemaker syndrome. This arises when intrinsic atrial impulses occur during or just after ventricular pacing, thus causing the atria to contract against closed AV valves and producing reflux of atrial blood through the superior vena cava and pulmonary veins. Symptoms may include headache, dizziness, fatigue, lethargy, neck throbbing, cough, dyspnea, chest "fullness," and, occasionally, orthostatic hypotension or syncope. Pacemaker syndrome is especially prevalent in patients who have intact retrograde conduction, where retrograde impulses stimulate atrial contraction immediately after ventricular pacing. In some series, more than 20% of patients who require frequent VVI pacing display some degree of pacemaker syndrome.

Pacemaker syndrome is resolved by changing over to a dual-chambered pacemaker. Patients with chronic atrial fibrillation are not subject to pacemaker syndrome.

Pacemaker tachycardia

The most common clinical problem inherent to DDD pacemakers is pacemaker tachycardia, in which (i) a premature ventricular complex causes a retrograde impulse to be transmitted to the atrium, where (ii) it is sensed by the atrial lead and interpreted by the pacemaker as an intrinsic atrial beat, so that (iii) the pacemaker then triggers a ventricular paced beat, which again (iv) transmits a retrograde impulse to the atrium, thus establishing a pacemaker-mediated "reentrant tachycardia" (Figure 5.24). In the typical case, pacemaker tachycardia occurs at the maximum programmed pacing rate.

A number of methods have been used to control pacemaker tachycardia.

- Lengthening the postventricular atrial refractory period (PVARP) can essentially "blind" the atrium for a time after a ventricular event, to reduce the odds that a retrograde P wave will be sensed. Unfortunately, increasing the PVARP also reduces the maximum tracking rate the pacemaker will allow.

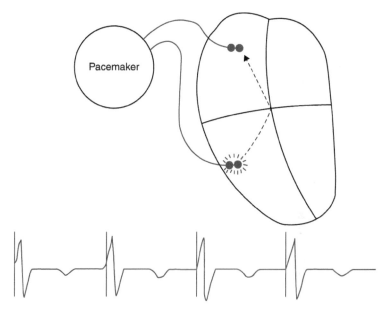

Figure 5.24 Pacemaker tachycardia. With DDD pacemakers, the potential for a reentrant tachycardia exists, the pacemaker itself serving as the antegrade limb of the reentrant circuit. Pacemaker tachycardia is most often initiated by a PVC, which conducts retrogradely to the atrium. The atrial electrode of the pacemaker senses the retrograde atrial impulse and initiates the AV escape interval of the DDD pacemaker. At the end of the AV interval, a ventricular pacing spike is delivered. If this paced ventricular impulse again conducts retrogradely to the atrium, an incessant tachycardia can result.

- The sensitivity of the atrial lead can be reduced, so that SA nodal impulses can still be detected but retrograde P waves (which often have relatively small amplitudes) cannot.
- Many modern pacemakers incorporate a feature that automatically lengthens PVARP for one cycle following a premature ventricular complex, which can inhibit the initiation of pacemaker tachycardia.
- Special algorithms, available in some pacemakers, can automatically withhold a single ventricular paced impulse after a certain number of beats, whenever the pacemaker is pacing at the maximum tracking rate. This single inhibited ventricular impulse will terminate pacemaker tachycardia.

In general, by using one or more of these strategies, pacemaker tachycardia can be managed adequately.

Inappropriate rate tracking

In the past, DDD pacing was often difficult to manage in patients with episodic atrial tachyarrhythmias, since the pacemaker would track the atrial tachycardia and pace the ventricle at inappropriately high rates. Because patients with sick sinus syndrome often develop these arrhythmias, inappropriate rate tracking was once a major problem.

This has been largely resolved by including mode-switching features in modern pacemakers. Under mode-switching, when an atrial tachyarrhythmia occurs, the pacemaker automatically switches to a nonatrial tracking mode, most commonly the VVI (or VVIR) mode. When the atrial arrhythmia terminates, the pacemaker switches back to the DDD (or DDDR) mode.

Ventricular dyssynchrony

In patients with heart failure, left bundle branch block is associated with worse outcomes because it produces ventricular dyssynchrony. The dyssynchrony occurs because the ventricular septum contracts earlier than the left ventricular free wall. Consequently, left ventricular emptying becomes inefficient.

Right ventricular pacing is analogous to left bundle branch block, since it stimulates the right ventricle before the left ventricle. At least two clinical trials – the DAVID trial (Wilkoff BL et al., JAMA 2002;288:3115) and the MOST trial (Sweeney MO et al., Circulation 2003;107:2923) – have demonstrated that, in patients with heart failure or at increased risk of heart failure, the more time spent in right ventricular pacing, the higher the risk of developing worsening heart failure. This risk has not been demonstrated in patients with normal left ventricles.

Consequently, it is now recommended that in patients with heart failure, or whose left ventricular ejection fractions are less than 0.4, biventricular pacing ought to be strongly considered if they are expected to require right ventricular pacing more than 40% of the time.

Other complications of pacemaker therapy

In addition to the problems that can arise as a result of pacing therapy itself, permanent pacemakers can produce complications related to the pacemaker system – that is, to the pacemaker generator, the leads, and the surgical procedures required to insert them.

Complications related to the implantation surgery include right ventricular perforation, perforation with tamponade, pneumothorax, pocket hematomas, pocket erosion, and pacemaker system infection. Lead complications include lead fracture, lead dislodgment, insulation deterioration, and diaphragm or pocket stimulation. Pacemaker system infection may occur with implantation surgery or with subsequent generator replacements. There is some data suggesting that leads across the tricuspid valve may occasionally cause valve injury and tricuspid regurgitation.

Leadless pacemakers

In an effort to reduce or eliminate some of these potential complications, several pacemaker manufacturers have developed "leadless" pacemakers. These devices are cylindrical, self-contained capsules that can be implanted in the right ventricle by means of a minimally invasive, catheter-based insertion system, and that function as VVIR pacemakers. They stay in place with a fixation mechanism (either tines or a helix), and are projected to last from 7 to 12 years. They are designed to be extractable.

Their chief advantage is that they do not employ pacemaker leads or require a pocket. Eliminating these two features of the pacemaker system is expected to greatly reduce the opportunity for pacemaker complications, including infections.

Early studies have shown that the devices operate as they are designed to do. There is a somewhat higher incidence of right ventricular perforation and tamponade during placement than is typically seen with right ventricular pacing leads, and there is a small risk of early embolization. However, the risk of pneumothorax is eliminated (since these devices are inserted via the femoral vein), and the risk of early infections has likewise been virtually eliminated. Postmarketing studies will be required to document the expected long-term reduction in overall pacemaker system complications.

Deciding which pacemaker to implant

The choice of which kind of pacemaker to implant – a single-chambered or dual-chambered pacemaker – is largely an empiric one. Randomized trials designed to detect a significant difference in outcomes between these two general types of pacemaker have largely failed to do so. Specifically, the risk of mortality and stroke is not measurably improved for one type of pacemaker over the other.

In general, however, most electrophysiologists feel that maintaining AV synchrony still provides significant benefits. Avoiding overt or subtle pacemaker syndrome is one such benefit. Another is that the incidence of atrial fibrillation appears reduced with dual-chambered pacing (possibly because the atrial stretching that occurs when the atria contract against closed AV valves may increase the likelihood of atrial fibrillation). Thus, maintaining AV synchrony seems to have real benefits in many patients and should be a major consideration in selecting the appropriate pacemaker for a patient.

The other major consideration is maintaining rate responsiveness, since the ability to perform physical activity is strongly dependent on the ability to increase the heart rate appropriately with exercise.

Keeping these two major considerations in mind (i.e., maintaining both AV synchrony and rate responsiveness), the appropriate pacemaker can usually be selected by answering two fairly simple questions (Figure 5.25). The first is: "Is there chronic atrial fibrillation?" If so, maintaining AV synchrony becomes moot and a single-chambered VVIR pacemaker should be used. In virtually all other cases, a dual-chambered pacemaker is preferable.

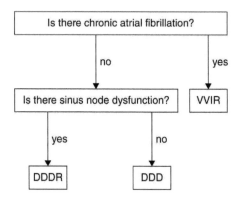

Figure 5.25 Decision tree for the selection of a pacemaker.

Is the electrophysiology study helpful in selecting the right pacemaker?

One circumstance in which electrophysiologic testing may be helpful is when considering an AAIR pacemaker. In patients with pure SA nodal disease and normal AV conduction, an AAIR pacemaker will result in both AV synchrony and rate responsiveness and would be a very reasonable choice, especially since it reduces the risk of tricuspid valve injury. Unfortunately, at least one-third of patients with SA nodal disease have concomitant AV conduction disease. Thus, electrophysiologic testing might be considered prior to the use of AAI pacing, in order to rule out subtle conduction abnormalities. Indeed, one advantage of avoiding the AAI mode altogether is that doing so virtually eliminates the need to ever do electrophysiologic testing in deciding which pacemaker to implant.

6

The Electrophysiology Study in the Evaluation of Supraventricular Tachyarrhythmias

The electrophysiology (EP) study has revolutionized our understanding of supraventricular tachyarrhythmias. Maneuvers and observations in the electrophysiology laboratory allow us to make precise diagnoses, which then guide therapy.

The study of supraventricular tachyarrhythmias is the most challenging and intellectually satisfying type of EP study.

In this chapter, we will review the various types of supraventricular tachyarrhythmia and describe how the EP study helps to elucidate the mechanisms and most appropriate therapy for them.

General classification of supraventricular tachyarrhythmias

As described in Chapter 2, most supraventricular tachyarrhythmias are caused by abnormal automaticity, triggered activity, or reentry.

Automatic supraventricular tachyarrhythmias

Automatic supraventricular tachyarrhythmias are relatively uncommon, except in acutely ill patients. When they do occur, they are usually associated with fairly obvious metabolic disturbances, the most common being myocardial ischemia, acute exacerbations of chronic lung disease, acute alcohol ingestion, and electrolyte disturbances.

Fogoros' Electrophysiologic Testing, Seventh Edition. Richard N. Fogoros and John M. Mandrola.
© 2023 John Wiley & Sons Ltd. Published 2023 by John Wiley & Sons Ltd.

Automatic atrial tachycardia

Automatic atrial tachycardia usually arises from an ectopic automatic focus located somewhere within the atrial myocardium. Characteristically, automatic atrial tachycardias display the typical warm-up phenomenon seen with automatic rhythms (i.e., the rate accelerates after its initiation). The peak rate is usually less than 200 beats/min. There is a discrete P wave before each QRS complex, and the P wave configuration generally differs from the sinus P wave (depending on the location of the automatic focus within the atria). Because the atrioventricular (AV) node is not necessary for maintenance of the arrhythmia, AV block is commonly seen during automatic atrial tachycardia; interventions that affect AV conduction may produce block but do not affect the tachycardia itself.

Triggered activity and microreentry can also cause focal atrial tachycardia. Regardless of mechanism, the origin of focal atrial tachycardias is not random, so ablation is often a good therapeutic option. In the right atrium, focal sites tend to occur along the crista terminalis, tricuspid annulus, and perinodal regions, and in the left atrium, the pulmonary vein ostia and mitral annulus are the most common areas.

Digitalis toxicity

Digitalis toxicity often presents as atrial tachycardia with AV block and, while the mechanism is felt to be triggered automaticity, this arrhythmia is clinically indistinguishable from standard automatic atrial tachycardia. Thus, any unexplained atrial tachycardia with block should prompt a search for digitalis toxicity. Digitalis toxicity has become far less common in recent years, owing to increased awareness and testing of blood levels.

Multifocal (or chaotic) atrial tachycardia

Multifocal (or chaotic) atrial tachycardia (Figure 6.1) is a form of automatic atrial tachycardia characterized by multiple (usually at least three) P-wave morphologies and irregular PP intervals. It is thought to be due to multiple atrial automatic foci that are firing at differing rates. Multifocal atrial tachycardia is often seen with acute pulmonary disease and may be related to theophylline use.

Inappropriate sinus tachycardia (IST)

Inappropriate sinus tachycardia (IST) is a unique type of automatic tachycardia originating in the sinus node. Consequently, except for

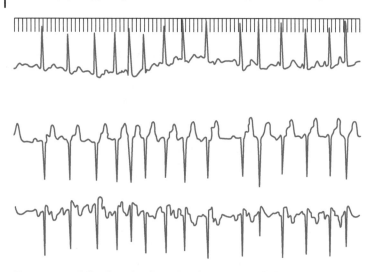

Figure 6.1 Multifocal atrial tachycardia. This is an irregularly irregular rhythm with multiple (but discrete) P-wave morphologies. It is thought to be due to multiple atrial automatic foci.

the clinical setting, IST is identical to normal sinus tachycardia. Patients with IST have sinus rates that are abnormally high at rest (usually around 100 beats/min, though during sleep the rates may drop to the mid-80s or even lower) and invariably increase rapidly with even minimal exertion. They have no identifiable reason for secondary sinus tachycardia, such as anemia, infection, hyperthyroidism, pheochromocytoma, substance abuse, or cardiopulmonary disease. Their sinus tachycardia is therefore "inappropriate."

While IST can occur in anybody, the typical sufferer is a woman in her 20s or 30s who has been having symptoms for months to years. Prior to the onset of IST, which often follows a viral illness or physical trauma, most of these patients will have been in excellent health. Patients with IST often have debilitating palpitations, and may have several other associated symptoms including orthostatic hypotension, blurred vision, dyspnea, tingling, and gastrointestinal disturbances.

The cause of IST is unclear. Several lines of evidence suggest it may be a primary sinoatrial (SA) nodal disorder. First, the intrinsic heart rate (see Chapter 5) in patients with IST tends to be elevated, suggesting that even in the absence of autonomic influence, the SA node displays enhanced automaticity. Second, patients with IST tend to have an abnormally enhanced heart rate response to epinephrine, similar to their abnormal exercise response. And third, at least some evidence exists that the SA node in patients with IST is structurally abnormal. It is important to know whether IST is a primary SA nodal disorder because if it is, ablation of the SA node ought to cure the condition (ablation therapy is discussed beginning in Chapter 8). Accordingly, electrophysiologists have tested this theory by performing SA nodal ablations in hundreds of patients with IST. The outcome is very interesting. The immediate response is usually quite favorable – over 90% of patients no longer have IST immediately after SA nodal ablation. Unfortunately, in about 80% of patients who have such "successful" ablations, the IST recurs within 6–9 months.

Repeat electrophysiologic testing usually shows regeneration of SA nodal function, complete with its IST-like behavior, though this regenerated SA nodal activity is often found inferior to the original site of ablation, along the crista terminalis. Repeated ablations usually yield the same results: early success and late failure. These findings speak against IST being a pure SA node disorder.

There is actually quite a bit of evidence that IST may often be one of the dysautonomias. It shares many of the characteristics of dysautonomia, including that its onset is frequently preceded by a viral illness or trauma and that the patient profile is typical, and "extra" symptoms frequently occur which are consistent with other forms of dysautonomia. (Indeed, many IST patients might have been labeled as suffering from irritable bowel syndrome, postural orthostatic tachycardia syndrome, chronic fatigue syndrome, or posttraumatic stress disorder if they had seen someone other than an electrophysiologist). Further, the fact that something seems to cause the successfully ablated SA nodes to regenerate suggests a more systemic problem than intrinsic SA nodal disease. Finally, even during transiently successful SA nodal ablations, the other symptoms consistent with dysautonomia typically persist in patients with IST.

Treating IST is challenging. The mainstay of treatment is pharmacologic therapy with β-blockers, calcium blockers, type Ic antiarrhythmic agents, and ivabradine. Usually, a combination of drugs is required to achieve an adequate slowing of the heart rate. Patients also often respond to long-term aerobic exercise training. In patients who remain largely disabled by symptoms of IST despite noninvasive efforts at control, SA nodal ablation could be considered despite its drawbacks.

For the non-IST forms of automatic supraventricular tachycardia, the basic principle of therapy is to attempt to reverse the underlying cause. Digitalis toxicity should be suspected in any patient who has been taking this drug, and digitalis should be withheld until toxic levels are ruled out. If the ventricular response is rapid enough to produce hemodynamic instability, the ventricular rate can usually be slowed with digitalis (if toxicity has been ruled out), verapamil, or β-blockers. In addition, if rapid 1 : 1 conduction is occurring during an automatic atrial tachycardia, an immediate slowing of the ventricular response can sometimes be accomplished by pacing the atria even faster than the rate of the tachycardia – fast enough to produce 2 : 1 or 3 : 1 AV block.

Because these arrhythmias are not reentrant, they cannot be pace-terminated and usually do not respond well to direct current (DC) cardioversion. Class Ia antiarrhythmic drugs can be used in an attempt to terminate the arrhythmias but, unless the underlying cause is reversed, these drugs tend to be relatively ineffective. The EP study is not helpful in patients with automatic supraventricular tachyarrhythmias, unless an ablation procedure is contemplated.

Reentrant supraventricular tachyarrhythmias

The vast majority of supraventricular tachyarrhythmias seen in ambulatory patients are due to reentry. In contrast to automatic atrial tachycardias, reentrant supraventricular tachycardias are seen in patients who are not acutely ill. Further, in contrast to reentrant ventricular tachyarrhythmias (see Chapter 7), reentrant supraventricular tachycardias are usually seen in patients who are free of chronic heart disease. While reentrant circuits in the ventricle generally do not appear unless disease of the ventricular myocardium is present, the reentrant substrate for supraventricular arrhythmias tends to be congenital. Overt heart disease is therefore not necessary in order for a patient to develop these arrhythmias. The typical patient with reentrant supraventricular tachycardia is young and healthy.

There are five general categories of reentrant supraventricular tachyarrhythmia: AV nodal reentry, bypass tract-mediated macroreentry, intraatrial reentry, SA nodal reentry, and atrial flutter/atrial fibrillation (AF). Some clinicians still tend to lump these reentrant arrhythmias (except for atrial flutter and atrial fibrillation) together into one large group called PAT (paroxysmal atrial tachycardia – generally, any regular, narrow-complex tachycardia with sudden onset and sudden termination). The term PAT, however, is a vestige from the days when the mechanisms for supraventricular arrhythmias were poorly understood. The EP study has now made it clear that PAT is almost always due to one of the categories of reentrant supraventricular tachyarrhythmia just listed. We now favor the term paroxysmal supraventricular tachycardia (PSVT) except for cases in which it is known to be due to true "atrial tachycardia." In many cases, the knowledgeable clinician can tell which type of supraventricular tachyarrhythmia they are dealing with (and therefore what type of therapy to use), merely by keeping these categories in mind while examining a 12-lead electrocardiogram (ECG) of the arrhythmia.

AV nodal reentrant tachycardia

AV nodal reentrant tachycardia is the most common type of reentrant supraventricular tachycardia and is the operative mechanism in up to 60% of patients presenting with PSVT. In AV nodal reentry, the reentrant circuit is usually said to be enclosed within the AV node (Figure 6.2a). In patients with AV nodal reentry, the AV node is functionally divided into two longitudinal pathways (dual AV nodal

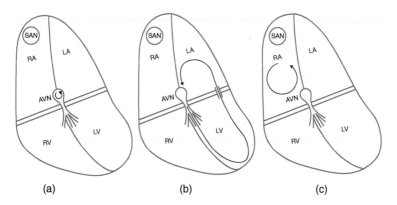

(a) (b) (c)

Figure 6.2 The three most common reentrant supraventricular tachycardias. (a) AV nodal reentrant tachycardia. In this arrhythmia, the reentrant circuit is small and is thought to be localized entirely within the AV node. (b) Bypass tract-mediated macroreentrant tachycardia. An AV bypass tract serves as one pathway (usually the retrograde) and the normal AV conduction system serves as the other pathway of this large (hence, macroreentrant) reentrant circuit. (c) Atrial reentrant tachycardia. In this arrhythmia, the reentrant circuit is contained within the atrial myocardium.

pathways) which form the reentrant circuit. Because, for all practical purposes, the reentrant circuit in AV nodal reentry involves the AV node exclusively, this arrhythmia responds well to autonomic maneuvers and drugs that affect the AV node (digitalis, calcium blockers, and β-blockers).

Bypass tract-mediated macroreentrant tachycardia

Bypass tract-mediated macroreentrant tachycardia is the next most common type of arrhythmia presenting as PSVT (30%). In macroreentrant tachycardia, an AV bypass tract is present. (The majority of patients presenting with macroreentrant tachycardia do not have overt Wolff–Parkinson–White syndrome. Instead, they have concealed bypass tracts – bypass tracts that are incapable of conducting in the antegrade direction and therefore generate no δ waves.) In these patients, the bypass tract acts as one pathway (almost always the retrograde pathway) and the normal AV conducting system acts as the other (antegrade) pathway of the reentrant circuit (Figure 6.2b). Because this reentrant circuit is a large circuit involving the AV node, the His–Purkinje system, and the ventricular and atrial myocardia as well as the bypass tract, it is termed a *macroreentrant circuit*. Also, because the circuit consists of several types of cardiac tissue, it can be attacked on many levels by many types of drugs.

Intraatrial reentry

Intraatrial reentry accounts for only a small percentage of patients presenting with PSVT. In intraatrial reentry, the reentrant circuit is entirely within the atrial myocardium and does not involve the AV conducting system (Figure 6.2c). It resembles automatic atrial tachycardia in that discrete P waves, which usually differ from normal sinus P waves, precede each QRS complex, and AV block can occur without affecting the arrhythmia itself. It differs from automatic arrhythmias by its paroxysmal onset and offset and the fact that it can be induced and terminated by pacing.

Class Ia drugs may be effective. Because the AV node is not part of the reentrant circuit, drugs that block the AV node do not generally affect this arrhythmia.

SA nodal reentry

SA nodal reentry is a fairly uncommon arrhythmia in which the reentrant circuit is thought to be enclosed within the SA node. Discrete P waves identical to sinus P waves precede each QRS complex. SA nodal reentrant tachycardia is distinguishable from both normal sinus tachycardia and IST by its onset, which is paroxysmal and does not display warm-up, by its equally sudden termination, and by the fact that it is inducible and terminable with pacing. Because the reentrant circuit is enclosed within the SA node, autonomic maneuvers and drugs such as digitalis, calcium blockers, and β-blockers tend to ameliorate this arrhythmia.

Atrial flutter and atrial fibrillation

Finally, atrial flutter and atrial fibrillation are forms of reentrant atrial tachycardia. While these are technically atrial tachycardias north of the ventricle (*supra*), we generally do not call them either PAT or PSVT. In atrial flutter, the atrial rate is regular and in excess of 220 beats/min, and usually displays a typical saw tooth pattern (Figure 6.3). Atrial flutter can often be terminated by pacing. Atrial flutter is often accompanied by AV block, usually in a 2:1 pattern. In atrial fibrillation, the atrial activity is continuous and chaotic, and definite P waves cannot be distinguished (Figure 6.4). The ventricular response is irregular, reflecting the chaotic atrial activity. Both atrial flutter and atrial fibrillation are similar to intraatrial reentry (and to automatic atrial tachycardia) in that blocking the AV node does not directly affect these arrhythmias. In general, therapy is aimed at either "rhythm control," e.g., converting the patient to normal sinus rhythm (with class I or class III drugs or cardioversion, or both), or "rate

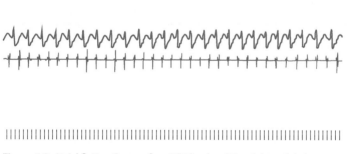

Figure 6.3 Atrial flutter. One surface ECG lead and the right atrial electrogram are shown. Note the rapid, regular atrial rate (cycle length approximately 200 ms) and the 3:2 ventricular response.

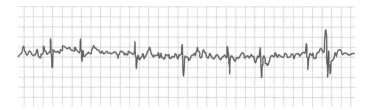

Figure 6.4 Atrial fibrillation. Note the chaotic atrial activity, absence of discrete P waves, and irregularly irregular ventricular response.

control," i.e., letting the atria continue to fibrillate and controlling the ventricular response with AV nodal blocking agents.

In summary, reentrant supraventricular tachyarrhythmias include several types of arrhythmia, whose therapies depend on the location and characteristics of the respective reentrant circuits. Once these arrhythmias are understood, the proper diagnosis can often be made (and proper therapy initiated) without resorting to invasive testing. The EP study, however, can be vital in managing patients with reentrant supraventricular tachyarrhythmias, especially because the majority of these arrhythmias can now be cured with transcatheter ablation techniques (see Chapter 9).

General outline of the EP study in reentrant supraventricular tachyarrhythmias

The key to studying supraventricular tachyarrhythmias in the EP laboratory is the capability of inducing these arrhythmias with programmed pacing techniques, while at the same time recording intracardiac electrograms from various key locations within the heart.

As noted in Chapter 2, inducing any reentrant rhythm requires the existence of an appropriate anatomic substrate to form a reentrant circuit. In supraventricular tachyarrhythmias, the reentrant circuits can incorporate SA or AV nodal tissue, bypass tracts, and atrial and ventricular myocardial tissue. By recording strategically placed intracardiac electrograms and studying the patterns of activation, examining the mode of initiation and termination of arrhythmias, and studying the response to programmed pacing, most supraventricular tachyarrhythmias can be fully characterized in the EP laboratory.

Specifically, the EP study seeks to determine the anatomic location and electrophysiologic characteristics of the reentrant circuit, the propensity of the circuit to sustain arrhythmias, the characteristics of those arrhythmias, and the response of the reentrant arrhythmias to various therapies.

Positioning the catheters

To localize the reentrant circuits in supraventricular tachyarrhythmias, it is important to record electrograms from all four major cardiac chambers, as well as from the His bundle region. These recordings can generally be obtained by positioning four electrode catheters: one in the right atrium, one in the right ventricle, one in the His bundle position, and one in the coronary sinus (to record both left atrial and left ventricular deflections (Figure 6.5). With catheters in these four positions, one can record electrograms from the most critical locations and introduce paced impulses from the right ventricle and from both atria (pacing from the coronary sinus catheter generally produces capture in the left atrium alone).

Evaluation of supraventricular tachyarrhythmias

Once the catheters are positioned, the characteristics of the arrhythmia can be deduced by answering four general questions.

- What is the mode of initiation and termination of the tachycardia?
- What are the patterns of antegrade and retrograde activation during sinus rhythm and during tachycardia?
- What is the evidence that atrial or ventricular myocardium is necessary to the reentrant circuit?
- What are the effects of autonomic maneuvers and drugs on the tachycardia?

These questions must be addressed for each type of supraventricular tachycardia that is induced during the study.

What is the mode of initiation and termination of the tachycardia?

In assessing the mode of initiation of tachycardia, the electrophysiologist addresses several points.

First, is the tachycardia more readily inducible from one location than another? As noted in Chapter 4, inducing a reentrant arrhythmia

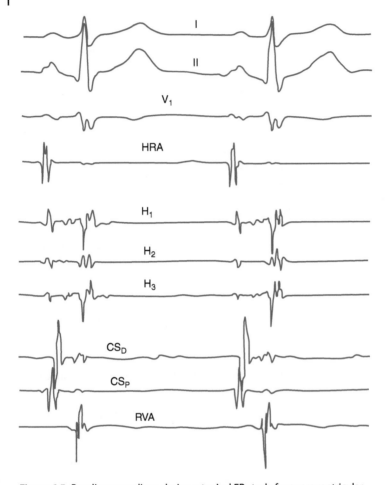

Figure 6.5 Baseline recordings during a typical EP study for supraventricular tachycardia. Surface leads I, II, and V_1 allow estimation of the QRS axis. The high right atrial (HRA) electrogram records activity near the SA node. The His bundle electrogram is recorded from several electrode pairs on the His catheter (three in this example). Two recordings are made from the coronary sinus (both of which record left atrial and left ventricular activity) – coronary sinus distal (CS_D) is recorded from the distal electrode pair on the coronary sinus catheter and coronary sinus proximal (CS_P) is recorded from the proximal pair of electrodes. Finally, a recording is made from the right ventricular apex (RVA). With this combination of recordings, the electrophysiologist can keep track of events in all four cardiac chambers, as well as in the normal AV conducting system.

requires the delivery of a premature impulse to the reentrant circuit at just the right moment. A major element influencing the inducibility of reentrant arrhythmias, then, is the distance between the pacing catheter and the reentrant circuit – the closer the catheter is to the circuit, the more likely it is that a paced premature beat will arrive at the circuit early enough to induce reentry. Thus, for instance, if a reentrant rhythm is significantly easier to induce with left atrial pacing (i.e., pacing from the coronary sinus) than it is with right atrial pacing, then the reentrant circuit may involve a left-sided bypass tract.

It is important to observe whether supraventricular tachycardia is readily inducible with ventricular pacing. Inducing tachycardia with ventricular pacing is readily accomplished in macroreentrant tachycardias, is relatively difficult in AV nodal reentry, and is rare with intraatrial reentry. (In intraatrial reentry, the arrhythmia can be induced by ventricular stimulation only indirectly and infrequently, by means of retrograde stimulation of the atrium.)

Another point relating to the mode of initiation of the tachycardia is the site of the conduction delay that typically occurs with the onset of reentrant supraventricular tachyarrhythmias. The reason for this conduction delay can be seen by reviewing the mechanism for inducing reentrant arrhythmias (see Figure 2.6). As described in Chapter 2, a reentrant circuit requires two roughly parallel pathways (labeled pathways A and B) connecting proximally and distally to common conducting tissues, forming an anatomic circuit. Pathway B has a longer refractory period than pathway A, and pathway A conducts impulses slower than pathway B. The initiation of reentry occurs when a premature impulse enters the circuit at a time when pathway B is still refractory from the previous normal impulse but pathway A has already recovered.

Note that, since pathway B conducts faster than pathway A, a normal (i.e., not premature) impulse will conduct via pathway B rather than pathway A (Figure 6.6a). When an early impulse initiates reentry, this impulse is blocked in pathway B (fast pathway) and instead conducts via pathway A (slow pathway). Thus, a beat that initiates reentry is commonly accompanied by conduction delay (Figure 6.6b). The electrophysiologist must pay particular attention to the occurrence of conduction delay in association with the onset of tachycardia. The site of this delay virtually always points to one of the pathways within the reentrant circuit.

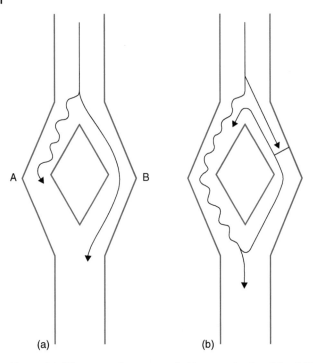

(a)   (b)

Figure 6.6 Why reentry is accompanied by a conduction delay. (a) In this generic reentrant circuit, a normal impulse travels from top to bottom by the fastest available pathway (pathway B). No conduction delay is seen. (b) When a premature impulse blocks in pathway B and initiates reentry, that impulse must travel from top to bottom via the slow pathway (pathway A). Thus, an observer watching the exit of the impulse from the circuit will see a conduction delay whenever reentry is initiated.

An additional issue relating to the mode of initiation is the tachycardia (or echo) zone. The tachycardia zone is the range of coupling intervals of premature beats that will initiate reentrant tachycardia. As one introduces a series of premature impulses with progressively shorter coupling intervals, one impulse will eventually encounter the reentrant circuit during the effective refractory period (ERP) of pathway B (i.e., the impulse blocks in pathway B). At this point, reentry is often initiated. The latest premature impulse that blocks in pathway B (if it were any later, the impulse would not encounter refractory tissue) usually defines the beginning of the tachycardia zone. If one now continues to introduce premature impulses with progressively shorter coupling intervals, reentry will typically be induced with each succeeding premature beat until the ERP of pathway A is finally encountered. At this point, the premature impulse blocks in both pathways of the reentrant circuit and no further reentry occurs. The ERP of pathway A thus defines the end of the tachycardia zone. Note that the width of the tachycardia zone is related to the difference between the refractory periods of the two pathways constituting the reentrant circuit. The wider the tachycardia zone, the more likely a premature impulse will fall within that zone and induce reentry. During the EP study for supraventricular tachycardia, one thus tries to identify the refractory periods (and thus the tachycardia zone) of the various pathways involved in the reentrant circuit. By doing so, one can attempt to tailor therapy to reduce the width of the tachycardia zone.

The mode of termination of the arrhythmia is somewhat less helpful than the mode of initiation in localizing the bypass tract. Nonetheless, careful observation of the precise mechanism of termination of reentry can offer clues as to the type of reentrant rhythm. This point will be discussed in detail later.

What are the patterns of antegrade and retrograde activation during sinus rhythm and during supraventricular tachycardia?

Abnormalities in the pattern of activation of impulses traveling from the atria to the ventricles and from the ventricles to the atria can help to localize portions of the reentrant circuit.

We have already discussed normal antegrade activation patterns (see Chapter 1). Impulses arising in the SA node traverse the atria in a radial fashion until they encounter the fibrous skeleton of the heart at the AV groove. There, the impulses are abolished, except in the AV conducting system (the AV node and His–Purkinje structures). Because of its electrophysiologic properties, impulses conduct relatively slowly through the AV node. Further, premature impulses conduct even more slowly (manifested in the His electrogram as a prolonged AH interval). Typically, if one introduces single atrial extrastimuli with progressively shorter coupling intervals, the delay in AV nodal conduction (and the AH interval) increases gradually. Eventually, the ERP of the AV node is reached and the early impulse is blocked.

This normal pattern of gradually increasing AH intervals with progressively premature atrial impulses is shown graphically in Figure 6.7.

This AV nodal conduction curve shows the normal smooth and continuous prolongation in AH intervals with progressively premature

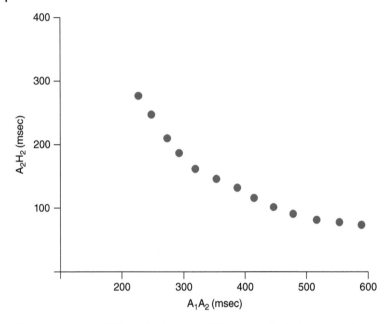

Figure 6.7 A normal AV conduction curve. With progressively shorter coupling intervals, premature atrial beats display a progressive conduction delay in the AV node. In this graph, the conduction intervals (A, A_2) are shown on the x-axis and the resulting AH intervals (A_2H_2) are shown on the y-axis. The normal AV conduction curve is smooth and continuous, as shown.

beats. This normal pattern can be disrupted by two general conditions that produce supraventricular tachycardias: dual AV nodal pathways and AV bypass tracts. These two conditions will be discussed in detail later.

When an impulse is conducted from the atria to the ventricles via the normal AV conducting system, ventricular activation follows a typical pattern. First, the intraventricular septum is depolarized, then the apices of the right and left ventricles, then the ventricular free walls, and finally the basilar portions of the ventricles. The area of the ventricles that is depolarized last is the left ventricular posterobasilar area. This normal pattern of ventricular activation is altered if there is a bypass tract that preexcites the ventricle. Studying the ventricular activation pattern in the EP laboratory can help to localize the ventricular insertion of a bypass tract.

The characteristics of normal retrograde conduction (i.e., the conduction of impulses from the ventricles to the atria that occurs during ventricular pacing) are important in evaluating supraventricular tachycardias. Normally, retrograde conduction occurs over the normal AV conducting system – the impulse travels from the ventricular myocardium to the Purkinje fibers, then to the His bundle, to the AV node, and finally to the atria, where it spreads in a radial fashion (i.e., from the atrial septum to the right and left atria). Although some retrograde conduction can be seen in most individuals, in most cases retrograde conduction is not as efficient as antegrade conduction. Thus, in most individuals, retrograde block occurs at longer coupling intervals than antegrade block (this is not always the case, however; for example, a substantial minority of patients with complete antegrade AV block have intact retrograde conduction).

In normal individuals, if one introduces progressively earlier extrastimuli from the ventricle and measures the retrograde conduction intervals, one will see a progressive prolongation of the VA (ventriculoatrial) interval (Figure 6.8), similar to the gradual prolongation in the AH interval that one sees with antegrade conduction. Normally, block will occur first in the His–Purkinje system. In practical terms, however, one is only rarely able to discern the H spike in the His electrogram during retrograde conduction, as it is usually hidden in the large V complex.

In studies of supraventricular tachyarrhythmias, the pattern of retrograde atrial activation is important. With normal retrograde conduction, the earliest atrial activation is seen in the His electrogram because that electrogram records the atrial activity near the AV node (i.e., the point of entry of the impulse into the atrial myocardium during normal retrograde conduction). The retrograde impulse then spreads radially across the atria, and the right atrial electrogram and left atrial electrogram are inscribed more or less at the same time (Figure 6.9a). This normal pattern of retrograde activation can be disrupted if an AV bypass tract is present. In this case, eccentric retrograde activation of the atria can occur. With a right-sided bypass tract, for instance, the right atrial electrogram will be inscribed earliest (Figure 6.9b); with a left-sided bypass tract, the left atrial electrogram will be inscribed earliest (Figure 6.9c). Mapping of retrograde atrial activation is one of the most useful methods for localizing AV bypass tracts.

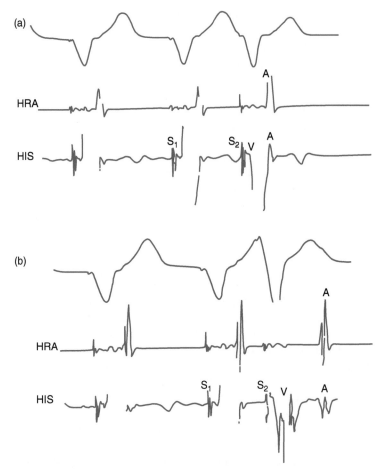

Figure 6.8 Normal VA conduction during right ventricular pacing. A surface ECG lead, a high right atrial (HRA) electrogram, and a His bundle electrogram are shown. (a) With a relatively long S_1–S_2 coupling interval, retrograde conduction to the atrium is rapid (the VA interval following the S_2 is short). Note that the retrograde atrial impulse is recorded in the His electrogram (near the AV node) before it reaches the high right atrium. This suggests retrograde conduction via the normal AV conducting tissues. (b) With a shorter coupling interval, retrograde conduction still occurs, but it is slower (the VA interval following the S_2 is longer than in the previous figure). This retrograde conduction delay with shorter coupling intervals is normal when retrograde conduction occurs via the normal AV conducting tissues.

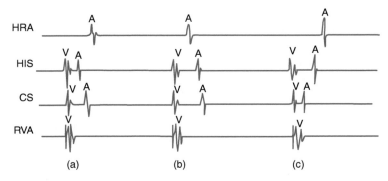

Figure 6.9 Patterns of retrograde atrial activation are important for localizing AV bypass tracts. This figure shows electrograms from the high right atrium (HRA), the His bundle, the coronary sinus (CS), and the right ventricular apex (RVA) during pacing from the RVA. (a) The normal pattern of retrograde atrial activation. This pattern is seen when retrograde conduction occurs via the normal AV conducting system or with septal bypass tracts. The atrial septum is activated first (His electrogram), followed by left atrial (CS electrogram) and right atrial activation. (b) Retrograde activation pattern with a right-sided bypass tract. The right atrium is activated first because retrograde conduction occurs via a right-sided bypass tract. The septal atrium and the left atrium are then activated. (c) Retrograde activation pattern with a left-sided bypass tract. The left atrium is activated first (CS electrogram) because retrograde conduction occurs via a left-sided bypass tract. The atrial septum and the right atrium are then activated.

What is the evidence that atrial or ventricular myocardium is necessary to the reentrant circuit?

Once a reentrant tachycardia has been induced, it can be helpful to attempt to deduce whether the atrial myocardium and ventricular myocardium are part of the reentrant circuit. One should always look for evidence of antegrade or retrograde block during the tachycardia. If either antegrade or retrograde block is seen to occur without affecting the cycle length of the tachycardia, macroreentry can mostly be ruled out. A caveat includes reentry within the AV node that is associated with 2 : 1 block in the His–Purkinje system.

For instance, in AV nodal reentrant tachycardia, retrograde stimulation of the atria occasionally occurs with a Wenckebach pattern (i.e., occasional retrograde beats are dropped). When this phenomenon is observed during a supraventricular tachycardia of constant cycle length, a reentrant circuit in which the atria are required for the maintenance of tachycardia can be ruled out.

The effect of bundle branch block on the cycle length of the tachycardia can also be instructive. In AV nodal reentry, bundle branch block does not change the reentrant circuit because the circuit does not involve the bundle branches. In macroreentry, however, the sudden occurrence of bundle branch block on the same side as the AV bypass tract (such as left bundle branch block [LBBB] occurring during a macroreentrant tachycardia involving a left-sided bypass tract) will increase the cycle length of the tachycardia and the time from ventricle to atrium (VA time) (Figure 6.10).

What are the effects of autonomic maneuvers and drugs on the tachycardia?

When attempting to define the anatomic substrate of, and effective therapy for, reentrant supraventricular tachyarrhythmias, it is often helpful to take advantage of the differential effects of autonomic maneuvers and drugs on various cardiac structures. As noted in

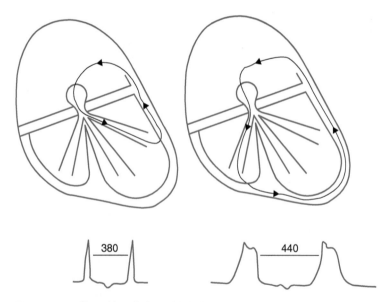

Figure 6.10 Effect of bundle branch block on macroreentrant tachycardia. In this figure, macroreentrant tachycardia involving a left-sided bypass tract is present. Initially, no bundle branch block is present, and the tachycardia cycle length is 380 ms. If LBBB occurs, it will now take longer for the reentrant impulse to reach the left-sided bypass tract, and the tachycardia cycle length is prolonged to 440 ms.

previous chapters, the AV node has rich autonomic innervation and is exquisitely sensitive to changes in both sympathetic and parasympathetic tone. In contrast, atrial and ventricular myocardial tissue responds moderately to changes in sympathetic tone but only minimally to changes in parasympathetic tone. Thus, vagal maneuvers, by increasing the refractory period and decreasing the conduction velocity of the AV node, can terminate reentrant arrhythmias in which the AV node is part of the reentrant circuit (such as AV nodal reentry and macroreentry). If the AV node is excluded from the reentrant circuit (as in intraatrial reentry), vagal maneuvers may increase heart block but will not directly alter the reentrant impulse.

Likewise, drugs that have a specific effect on the AV node (such as digitalis, calcium blockers, and β-blockers) can be effective in terminating or preventing reentrant arrhythmias that include the AV node as part of the circuit. In contrast, class Ia drugs have relatively little effect on the AV node but increase the refractory periods and slow conduction velocity in atrial and ventricular myocardium and in bypass tracts. Thus, reentrant circuits that involve these structures can be altered by class Ia drugs. The class Ic drugs slow conduction in all cardiac tissues, including the AV node. Although offering relatively little help in identifying the anatomic substrate, class Ic drugs can be helpful in treating many forms of supraventricular tachyarrhythmia.

General procedure for performing the EP study in patients with supraventricular tachyarrhythmias

When studying patients with supraventricular tachyarrhythmias, once the electrode catheters are in position, most electrophysiologists begin with ventricular stimulation to study the characteristics of retrograde conduction. Although it may seem odd to begin with ventricular pacing when studying supraventricular arrhythmias, there are two reasons for doing so. First, many patients who have supraventricular tachycardias (especially those with bypass tracts) have a propensity for developing atrial fibrillation with atrial pacing. Atrial fibrillation, since it entails continuous and chaotic atrial activity, virtually precludes meaningful evaluation of other reentrant supraventricular arrhythmias. By first performing ventricular stimulation, the electrophysiologist hopes to avoid the early induction of atrial fibrillation. Second, for AV nodal reentry and for bypass tract-mediated macroreentry (the two most common forms of reentrant supraventricular tachyarrhythmia), retrograde conduction is a prominent and necessary component of reentry. Thus, the characteristics of retrograde conduction and the retrograde activation pattern of the atrium with ventricular stimulation are important in characterizing these arrhythmias. It is therefore logical to evaluate these characteristics as early as possible.

Generally, retrograde conduction is evaluated using the extrastimulus and incremental pacing techniques. Single ventricular extrastimuli are introduced (either in sinus rhythm or following a train of paced beats) with gradually decreasing coupling intervals until the extrastimulus fails to capture the ventricle. With each extrastimulus, the electrophysiologist notes the presence or absence of retrograde stimulation of the atrium, the pattern of atrial activation, and the conduction time of the retrograde impulse (the VA interval; see Figure 6.8). The coupling interval at which retrograde conduction is blocked (the retrograde effective refractory period [ERP]) is also noted. Next, incremental trains are introduced with progressively shorter cycle lengths. Note is taken of the cycle length at which 1 : 1 retrograde conduction no longer occurs.

After ventricular stimulation is completed, pacing is performed from the high right atrium. The procedure here is similar to that described in Chapter 5 – atrial extrastimuli and incremental atrial pacing are used to assess the characteristics of AV conduction and of SA nodal function.

Next, similar stimulation is performed using left atrial pacing (i.e., with the coronary sinus catheter). This is done to look for evidence of a left-sided AV bypass tract.

When a bypass tract is suspected, pacing from multiple atrial sites is often performed (by moving the right atrial and/or coronary sinus catheters to various positions) to try to localize the bypass tract – the closer to the bypass tract one paces, the more preexcitation will occur.

For the vast majority of patients with reentrant supraventricular tachyarrhythmias, the reentrant arrhythmia will be induced during one or more of these pacing maneuvers. Whenever reentrant tachycardia is induced, the protocol is interrupted so that the characteristics of the arrhythmia can be studied. Specifically, the mechanism of the tachycardia is noted, the cycle length is recorded, an assessment of the patient's hemodynamic stability and level of symptoms is made, and atrial or ventricular stimulation is carried out to examine the effect of such stimulation on the arrhythmia.

If reentrant supraventricular tachycardia is not induced with standard pacing techniques, multiple extrastimuli are used and drug administration (such as an isoproterenol infusion) is implemented to try to bring out the arrhythmia.

If a bypass tract is known or suspected to be present, sometimes the electrophysiologist will induce atrial fibrillation. This is done to assess the ability of the bypass tract to conduct rapidly enough during atrial fibrillation to pose a lethal risk to the patient. But if the patient has symptomatic tachycardia and/or the accessory pathway (AP) has rapid conduction characteristics, AF induction can be omitted.

Although this general outline of the EP study for supraventricular tachyarrhythmias is fairly representative, no two electrophysiologists follow precisely the same protocol. In fact, no single electrophysiologist follows precisely the same protocol in every patient. Even within the same general category of arrhythmias, supraventricular arrhythmias show tremendous variability from patient to patient. Thus, every EP study has to be individualized. Electrophysiologists usually approach these patients with a general outline of a protocol, tailoring the study as they go, depending on the findings.

With this introduction, we will now review the electrophysiologic evaluation of specific types of supraventricular tachyarrhythmia.

The EP Study in AV nodal reentrant tachycardia

As we have noted, AV nodal reentrant tachycardia is the most common type of arrhythmia presenting as PSVT, probably accounting for 60% of all such arrhythmias. AV nodal reentry is seen in all age groups and occurs in both sexes equally. The incidence of underlying heart disease in patients with this arrhythmia is no greater than in the normal population.

Mechanism of AV nodal reentry

One can think of the AV node in patients with AV nodal reentrant tachycardia as being shaped like a doughnut (Figure 6.11). The AV node in these patients behaves functionally as if there were two separate pathways through the node. The two pathways (the alpha and beta pathways) are differentiated by their characteristic electrophysiologic properties. The alpha pathway (or slow pathway) usually has

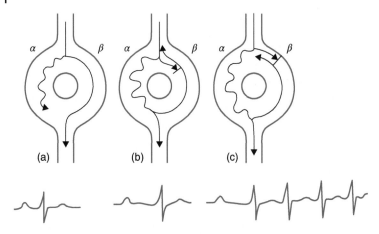

Figure 6.11 AV nodal reentrant tachycardia. (a) In AV nodal reentry, the AV node is functionally divided into two pathways (alpha and beta). The alpha pathway conducts more slowly than the beta, and the beta pathway has a longer refractory period than the alpha. A normal atrial impulse reaches the ventricles via the beta pathway. (b) A premature atrial impulse can find the beta pathway refractory at a time when the alpha pathway is not. In this case, the premature impulse conducts via the alpha pathway. Because conduction down the alpha pathway is slow, the resultant PR interval is prolonged. (c) If conditions are right, a premature impulse can block in the beta pathway and travel down the alpha pathway (as in (b)), then travel retrograde up the beta pathway and reenter the alpha pathway in the antegrade direction. A circuitous impulse is thus established within the AV node, and AV nodal reentrant tachycardia results. Note the prolonged PR interval in the beat that starts AV nodal reentry (caused by jumping from the beta to the alpha pathway). This conduction delay is typically seen in reentrant supraventricular arrhythmias.

a relatively short ERP and conducts slowly. The beta pathway (or fast pathway) usually has a relatively long ERP and conducts more rapidly. Patients whose AV nodes are arranged in such a fashion are said to have dual AV nodal pathways.

In patients with dual AV nodal pathways, a normally timed sinus impulse will conduct through the AV node via the beta pathway, since the beta conducts more rapidly than the alpha pathway (Figure 6.11a). However, a premature atrial impulse can arrive at the AV node at such a time that the beta pathway (with a relatively long ERP) is still refractory from the previous normal beat but the alpha pathway (with a relatively short ERP) is no longer refractory. This early impulse will then traverse the alpha pathway, reaching the His bundle after a prolonged conduction time through the AV node (since the alpha pathway conducts slowly [Figure 6.11b]). This AV nodal conduction delay is manifested by a prolonged PR interval on the surface ECG. If the beta pathway recovers by the time the impulse reaches the distal portion of the alpha pathway, the impulse may conduct retrogradely up the beta pathway (producing an atrial echo beat). If this retrograde impulse is then able to reenter the alpha pathway, a continuously circulating impulse can be established within the AV node. This is AV nodal reentrant tachycardia (Figure 6.11c).

Thus, in AV nodal reentrant tachycardia, the reentrant circuit can be visualized as being located within the AV node. In most cases, both the atria and ventricles are stimulated by impulses exiting from the circuit during each lap. Neither the atria nor the ventricles, however, are necessary for the maintenance of that reentrant circuit. It is thus possible to have block in the His bundle, preventing the ventricles from being stimulated, without affecting the reentrant circuit itself. It is also possible to have retrograde block, preventing the atria from being stimulated, but without affecting the arrhythmia.

There is evidence that in some patients the beta pathway may not be typical AV nodal tissue. In such patients, the beta pathway does not respond to AV nodal drugs (digitalis, calcium blockers, β-blockers) like the alpha pathway does. In these patients, the beta pathway may be more affected by class Ia drugs than is typical for AV nodal tissue.

Mode of initiation and termination of AV nodal reentry

Most often, AV nodal reentrant tachycardia is induced with atrial extrastimuli. If one introduces progressively earlier atrial premature impulses, impulses with relatively longer coupling intervals will conduct down the beta (fast) pathway, just as sinus beats do (Figure 6.12a). When the coupling interval of a premature impulse becomes shorter than the ERP of the beta pathway, however, that impulse blocks in the beta pathway and jumps to the alpha (slow) pathway (thus producing the typical conduction delay in the AV node). It is at this point that AV nodal reentry is usually first seen (Figure 6.12b). Premature impulses that are yet earlier will also induce AV nodal reentry, until the ERP of the alpha pathway is reached (at which point the premature impulse is blocked entirely). The tachycardia zone in AV nodal reentry is from the ERP of the beta pathway to the ERP of the alpha pathway. In this

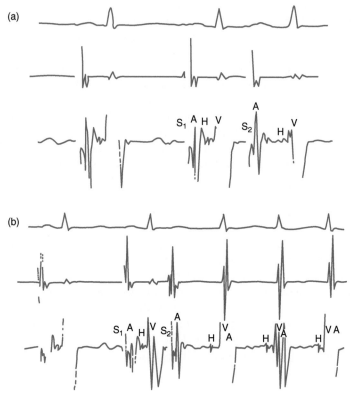

Figure 6.12 Initiation of AV nodal reentry with atrial extrastimuli. One surface ECG lead, one high right atrial electrogram, and one His bundle electrogram are shown. (a) An S_2 impulse conducts through the normal AV conducting system with a moderate prolongation in the AH interval. This response is normal and is similar to the normal conduction pattern shown in Figure 6.7. (b) With a slightly shorter S_1–S_2 coupling interval, a large jump in the resultant AH interval occurs (compared to the previous figure), and AV nodal reentry is initiated. The sudden increment in AH intervals represents a shift in conduction from the beta to the alpha pathway in this patient with dual AV nodal pathways. Note (in the last two beats in this figure) that during AV nodal reentry, the retrograde A spike (which is labeled on the His electrogram) occurs very soon after the V spike. This is because retrograde conduction occurs via the rapidly conducting beta pathway. On the surface ECG, the retrograde P wave is usually buried in the QRS complex (as in this figure) during AV nodal reentrant tachycardia.

arrhythmia, the tachycardia zone tends to be reproducible (that is, successive measurements will yield the same result).

AV nodal reentry is also commonly induced with incremental atrial pacing at the Wenckebach cycle length. At this cycle length, progressive prolongation in AV nodal conduction is seen until block occurs in the beta pathway and conduction is instead down the alpha pathway – at this point, AV nodal reentry is usually seen.

AV nodal reentry is less often, and less reproducibly, induced with ventricular pacing. Normally in patients with dual AV nodal pathways, ventricular pacing produces retrograde impulses that enter the AV node and begin traveling up both the beta and the alpha pathways (Figure 6.13a). Because conduction in the beta pathway is faster, the retrograde impulse reaches the atria via the beta pathway. Reentry is

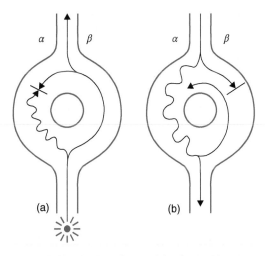

Figure 6.13 Initiation of AV nodal reentry with a ventricular paced beat. Because the reentrant circuit in AV nodal reentry is exposed to both the atria and the ventricles, it is possible that a premature ventricular beat (as well as a premature atrial beat) can initiate reentry. However, in practice this event is rare. (a) A ventricular paced impulse begins traveling up both the beta and the alpha pathways. The impulse reaches the atria via the beta pathway (since this pathway conducts rapidly) and cannot reenter the alpha pathway because it encounters the retrograde impulse traveling up it slowly. This is why AV nodal reentry is difficult to initiate with ventricular pacing. (b) If the events shown in (a) occur at just the right time, the following sinus beat can encounter the AV node at a time when the beta pathway is still refractory from the recent retrograde impulse. Thus, AV nodal reentry can be initiated indirectly by a premature ventricular impulse.

not induced, however – the impulse is not able to turn around and travel back down the alpha pathway because the alpha pathway has just been stimulated itself by the retrograde impulse and is still refractory. Relatively rarely, AV nodal reentry is induced by ventricular pacing if a ventricular extrastimulus can be interpolated between two sinus beats. In this case, the beta pathway can be rendered refractory by the retrograde impulse, so that the next sinus impulse blocks in the beta pathway and conducts down the alpha pathway, thus producing reentry (Figure 6.13b).

Termination of AV nodal reentrant tachycardia follows the typical pattern described in Chapter 4 (see Figure 4.12). Relatively late premature impulses can encounter refractory tissue and be prevented from entering the circuit (see Figure 4.12a). Early impulses may enter the circuit via the alpha pathway, resulting in a resetting of the tachycardia (see Figure 4.12b). Still earlier impulses can terminate the tachycardia (see Figure 4.12c). The ability to cause a premature impulse to reach the AV node early enough to terminate AV nodal reentry depends on the distance of the pacing catheter from the AV node and on the refractory and conduction characteristics (i.e., the functional refractory period [FRP] – see Chapter 4) of the intervening tissue. If terminating the tachycardia with single atrial or ventricular extrastimuli is not possible, the chances of terminating the arrhythmia can be improved by repositioning the catheter or, more commonly, by introducing multiple extrastimuli. This latter maneuver has the effect of reducing the FRP of intervening myocardial tissue.

Patterns of activation with AV nodal reentry

Dual AV nodal pathways are the rule in patients with AV nodal reentrant tachycardia. Because there are two pathways of conduction through the AV node, the AV nodal conduction curve can be expected to be abnormal. Figure 6.14 shows a typical AV nodal conduction curve in a patient with dual AV nodal pathways. With extrastimuli having relatively long coupling intervals, conduction through the AV node occurs via the beta pathway. As atrial extrastimuli are introduced with progressively shorter coupling intervals, the AH interval increases gradually at first, as it would in a normal AV node. At the point at which the ERP of the beta pathway is reached, however, conduction suddenly shifts to the alpha pathway, at which time there is a sudden increment in the AV nodal conduction time. This increment

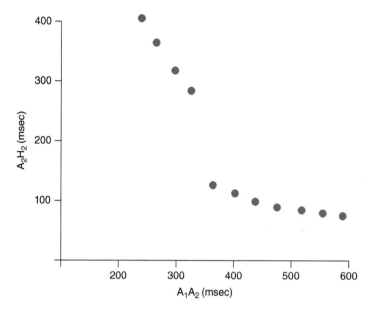

Figure 6.14 Atypical AV conduction curve from a patient with AV nodal reentrant tachycardia. Compare this curve to the normal curve in Figure 6.7. In AV nodal reentry, dual AV nodal pathways are present. Premature atrial impulses with longer coupling intervals conduct down the beta pathway. With earlier premature atrial impulses, the refractory period of the beta pathway is reached, and conduction jumps to the slower alpha pathway. It is at this point that AV nodal reentry may occur. On the AV conduction curve, this jump from faster to slower conduction is manifested by a sudden discontinuity in the curve. The sudden lengthening of the AH interval when conduction shifts from the beta to the alpha pathway is also seen in Figure 6.12.

is manifested by a sudden jump in the AH interval. The AV nodal conduction curves in patients with dual AV nodal pathways show a discontinuity – the discontinuity represents the point at which conduction shifts from the beta to the alpha pathway.

Occasionally, patients with dual AV nodal pathways will manifest their two pathways during normal sinus rhythm – these patients can be seen to have two distinct PR intervals during sinus rhythm. In other patients with dual AV nodal pathways, evidence for dual pathways is not seen during baseline electrophysiologic testing. In these patients, the ERPs of the alpha and beta pathways are similar (i.e., the tachycardia zone is extremely narrow). Such patients either have few arrhythmias or only have arrhythmias when autonomic stresses (such as a sympathetic surge) dissociate the refractory periods of the two pathways (in which case a differential effect of autonomic stresses on the two pathways must be postulated). When AV nodal reentry is suspected in patients who have no evidence for dual pathways during baseline testing, autonomic or pharmacologic maneuvers should be tried in an attempt to dissociate the pathways.

The pattern of ventricular activation during antegrade conduction is normal because stimulation of the ventricles in AV nodal reentry is via the normal His–Purkinje system. Likewise, the pattern of atrial activation during retrograde stimulation is also normal.

Evidence that atrial and ventricular myocardium are not required for AV nodal reentry

Most authorities feel that atrial and ventricular myocardium are not necessary for maintenance of AV nodal reentry. Although during electrophysiologic testing it is difficult to prove that atrial and ventricular tissues are not required to maintain AV nodal reentry, evidence is sometimes present spontaneously during AV nodal reentrant tachycardia. One should always be alert for the phenomenon of retrograde Wenckebach conduction during tachycardia. If the tachycardia cycle length is constant at the same time that the relationship of the retrograde P waves to the QRS complex is changing, or especially if occasional retrograde P waves are dropped, that is strong evidence that the atria are not required for the maintenance of the tachycardia. Likewise, if occasional antegrade block occurs without a change in the tachycardia cycle length, the ventricles are thus not required for maintenance of tachycardia. Finally, because the activation pattern of the ventricular myocardium has no bearing on the cycle length of the reentrant circuit, if bundle branch block should develop during AV nodal reentry, no change in the rate of the tachycardia should occur.

If these spontaneous events are not seen, extrastimuli from the atria and the ventricles can help to show that the atria and ventricles are not required. Capture of the atria near the AV node or capture of the His bundle without changing the tachycardia suggests that the reentrant circuit is localized to the AV node. In practice, it is difficult and impractical to prove that the atria and the ventricles are not necessary by using extrastimuli. Fortunately, it is also usually unnecessary because the diagnosis of AV nodal reentry rarely hinges on rigorous documentation that the atria and ventricles are not required.

Other observations in AV nodal reentry

Relationship of P Waves to QRS complexes during AV nodal reentry

One of the most useful observations made in the electrophysiology laboratory in patients with AV nodal reentry is the relationship between retrograde P waves and the QRS complexes on the surface ECG during the tachycardia. During AV nodal reentry, the atrium is stimulated in the retrograde direction by impulses exiting to the atria via the beta pathway. Because the beta pathway tends to conduct rapidly, retrograde atrial activation tends to occur during or just after ventricular depolarization. On the surface ECG, P waves thus tend either to be buried within the QRS complex or to occur just at the end of the QRS. In patients presenting with regular, narrow-complex tachycardia in which P waves cannot be discerned at all in a good-quality 12-lead ECG, one can make the diagnosis of AV nodal reentry with some confidence.

Atypical AV nodal reentry

In patients with atypical AV nodal reentry, the ERP of the alpha pathway is longer than that of the beta pathway. In these individuals, reentry occurs in the opposite direction (i.e., up the alpha pathway and down the beta pathway), and the P to QRS relationship is not typical of AV nodal reentry (because retrograde conduction occurs through the slow pathway). Patients with this unusual form of AV nodal reentry may have incessant tachycardia.

Treatment of AV nodal reentry

Because both pathways in AV nodal reentry involve AV nodal tissue, drugs and maneuvers that increase the refractory period and slow the conduction velocity of AV nodal tissue are very effective at terminating the arrhythmia. In addition to maneuvers that increase vagal tone (Valsalva maneuver, carotid sinus massage, and ice-water immersion), the digitalis agents, calcium blockers, and β-blockers tend to be effective. In most instances, these agents work by producing Wenckebach conduction in the slow pathway. They thus cause termination of reentrant tachycardia after a few cycles, when an impulse that has conducted retrogradely through the beta pathway fails to reenter the alpha pathway.

Because occasionally the alpha and beta pathways respond differently to various agents, it is sometimes possible to potentiate tachycardia with drugs. For instance, in some patients, the beta pathway is relatively unaffected by drugs that normally depress AV nodal function. Thus, a drug might slow conduction in the alpha pathway without prolonging refractoriness in the fast pathway. In this case, any premature impulse traveling down the alpha pathway would tend to be so delayed that the beta pathway would be much more likely to have recovered by the time the impulse reached it. Reentry, then, would tend to be easier to start and more difficult to stop.

Patients in whom standard AV nodal drugs seem to be ineffective may respond to class Ia or class Ic drugs. The beta pathway in such patients seems to behave less like AV nodal tissue and more like atrial or ventricular myocardial tissue.

Techniques for performing transcatheter ablation of the slow (alpha) pathway in patients with AV nodal tachycardia are now quite advanced (see Chapter 9). Transcatheter ablation of AV nodal reentry can now be performed successfully in well over 95% of patients who undergo this procedure. Ablation should be strongly considered in any patient with AV nodal reentry who has frequent or disabling episodes.

Bypass tract-mediated supraventricular tachyarrhythmias

As described in Chapter 1, there is normally only one way for electrical impulses to travel from the atria to the ventricles – the normal AV conduction system. Of every thousand individuals, however, several are born with a second electrical connection between the atria and the ventricles. These extra connections are called bypass tracts (or accessory pathways), because they offer a potential route for electrical impulses to bypass all or part of the normal AV conduction system. Bypass tracts consist of tiny bands of myocardial tissue that most commonly insert in atrial muscle on one end and in ventricular muscle on the other. They tend to occur sporadically, although patients with Ebstein's anomaly and mitral valve prolapse have a somewhat higher incidence than the general population.

The electrophysiologic characteristics of these bypass tracts vary, but they generally behave much more like myocardial tissue than AV nodal tissue. Thus, they do not display slowing of conduction with premature impulses as the AV node does. Also, when stimulated rapidly, bypass tracts develop block in the manner of His–Purkinje tissue rather than AV nodal tissue. That is, the block is sudden (of the Mobitz II variety) instead of gradual (i.e., Wenckebach conduction does not occur).

Bypass tracts are generally invisible to the naked eye (significantly, surgeons cannot see them when attempting surgical disruption) and therefore must be located by their electrophysiologic effects alone. Bypass tracts can occur virtually anywhere along the AV groove, except in the space between the aortic valve and the mitral valve, and can also occur more or less parallel to the AV conducting system in the septal area. There are four general types of bypass tract (Figure 6.15): AV bypass tracts (the "typical" bypass tracts, in which the tract is located along the AV groove and connects atrial and ventricular muscle; tract A in Figure 6.15); AV nodal bypass tracts (which connect the low atrial myocardium to the His–Purkinje system; tract B); bypass tracts that connect the distal atrial myocardium (near the AV node) to the right bundle branch (so-called "Mahaim" tracts; tract C); and bypass tracts that connect the His or Purkinje fibers

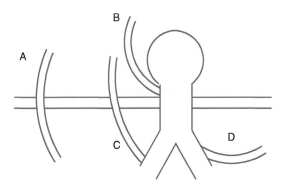

Figure 6.15 Four types of bypass tract. Tract A is an AV bypass tract, connecting atrial myocardium to ventricular myocardium. Tract B is an AV nodal bypass tract, connecting atrial myocardium to the His–Purkinje system. Tract C is a "Mahaim" tract, connecting the distal atrium (near the AV node) to the right bundle branch. Tract D connects the distal conducting system to the ventricular myocardium.

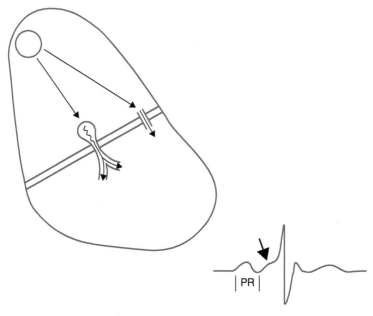

Figure 6.16 Preexcitation. In this example, there is a left-sided AV bypass tract. An impulse arising from the SA node stimulates the ventricles via both the normal conducting system and the bypass tract. Thus, the resulting QRS complex represents a fusion beat between normal and eccentric activation. Because conduction through the bypass tract does not display the normal conduction delay seen in the AV node, earliest ventricular activation classically occurs via the bypass tract. Hence, the PR interval is shorter than normal, and the QRS complex has a slurred onset known as a delta wave (thick arrow). Patients whose bypass tracts conduct antegradely, as shown, are said to have Wolff–Parkinson–White syndrome.

to ventricular myocardium (tract D). AV bypass tracts are by far the most common variety.

Bypass tracts may or may not conduct in the antegrade direction. When they do (in which case the patient is said to have Wolff–Parkinson–White syndrome), the surface ECG often shows preexcitation of the QRS complex (Figures 6.16 and 6.17). Preexcitation refers to antegrade conduction over a bypass tract that stimulates the ventricle prematurely. This ventricular stimulation is premature because the bypass tract conducts rapidly, like most myocardial tissue. Thus, an impulse traveling over the bypass tract does not display the delay seen when an impulse encounters the AV node. Preexcitation is usually manifested by a short PR interval and a slurring of the onset

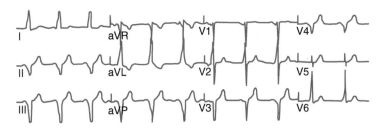

Figure 6.17 A typical 12-lead ECG from a patient with an AV bypass tract. Note the short PR interval and the delta wave visible on most leads.

of the QRS complex (which is termed a "delta wave"). In patients whose bypass tracts are capable of antegrade conduction, most QRS complexes are actually fusion beats between ventricular stimulation via the normal AV conduction system and ventricular stimulation via the bypass tract. The degree of preexcitation then depends on several factors, including the AV nodal conduction time (the slower AV nodal conduction, the larger the delta wave), the conduction velocity and the refractory period of the bypass tract itself (more preexcitation occurs in tracts with rapid conduction velocity and shorter refractory periods), and the proximity of the bypass tract to the SA node (the atrial impulse reaches a right-sided bypass tract earlier than it reaches a left-sided bypass tract, and thus right-sided bypass tracts tend to preexcite more).

In many patients who present with supraventricular tachycardia mediated by bypass tracts, the bypass tracts are incapable of antegrade conduction. Instead, they conduct in the retrograde direction only. Such bypass tracts are called concealed bypass tracts, because they never manifest delta waves or short PR intervals and are totally unapparent on the ECG when the patient is in normal sinus rhythm.

Bypass tracts are clinically significant for three reasons. First, they can confuse the clinician. Delta waves can masquerade as Q waves and lead to the false diagnosis of myocardial infarction. Marked preexcitation that occurs during an atrial tachycardia can lead to the mistaken diagnosis of ventricular tachycardia. Second, bypass tracts often act as one pathway of a macroreentrant circuit (the normal AV conduction system acting as the second pathway). Thus, macroreentrant supraventricular tachycardia is common in patients with bypass tracts. Third, bypass tracts can bypass the normal protective mechanism of the AV node during atrial tachyarrhythmias (specifically, during atrial flutter or fibrillation). In bypass tracts with short antegrade refractory periods, extremely rapid ventricular rates can result during atrial tachyarrhythmias. This problem is life-threatening. Concealed bypass tracts, without antegrade conduction, pose no increased risk during flutter or fibrillation.

The EP study can play a major role in characterizing the significance of bypass tracts and developing appropriate therapy. The EP study can be used to determine the characteristics of the pathways of a macroreentrant circuit and can help to select effective therapy for macroreentrant arrhythmias. In addition, it can help to determine the potential of the bypass tract to mediate lethal arrhythmias (the potential for lethal arrhythmias is not an issue in patients with concealed bypass tracts, since it depends on efficient antegrade conduction). Finally, and most importantly, the EP study can be used to precisely localize and ablate the bypass tract (see Chapter 9).

The EP study in bypass tract-mediated macroreentry

The mechanism of macroreentrant supraventricular tachycardia

Macroreentrant "supraventricular" tachycardia is actually a misnomer because the reentrant circuit involves ventricular as well as supraventricular structures. The mechanism of this arrhythmia is illustrated in Figure 6.18. A bypass tract acts as one of the pathways of the reentrant circuit. Like pathway B in our model of reentry, the bypass tract conducts rapidly and often has a relatively long refractory period. The pathway A of the reentrant circuit is formed by the normal AV conduction system, which displays the characteristics of slow conduction and a relatively short ERP. In short, in a heart containing a bypass tract, the characteristics of an ideal reentrant circuit are often present (Figure 6.18a). A macroreentrant rhythm can then often be started simply by introducing an atrial premature impulse at a time when the bypass tract is still refractory from the previous impulse but when the AV node has recovered (Figure 6.18b,c). The macroreentrant tachycardia has a normal QRS complex because antegrade conduction is via the normal AV conduction system.

Mode of initiation and termination of macroreentry

Bypass tract-mediated macroreentrant supraventricular tachyarrhythmias can usually be both initiated and terminated with either atrial or ventricular pacing.

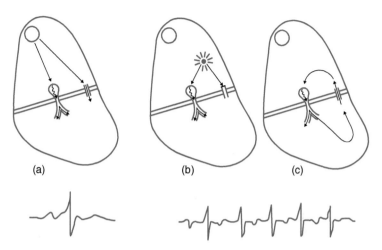

(a)   (b)   (c)

Figure 6.18 Bypass tract-mediated macroreentry. In this illustration, a left-sided AV bypass tract is present. (a) A normal impulse arising in the SA node stimulates the ventricle via both the normal conducting system and the bypass tract, as in Figure 6.16. The resulting ECG shows the typical short PR interval and delta wave. (b) A premature atrial complex occurs during the refractory period of the bypass tract (which typically has a longer refractory period than the AV node). The impulse thus blocks in the bypass tract and reaches the ventricle solely via the normal conducting pathway, and with a normal PR interval (depending on the site of origin of the premature atrial contraction [PAC]) and a normal (i.e., no delta wave) QRS complex. (c) Because the PAC has blocked antegradely in the bypass tract, the bypass tract may no longer be refractory by the time the impulse reaches the ventricles by way of the normal conducting system. In this case, the bypass tract may be able to conduct the impulse retrogradely back to the atrium. Thus, a reentrant impulse is established, which travels antegradely down the normal conducting system and retrogradely up the bypass tract. This form of macroreentry is extremely common in patients with AV bypass tracts.

In the presence of a bypass tract, macroreentry is often inducible with a single atrial extrastimulus. In the case of a bypass tract that is capable of antegrade conduction, a typical response to a series of single premature atrial impulses with progressively shorter cycle lengths is shown in Figure 6.19. Premature impulses with relatively long coupling intervals may show only moderate preexcitation (Figure 6.19a). As coupling intervals are shortened, conduction in the AV node is prolonged, so that the resultant QRS complexes show progressively more preexcitation (i.e., impulses have more time to depolarize the ventricles via the bypass tract [Figure 6.19b]). When the coupling

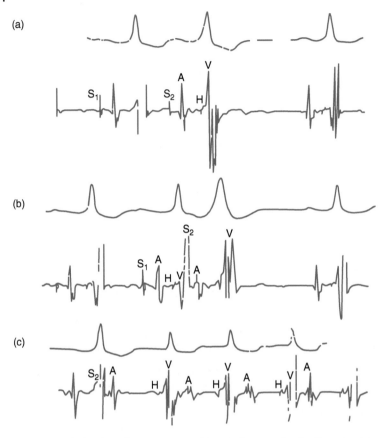

Figure 6.19 Induction of macroreentry with a single extrastimulus from the right atrium (i.e., by the mechanism illustrated in Figure 6.18). A surface ECG lead and the His bundle electrogram are depicted. (a) At a relatively long S_1–S_2 coupling interval, the premature atrial impulse conducts down both the normal conducting system and the bypass tract. The resultant QRS complex resembles the QRS complex in sinus rhythm (the last complex in (a)). (b) A premature atrial impulse with a shorter coupling interval encounters more delay in the AV node than was present in (a). Thus, the resultant QRS complex shows more preexcitation (more of the ventricle is depolarized via the bypass tract, while the impulse slowly wends its way through the AV node). The H spike is not visible during the premature beat in (b) because the His bundle is not stimulated until well into ventricular depolarization. (c) An even earlier atrial premature beat now encounters the refractory period of the bypass tract. Thus, the premature impulse reaches the ventricles entirely through the normal conducting system. Note the relatively long AH interval following the S_2 impulse, and the narrow (nonpreexcited) QRS complex. The impulse then returns to the atria retrogradely via the bypass tract, and macroreentrant tachycardia is established.

interval is shorter than the ERP of the bypass tract, the impulse suddenly blocks in the bypass tract and conducts entirely via the normal AV conduction system. The resultant QRS complex shows no preexcitation (Figure 6.19c). If conduction of this impulse through the normal AV conduction system is slow enough, the bypass tract may have enough time to recover so that the impulse can conduct retrogradely back to the atria, thus initiating macroreentry. The conduction delay seen with the onset of macroreentrant tachycardia represents the shift in AV conduction from the bypass tract to the AV node. The beginning of the tachycardia zone in macroreentry is thus related to the ERP of the bypass tract. In general, with even earlier premature atrial stimuli, macroreentry will be reproducibly inducible until the ERP of the AV conduction system is reached (the end of the tachycardia zone).

In the case of concealed bypass tracts (which are not capable of antegrade conduction), the initiation of macroreentry is somewhat more difficult to visualize. If there were truly no antegrade conduction down the bypass tract, one would expect every normally conducted sinus beat to conduct retrogradely back up the bypass tract and thus to initiate reentry. Because this is not the case, sinus beats must partially penetrate the bypass tract in the antegrade direction, rendering it refractory to subsequent retrograde conduction (Figure 6.20). (This phenomenon of conduction into a structure that cannot be directly observed but that one can deduce because of its effect on subsequent refractoriness is called *concealed conduction* or *concealed penetration*.)

To initiate macroreentry with atrial extrastimuli in patients with a concealed bypass tract, the extrastimulus must occur early enough that concealed conduction into the bypass tract is blocked (i.e., the extrastimulus must occur during the antegrade ERP of the concealed bypass tract [Figure 6.20]). In addition, the extrastimulus must occur early enough to cause sufficient delay in AV conduction so that the bypass tract has time to recover from concealed conduction. Induction of macroreentry in patients with concealed bypass tracts is facilitated by pacing near the bypass tract. Concealed conduction into the bypass tract then occurs early, and the bypass tract has more time to recover for subsequent retrograde conduction.

With either typical or concealed bypass tracts, macroreentry can also be induced with incremental atrial pacing, as long as pacing is rapid enough to cause complete or intermittent antegrade block in the bypass tract.

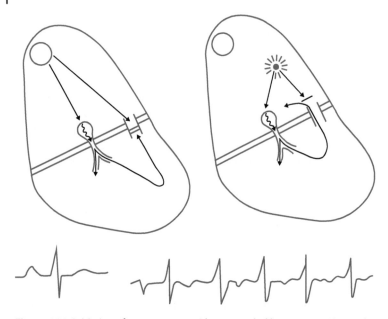

Figure 6.20 Initiation of macroreentry with a concealed bypass tract. No atrial impulses are capable of reaching the ventricles via a concealed bypass tract. However, some antegrade penetration of the bypass tract must be occurring, otherwise every atrial impulse would initiate reentry. This hidden conduction into the concealed bypass tract (called concealed penetration) is depicted in the first panel. Concealed antegrade penetration renders the bypass tract refractory to retrograde conduction and prevents reentry. Note that with a concealed bypass tract, the PR interval is normal and there is no delta wave. In the second panel, a premature atrial impulse occurs during the refractory period of the bypass tract, preventing concealed penetration from occurring. Because the bypass tract is not stimulated in the antegrade direction, the impulse may now conduct retrogradely back up the bypass tract and thus initiate reentry.

As opposed to AV nodal reentry, bypass tract-mediated macroreentry is often easy to induce with ventricular pacing. This is because retrograde conduction via the normal AV conduction system is often inefficient and therefore quick to block. Ventricular impulses that block retrogradely in the His bundle but conduct up the bypass tract will often induce reentry.

Termination of macroreentrant tachycardia can be accomplished with either atrial or ventricular extrastimuli. Atrial premature beats generally terminate macroreentry when they occur early enough to block antegradely in the AV node. Likewise, ventricular premature beats terminate macroreentry most commonly by preexciting the atrium (retrogradely via the bypass tract) early enough to produce antegrade block in the AV node.

Patterns of atrial and ventricular activation in bypass tract-mediated reentry

In bypass tracts that are capable of antegrade conduction, the ventricular activation patterns in sinus rhythm or with premature atrial complexes will be abnormal to the extent that preexcitation occurs. If one could record intracardiac electrograms along the ventricular side of the AV groove, the earliest ventricular activation would be seen at the ventricular insertion of the bypass tract. Because bypass tracts usually conduct rapidly and with constant conduction times until block occurs, the AV interval (or the PR interval) remains relatively constant with progressively premature atrial impulses until the ERP of the bypass tract is reached. The AV conduction curve is thus flat until block in the bypass tract occurs and AV conduction shifts to the AV node (Figure 6.21).

In patients with concealed bypass tracts, no preexcitation is seen. In these patients, the AV conduction curve is normal, unless there are coincidental dual AV nodal pathways.

Retrograde activation of the atrium is abnormal in patients who have left-sided or right-sided bypass tracts (see Figure 6.9). Often, with ventricular paced beats that have relatively long coupling intervals, atrial fusion occurs between normally conducted retrograde impulses and impulses that conduct up the bypass tract. With shorter coupling intervals, conduction up the normal pathways is delayed or blocked and retrograde activation patterns are frankly abnormal.

In patients who have anterior septal bypass tracts, the retrograde activation pattern of the atrium appears normal because the atrial insertion of these tracts is near the AV node. In these patients, however, progressively earlier ventricular paced beats do not result in a progressive delay in retrograde conduction time, as one would expect to see in retrograde conduction via the normal AV conduction system. The normal delay in retrograde atrial activation with progressively earlier ventricular stimulation is shown in Figure 6.8.

Requirement of the atria and ventricles in macroreentry

The reentrant circuit in macroreentrant tachycardia includes atrial and ventricular myocardium. Any instance of antegrade or retrograde

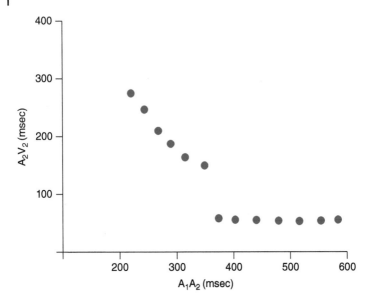

Figure 6.21 Atypical AV conduction curve in a patient with an AV bypass tract. At longer coupling intervals, premature atrial impulses are conducted to the ventricles via the bypass tract. Because the bypass tract does not typically display slowing in conduction with premature beats, this portion of the curve is flat. When the refractory period of the bypass tract is reached, AV conduction shifts to the normal AV conducting system. Thus, the curve is discontinuous. At the point where the curve shifts, the delta wave disappears from the resulting QRS complex. Also at this point, macroreentry is likely to occur. Intracardiac electrograms displaying this phenomenon are shown in Figure 6.19.

block occurring during the tachycardia, without producing a change in the tachycardia, rules out macroreentry, because a single blocked impulse in either direction should immediately terminate the arrhythmia. During tachycardia, premature atrial or ventricular extrastimuli can readily reset the tachycardia – this phenomenon can be used as evidence that the atria and ventricles are part of the circuit. An appropriately timed premature ventricular stimulus during tachycardia can often be shown to preexcite the atrium, which is strong evidence that retrograde stimulation via a bypass tract is operational (Figure 6.22). During macroreentry, the development of bundle branch block on the same side of the heart as the bypass tract will increase the cycle length of the tachycardia, strongly suggesting that the ventricles are part of the circuit (see Figure 6.10).

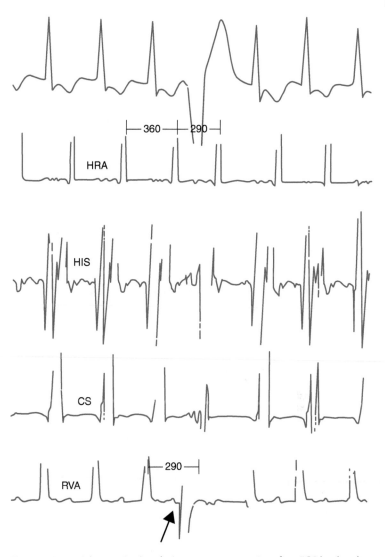

Figure 6.22 Atrial preexcitation during macroreentry. A surface ECG lead and intracardiac electrograms from the high right atrium (HRA), His bundle, coronary sinus (CS), and right ventricular apex (RVA) are shown. Macroreentrant tachycardia is present, with a cycle length of 360 ms. During the tachycardia, a single extrastimulus is delivered to the RVA at a coupling interval of 290 ms (arrow). This ventricular stimulation results in a premature retrograde atrial impulse at the same coupling interval (290 ms), best seen in the HRA electrogram. Preexcitation of the atrium with ventricular pacing during supraventricular tachycardia is strong evidence that an AV bypass tract is present.

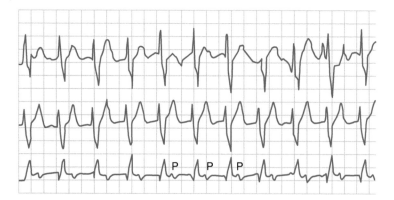

Figure 6.23 Macroreentrant tachycardia. Three surface EGG leads are shown, but P waves are best seen on the bottom tracing. The PR interval is typically longer than the RP interval.

Relationship of P to QRS during macroreentrant tachycardia

Unlike AV nodal reentry, in which the atria and ventricles are depolarized nearly simultaneously, in macroreentry the atria and ventricles are depolarized sequentially. Thus, distinct retrograde P waves are virtually always seen. P waves tend to be less than halfway between successive QRS complexes (the RP interval is shorter than the PR interval) because retrograde conduction via the bypass tract tends to be faster than antegrade conduction via the normal AV conducting system (Figure 6.23). The retrograde P wave axis depends on the location of the AP. Since most pathways are left sided or posterior septal, the P waves will be negative in the inferior leads (II, III, and AVF).

Treatment of macroreentrant supraventricular tachycardia

In theory, the main goal of pharmacologic therapy in macroreentry ought to be to reduce the width of the tachycardia zone. Drugs that increase the refractory period of the AV node (digitalis, calcium blockers, and β-blockers) can decrease the width of the tachycardia zone. In practice, however, the best results are often obtained not so much by narrowing the tachycardia zone as by increasing AV nodal block, thus resulting in Wenckebach conduction whenever tachycardia begins. This is effective therapy because a single blocked beat immediately terminates the tachycardia.

Another approach is to attempt to increase the retrograde refractory period of the bypass tract with class Ia drugs. Unfortunately, class Ia drugs also usually increase the antegrade refractory period of the bypass tract, which has the effect of increasing the tachycardia zone. Thus, class Ia drugs tend to be beneficial only when they have an extreme effect on the bypass tract, achieving "pharmacological ablation." If the effect of the drug is only moderate, macroreentry is often potentiated.

In general, the best results with drug therapy are obtained by using drugs that affect AV nodal conduction and refractoriness, either alone or in combination with class Ia drugs. Class Ic drugs such as flecainide and propafenone are often effective in treating macroreentrant tachycardia. Amiodarone is likewise effective, but most electrophysiologists consider it potentially too toxic to use in patients with nonlethal arrhythmias.

One important note about drug therapy is the treatment of AF with rapid conduction over an AP. The ECG has rapid, irregular, and wide QRS complexes. This should not be treated with AV node blocking agents as it would have no effect on rate since conduction is over the AP, and may speed conduction by lowering blood pressure (BP) and causing sympathetic stimulation. The most appropriate drugs in these settings are sodium channel blockers such as procainamide or amiodarone.

Today, however, drug alternatives are considered suboptimal, since most bypass tracts can be ablated in the electrophysiology laboratory with a high degree of success.

Localization of bypass tracts

Defining the location of bypass tracts is important if transcatheter ablation of the tract is contemplated. As noted, bypass tracts can occur anywhere along the AV groove (except in the space between the aortic and mitral valves). The good news is that AV bypass tracts are thought of as occurring in one of five general locations: left free wall, right free wall, posterior septum, anterior septum, or midseptum. Defining the location of a bypass tract is accomplished by studying the 12-lead ECG and by intracardiac mapping in the EP laboratory.

The location of bypass tracts as determined by intracardiac mapping has been correlated with the findings on the 12-lead ECG. The ECG patterns that have emerged match reasonably well with the five general locations of bypass tracts and are described in Chapter 9.

In the EP laboratory, bypass tracts are localized by studying the patterns of ventricular activation during preexcitation and of atrial activation during retrograde conduction. Left-sided and posterior septal tracts are the easiest to localize. The coronary sinus catheter lies in the AV groove between the left atrium and the left ventricle, and the os of the coronary sinus lies in the posterior septal region. By recording electrograms from multiple electrode pairs from an electrode catheter in the coronary sinus, early activation of the left atrium during retrograde conduction (and of the left ventricle during preexcitation) can be precisely localized. Right free wall and anterior septal tracts are more difficult to localize precisely, because there is no structure analogous to the coronary sinus that allows mapping of the right AV groove. Nonetheless, in the past few years electrophysiologists have become quite adept at precisely localizing bypass tracts. See Chapter 9 for details.

Atrial flutter/fibrillation in patients with bypass tracts

For reasons that are not well understood, patients with bypass tracts seem more predisposed to develop atrial flutter and fibrillation than the general population. Because some bypass tracts have the propensity for rapid conduction, an exceedingly rapid ventricular response can be seen in the presence of these arrhythmias (obviously, this is not a problem in patients with concealed bypass tract, which conduct only from ventricle to atrium). Patients who have rapidly conducting bypass tracts with short antegrade refractory periods are capable of conducting in excess of 300 beats/min (Figure 6.24). It can therefore be helpful during EP testing to assess the antegrade refractory period and the conduction velocity of the bypass tract during atrial fibrillation.

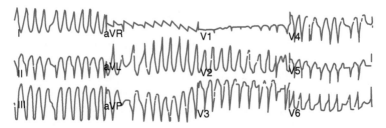

Figure 6.24 Atrial fibrillation in a patient with an AV bypass tract. Some patients with AV bypass tracts may experience extremely rapid conduction down the bypass tract during atrial tachyarrhythmias. The resulting QRS complexes are wide because ventricular stimulation is almost entirely via the bypass tract. This is a life-threatening arrhythmia.

During the EP study, the refractory periods of the bypass tract are measured in sinus rhythm and with atrial pacing. It is important to keep in mind, however, that bypass tracts respond to rapid stimulation like atrial or ventricular myocardium and not like AV nodal tissue – the faster the tract is stimulated, the shorter its refractory periods and the faster its conduction. Thus, the only way to know for sure how fast the tract can conduct during atrial fibrillation or atrial flutter is to attempt to induce these arrhythmias during the study. Further, because bypass tracts tend to respond somewhat to sympathetic stimulation, it is best to test the effect of AF on the bypass tract during an isoproterenol infusion. In general, bypass tracts are considered to be benign when the shortest preexcited RR interval during atrial fibrillation is greater than 270 ms. If the RR intervals are shorter than this, most electrophysiologists feel compelled to ablate the AP.

In patients who have potentially lethal bypass tracts, the addition of a class Ia drug, by increasing the antegrade ERP of the bypass tract and thus widening the tachycardia zone, can make macroreentry much more likely to occur. In these patients, the addition of a drug that affects the AV node can often be of benefit (using a β-blocker in this instance can both reduce macroreentry and counter the effect of sympathetic stimulation on the antegrade ERP of the bypass tract).

Some drugs, particularly digitalis and verapamil, can actually reduce the antegrade ERP of bypass tracts, rendering the tracts more dangerous. These drugs should generally be avoided in patients with preexcitation. If they are to be used, their effect on the antegrade ERP of the bypass tract should be specifically measured in the EP laboratory.

Given all the drawbacks to using chronic antiarrhythmic drug therapy in patients with potentially malignant bypass tracts, the treatment of choice for most of these patients is radiofrequency ablation of the bypass tract. Not only does ablation eliminate the bypass tract, it also eliminates the necessity of taking chronic daily antiarrhythmic drug therapy. This factor is especially important considering that the majority of patients presenting with bypass tracts are relatively young.

Uncommon varieties of bypass tracts

AV nodal bypass tracts

AV nodal bypass tracts (tract B in Figure 6.15) are relatively rare bypass tracts that connect the low septal atrium to the distal conducting system (usually to the His bundle), thus bypassing the AV node. On the surface ECG, patients with AV nodal bypass tracts display short PR intervals and normal QRS complexes. The His electrogram in patients with such bypass tracts reveals a short AH interval.

These bypass tracts display the same electrophysiologic characteristics as the bypass tracts we have been discussing; that is, they behave like myocardial tissue rather than AV nodal tissue. Although patients with AV nodal bypass tracts can occasionally have reentrant arrhythmias that use the bypass tract as the retrograde pathway and the normal AV node as the antegrade pathway, the major clinical problem with these tracts is their propensity to conduct impulses to the ventricle extremely rapidly during atrial fibrillation. Drug therapy to prevent rapid conduction during atrial tachyarrhythmias consists of class Ia or Ic drugs, because these tracts do not respond to the usual AV nodal blocking agents. But again, ablation of these tracts is generally the treatment of choice.

Mahaim bypass tracts

Mahaim bypass tracts (tract C in Figure 6.15) form connections between atrial muscle and the right bundle branch (atriofascicular tracts) or between atrial muscle and ventricular muscle (AV fibers). These tracts, which are discussed in more detail in Chapter 9, do not have typical bypass tract electrophysiology but instead display the kind of decremental conduction seen in AV nodal tissue. Reentrant tachycardia, when it occurs with Mahaim tracts, uses the tract in the antegrade direction and the normal conducting system in the retrograde direction. Since right bundle branch preexcitation occurs in tachycardia mediated by these tracts, the tachycardia displays a LBBB configuration.

Fasiculoventricular bypass tracts

Fasiculoventricular bypass tracts (tract D in Figure 6.15) connect the His bundle or the Purkinje fibers to ventricular myocardium. They are extremely rare and because they almost never mediate reentrant arrhythmias, they have little clinical significance. Their only manifestation is a short HV interval.

Multiple Bypass Tracts

Approximately 10% of patients with bypass tracts have more than one. Multiple bypass tracts, when present, can be difficult to diagnose in the EP lab because one bypass tract almost always predominates and prevents other tracts from manifesting themselves. Additional tracts become clinically significant most often following ablation of a bypass tract – successful ablation of the target bypass tract allows the hidden tract to become apparent. Multiple bypass tracts are more likely to be present if the 12-lead ECG shows atypical delta waves (including delta waves that appear to shift axis over time) or preexcited tachycardias. Multiple tracts are also likely if either multiple routes of atrial activation or mismatch of antegrade and retrograde activation during macroreentrant tachycardia are seen during electrophysiologic testing.

The EP study in intraatrial reentry

Intraatrial reentry is the mechanism of arrhythmia in a minority of patients presenting with supraventricular tachycardias. In intraatrial reentry, the reentrant circuit is entirely contained within the atrial myocardium. Superficially, intraatrial reentry resembles automatic atrial tachycardia because distinct P waves precede each QRS complex, P wave morphology almost always differs from normal sinus P waves, and AV block can occur without affecting the arrhythmic mechanism. Unlike automatic atrial reentry, however, intraatrial reentry is inducible and terminable with pacing.

The incidence of intraatrial reentry has increased substantially with the advent of atrial fibrillation ablation – especially when lines of block are attempted. Lines of block that develop conduction "leaks" set the stage for reentry within the atria, most often the left atrium.

Induction of intraatrial reentry is accomplished with atrial pacing. Invariably, whether the arrhythmia is induced with a single extrastimulus or with incremental atrial extrastimuli, induction occurs only when a premature impulse is early enough to produce intraatrial conduction delay (i.e., during the relative refractory period [RRP] of the atrium). The requirement for intraatrial conduction delay is further evidence that the arrhythmia being induced is reentrant in mechanism and that the atrial myocardium forms at least part of the reentrant circuit.

During intraatrial reentry, the atrial activation pattern typically differs from the normal atrial activation pattern because the atria are usually activated from a different location than during sinus rhythm. If the site of intraatrial reentry is near the SA node, however, the activation pattern can be indistinguishable from normal. In these cases, intraatrial reentry can often be distinguished from SA nodal reentry by the necessity of intraatrial conduction delay for initiation of the arrhythmia.

Because intraatrial reentrant circuits are contained entirely in atrial tissue, AV nodal block or block in the more distal conducting system can often be observed to occur without affecting the reentrant mechanism, thus demonstrating that the arrhythmia does not require the ventricular myocardium.

The pharmacologic treatment of intraatrial reentry requires drugs that affect the atrial myocardium; namely, antiarrhythmic drugs in classes Ia, Ic, and III. Drugs that affect primarily the AV node do not affect this arrhythmia (except perhaps to induce heart block). Transcatheter ablation of intraatrial reentry, using radiofrequency energy, has become the treatment of choice. Modern-day mapping catheters and systems have made ablation of intraatrial reentry much more feasible.

The EP study in SA nodal reentry

SA nodal reentry is a rare form of reentrant supraventricular tachycardia in which the reentrant circuit is enclosed entirely within the SA node. Because SA nodal tissue is electrophysiologically similar to AV nodal tissue, the mechanism of SA nodal reentry is believed to be the same as that of AV nodal reentry. Most likely, there are dual tracts within the SA node that form a potential reentrant circuit. The P-wave morphology on the surface ECG and the atrial activation pattern during SA nodal reentry are normal. SA nodal reentry is distinguished from standard sinus tachycardia by its paroxysmal onset and termination and by the ability to induce and terminate the arrhythmia by pacing.

Inducing and terminating SA nodal reentry is possible with atrial pacing, using either single extrastimuli or incremental pacing. Unlike in intraatrial reentry, conduction delay within the atrial myocardium is not necessary for the induction of SA nodal reentry. It is likely that the conduction delay necessary for the initiation of reentry occurs in one of the dual pathways presumably enclosed within the SA node, where it cannot be demonstrated.

Treatment of SA nodal reentry is similar to the treatment of AV nodal reentry. This arrhythmia responds to vagal maneuvers and to drugs that decrease conduction and increase refractoriness in the SA and AV nodes (digitalis, calcium blockers, β-blockers). SA nodal ablation can also be performed, but a permanent pacemaker may be required as a consequence.

The EP study in atrial flutter and atrial fibrillation

Atrial flutter and atrial fibrillation are felt to be reentrant supraventricular tachyarrhythmias in which the reentrant circuits are located entirely within the atrial myocardium. Both are inducible with single atrial extrastimuli or incremental atrial pacing during the atrial RRP (i.e., during pacing with coupling intervals short enough to produce intraatrial conduction delay). In atrial flutter, distinct P waves are seen, classically in a sawtooth pattern. In atrial fibrillation, atrial activity is continuous and chaotic, hence distinct P waves are not seen. In both arrhythmias, second-degree AV block is the rule.

Atrial flutter

Patients who have paroxysms of atrial flutter often have normal hearts, whereas patients with chronic atrial flutter more commonly have underlying heart disease that causes atrial distention or dilation. Most often, chronic atrial flutter eventually converts to chronic atrial fibrillation.

Patients in whom atrial flutter is inducible during EP testing tend to have demonstrable intraatrial conduction abnormalities. In these patients, atrial flutter is usually induced with atrial pacing at cycle lengths that are short enough to produce intraatrial conduction delays.

As already noted, these same characteristics are also typical for intraatrial reentrant tachycardias. It is probably legitimate to think of intraatrial reentry, atrial flutter, and atrial fibrillation as forming a spectrum of arrhythmias that have the same essential mechanism – that is, intraatrial reentry. Atrial flutter is distinguished from intraatrial reentrant tachycardia by its rate (flutter occurs from 220 to 350 beats/min, whereas intraatrial reentrant tachycardia occurs from 120 to 220 beats/min) and by its mode of termination. Whereas intraatrial reentrant tachycardia can often be terminated with single programmed atrial premature impulses, atrial flutter cannot. Atrial flutter

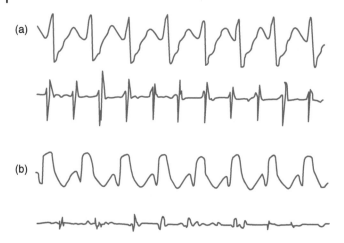

Figure 6.25 Two types of atrial flutter. A surface ECG lead and a right atrial electrogram are shown in both panels. (a) Typical atrial flutter displays a constant amplitude and cycle length on the intracardiac electrogram. This type of flutter is relatively easy to terminate with pacing. (b) Atypical flutter shows a somewhat variable cycle length and amplitude on the intracardiac electrogram. This type of flutter may be intermediate between atrial flutter and atrial fibrillation and is relatively difficult to terminate with pacing.

generally requires rapid atrial pacing for several seconds at rates from 20% to 50% faster than the flutter rate to terminate the arrhythmia.

The intraatrial electrogram recorded during atrial flutter normally shows rapid regular deflections with uniform cycle lengths and amplitude; the deflections correlate with the P waves on the surface ECG (Figure 6.25a). If this typical pattern is seen, the atrial flutter can often be terminated with rapid atrial pacing. In some cases of flutter, however, the intraatrial electrogram shows variability in the cycle length and amplitude of the atrial deflections. This second type of flutter is probably actually a form of atrial fibrillation (Figure 6.25b). Some experts may call this "coarse" AF. The best way to decipher "coarse" AF from atrial flutter is that in atrial flutter, there is no change in the p-wave or flutter morphology over the course of the ECG.

When vigorous attempts to pace-terminate the typical form of atrial flutter are made, two basic responses are commonly seen. The rhythm may be converted to sinus rhythm or to atrial fibrillation. Generally, atrial fibrillation is more likely to result when faster pacing rates are used (paced cycle lengths approaching 150% of the atrial flutter cycle length). When atrial fibrillation is the result of pace-termination of atrial flutter, the fibrillation usually spontaneously converts to sinus rhythm within 24 hours.

Treatment of Atrial Flutter

In general, the treatment of atrial flutter consists of restoring and maintaining sinus rhythm. Restoring sinus rhythm is most readily accomplished either by pace-termination of the flutter or by DC cardioversion. The major dilemma with atrial flutter is that antiarrhythmic drugs that slow conduction (type Ia and Ic) often perpetuate flutter. When long-term rhythm control is desired, catheter ablation is the treatment of choice. Transcatheter ablation of this arrhythmia (described in Chapter 12) should be strongly considered for any patient in whom chronic antiarrhythmic drug therapy would otherwise be contemplated.

Atrial fibrillation

Atrial fibrillation can be paroxysmal, persistent, long-standing persistent and permanent. Although atrial fibrillation (AF) is thought to be a reentrant arrhythmia of the atrial myocardium, its continuous and chaotic atrial activity precludes both meaningful analysis by recording intraatrial electrograms and pace-termination of the arrhythmia. Thus, although AF can be induced by pacing, it cannot be terminated by pacing. The exact mechanisms of AF remain elusive.

During standard EP testing of the SA node and AV conduction, a few seconds of AF are induced in a handful of normal patients. The induced AF is likely to terminate spontaneously within seconds, unless the patient has a history of spontaneous AF.

Experts used to think paroxysmal AF was a condition of normal hearts – so-called "lone" AF. Recent studies, however, have suggested that most patients with AF have underlying atrial substrate abnormalities of conduction and voltage. These studies have cast doubt on the existence of lone AF.

Treatment of atrial fibrillation

Atrial fibrillation is one of the most common cardiac arrhythmias seen in medical practice; it is unfortunate that it is also one of the most difficult to treat. The difficulty stems from the fact that patients who experience AF can differ vastly in symptoms and degree of heart disease.

Treatment of AF must be tailored to the individual patient – which sounds easy but is hard in practice.

The approach to treating AF can be visualized as the four legs of a table.

The first leg is stroke prevention. When stroke risk is deemed high enough (which is a matter of debate), clinicians recommend oral anti-coagulants.

The second leg is relatively newly discovered and is called risk factor modification. It is now recognized that cardiometabolic risk factors, such as obesity, hypertension, diabetes, sleep apnea, lack of fitness, and excess alcohol intake, contribute to structural, electrical, and autonomic abnormalities that promote AF.

The third leg of the table involves control of the ventricular rate. This is accomplished by administering drugs that affect AV nodal conduction and refractoriness (digitalis, calcium blockers, β-blockers). These drugs can be used in combination to achieve adequate rate control. When drugs fail to control rate, there is a more drastic (though effective and relatively safe) method for doing so – ablating the AV conduction system to produce complete heart block, and then inserting a permanent rate-responsive pacemaker. This option guarantees excellent rate control, and in patients whose symptoms are related to persistently high heart rates, it often creates a dramatic improvement in quality of life. This method of rate control is discussed in detail in Chapter 9.

The fourth leg of the table is rhythm control. Rhythm control isn't one therapy, it is the idea that we will try to establish and maintain sinus rhythm. Clinicians have three tools to pursue rhythm control: cardioversion, antiarrhythmic drugs, and catheter ablation. Cardioversion with a synchronized DC shock is highly effective at converting AF to sinus rhythm. The problem, of course, is that many (or most) patients will revert back to AF. Antiarrhythmic drugs will increase the chance of maintaining sinus rhythm once established. A general rule of thumb is that IC agents (sodium channel blockers propafenone and flecainide) are best used for paroxysmal AF, and the type III drugs (sotalol, dofetilide, amiodarone) are most useful for patients with persistent forms of AF.

Rhythm control versus rate control

One of the hardest decisions clinicians have to make in treating patients with AF is whether or not to pursue rhythm control. While observational studies suggest that having AF associates with higher risks for heart failure, stroke, and mortality, it is not clear that pursuing rhythm control modifies these long-term risks. (More on that to follow.) Rhythm control also places a substantial burden on patients in the form of more drugs and/or procedures as well as the potential for increased costs. And if that isn't complicated enough, overriding these consideration is what we will call the time penalty. That is, if one makes the decision to leave a patient in AF and pursue rate control, the AF may become irreversible after 1–2 years.

Does rhythm control reduce hard outcomes?

It might seem intuitive that if one were able to establish sinus rhythm, outcomes would be improved. But it is, in fact, complicated. Older studies done two decades ago, in an era when rhythm drugs were the only option, failed to show any improvement in outcomes. These studies were criticized because at that time, clinicians often stopped anticoagulants when sinus rhythm was established. We now know, in large part because of these studies, that anticoagulants should be continued.

More contemporary studies of rhythm control, which incorporated the use of catheter ablation, have been mixed. A large well-conducted trial called the CABANA (Packer DL et al., Am Heart J. 2018;199:192–199) compared rhythm drugs to catheter ablation in older patients with symptomatic AF and found no difference in hard outcomes. CABANA has been hotly debated because many patients in the drug arm crossed over to ablation and approximately 10% of patients in the ablation arm did not have ablation.

A trial comparing rhythm drugs to catheter ablation in patients with AF and heart failure called CASTLE-AF (Brachmann J et al., JACC Clin Electrophysiol. 2021;7(5):594–603) found significant reductions in heart failure hospitalizations and death in the ablation arm of the study. CASTLE-AF has also been debated, for two main reasons: one is because the investigators screened many more patients than they enrolled, suggesting a highly select group of patients that may not be representative of typical patients with heart failure and AF. The second criticism of CASTE-AF was that the number of events was low, which decreases confidence in the results.

Most recently, a European trial called EAST-AFNET 4 (Kirchhof P et al., N Engl J Med 2020;383:1305–1316) studied the use of early rhythm control vs standard care (mostly rate control). Rhythm control in this trial was mostly with rhythm drugs; about one in five patients had catheter ablation. EAST-AFNET 4 reported improved clinical outcomes in the rhythm control arm. Here the main criticism was potential bias in that patients in the early rhythm control arm had more interactions with clinicians – a form of performance bias.

Two clear reasons to pursue rhythm control

The two most obvious reasons to pursue rhythm control are if it is (i) causing symptoms and (ii) feasible. The matter of symptoms is more complex than it seems. Many patients report no palpitations or sensation of irregular beatings. A cursory history could lead a clinician to falsely conclude that this person has no symptoms. More detailed questions are needed. Patients with AF will often describe a sensation of fatigue, low power, low vigor, increased work of breathing with exercise and reduced exercise capacity. The problem is that fatigue and low power can have many causes.

The matter of feasibility of rhythm control is also complicated. Patients with massively dilated atria by echo or long duration of AF may be impossible to maintain in sinus rhythm (SR). But there is no definite measurement that tells us when rhythm control is impossible. Large atria sometimes do fine with rhythm control.

We often use a trial of rhythm control to assess both symptoms and feasibility. A cardioversion can be done and even if SR lasts a few weeks, a patient can report whether or not they felt better. We may also gain confidence that rhythm control could be feasible if SR lasts a few weeks.

Evaluation of patients with supraventricular tachyarrhythmias – when is electrophysiologic testing necessary?

Although the study of supraventricular tachyarrhythmias is probably the most intellectually stimulating and satisfying type of EP study one can perform, the fact is that many patients with supraventricular tachycardias can be managed adequately without invasive testing. Electrophysiology studies are often not necessary for two reasons. First, the surface ECG and response to vagal maneuvers can often cinch the diagnosis. Second, in the vast majority of cases, supraventricular tachyarrhythmias are not life-threatening. This makes the decision on how to treat the tachycardia (no treatment other than education on vagal maneuvers, drug therapy, and ablation) a preference-sensitive decision. Once the clinician removes fear through education, patients will weigh the choices of therapy in varied ways. Some may desire the near certain cure with ablation but others may be fine with terminating episodes with vagal maneuvers.

The examination of the surface ECG greatly aids in diagnosing the mechanism of supraventricular tachycardia. Atrial flutter and atrial fibrillation can be diagnosed almost immediately from the ECG and do not present a diagnostic problem. In the other types of supraventricular tachycardia, the relationship of P waves to QRS complexes and the morphology of P waves during tachycardia can be most helpful. Figure 6.26 shows the essential characteristics of the P waves in the four types of reentry that are commonly lumped under the heading "PSVT."

In the majority of patients with AV nodal reentry (the most common form of PSVT), the retrograde P waves occur during the QRS complex and are therefore invisible on the 12-lead ECG. In nearly every other kind of PSVT, P waves can usually be identified on careful inspection

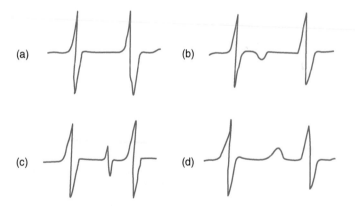

Figure 6.26 Typical P-wave relationships in four types of supraventricular tachycardia. Surface ECG lead II is depicted. (a) In AV nodal reentrant tachycardia, the P wave is usually buried within the QRS complex and is not discernible. (b) In bypass tract-mediated macroreentry, the inferior leads usually show a negative P wave, with the RP interval shorter than the PR interval. (c) In intraatrial reentry, discrete P waves are almost always seen. The P-wave morphology can have any configuration, and the PR interval is normal or short. (d) In SA nodal reentry, P waves and the PR interval appear normal.

of the ECG. Therefore, if there are no P waves, AV nodal reentry is the likely diagnosis.

In bypass tract-mediated macroreentry (the next most common type of PSVT – approximately 90% of patients presenting with PSVT have either this or AV nodal reentry), P waves virtually always can be seen. Because the P waves are generated retrogradely during this tachycardia, they are always negative in the inferior leads. Generally, the RP interval is less than the PR interval. Because the RP interval is relatively short, the retrograde P wave is often mistaken for a bump on the T wave by the unwary observer.

In intraatrial reentry, P waves are invariably seen on the 12-lead ECG. The PR interval is usually shorter than the RP interval and therefore the P waves are more obvious than in macroreentry. The P-wave morphology is variable from patient to patient and depends entirely on the location of the reentrant circuit within the atrium.

In SA nodal reentry, the P-QRS morphology is almost exactly identical to that seen in normal sinus rhythm. Thus, this arrhythmia is much more likely to be mistaken for sinus tachycardia than any of the other forms of reentrant supraventricular tachycardia.

Vagal maneuvers are also helpful in resolving these arrhythmias. Increased vagal tone commonly either decreases the rate of or terminates AV nodal reentry and macroreentry, because the AV node is part of the reentrant circuit in both of these arrhythmias. Likewise, vagal maneuvers may slow or terminate SA nodal reentry. In intraatrial reentry, however, vagal maneuvers have no effect on the cycle length of the tachycardia, but they may prolong the PR interval or produce AV block without changing the tachycardia.

Normally, EP testing needs to be performed in patients with supraventricular tachyarrhythmias in three general situations. First, electrophysiology studies can be helpful in patients whose arrhythmias appear refractory to treatment. In such patients, the arrhythmias usually have not responded to therapy, either because the mechanism of the arrhythmia is unknown or misunderstood, or because the reentrant circuit has unusual characteristics and does not respond to treatment in the usual way. Invasive studies can help by identifying the exact mechanism of the arrhythmias and by fully characterizing the various portions of the reentrant circuit. Pharmacologic or non-pharmacologic therapy can then be chosen based on that information.

Second, electrophysiology studies are indicated in patients with bypass tracts that are suspected to be capable of mediating life-threatening arrhythmias. Such patients would include those who have already demonstrated the propensity of the bypass tract to conduct dangerously rapidly during atrial fibrillation or flutter. Many electrophysiologists advocate invasive studies in any young patient with a bypass tract who has had symptomatic arrhythmias of any type. Some even recommend studying young patients who have preexcitation on an ECG, on the premise that any bypass tract that conducts antegradely may have lethal potential until proven otherwise. The idea here is that a 50 year old with preexcitation has a lower risk for rapid conduction because he or she has lived with the pathway for half a century. A teenager with preexcitation, however, has not lived long enough in harmony with the AP.

Third, and most commonly, EP studies are done for the purpose of performing transcatheter ablation. To ablate a tachycardia focus, one must know its mechanism and locale. EP studies do this – the exception being atrial fibrillation.

7

The Electrophysiology Study in the Evaluation and Treatment of Ventricular Arrhythmias

Ventricular tachyarrhythmias and sudden death

Sudden death (death that is instantaneous and completely unexpected) has long been a major public health problem in the United States. If this statement seems surprising, consider that each year, approximately 400 000 Americans die suddenly, and that sudden death is the most common form of death in the United States. Although most Americans are touched by sudden death, few realize that the majority of these deaths are due to electrical disturbances of the heart and are therefore, at least in theory, preventable

Consider a typical sudden cardiac death: a 59-year-old man who has suffered a myocardial infarction within the past 12 months has recovered, is now feeling well, and is leading a happy and productive life. He has followed his physician's advice and has altered his lifestyle in an exemplary fashion – he has stopped smoking, is on a heart-healthy diet, and has joined an exercise program. He is back at work, and his new sense of mortality has resulted in a broader and more tolerant perspective on everyday job-related stresses. In many ways, he feels better than he has in years.

Then one day, while watching television with his wife, he gasps softly and slumps over. An ambulance is called, but within minutes he is dead. The grieving widow is told by the emergency room physician (who has never seen the victim before) that her husband has died of a heart attack. Later, the victim's personal physician is only too quick (often through the honest desire to allay any feelings of guilt among surviving family members) to corroborate the "inevitability" of the event.

Fogoros' Electrophysiologic Testing, Seventh Edition. Richard N. Fogoros and John M. Mandrola.
© 2023 John Wiley & Sons Ltd. Published 2023 by John Wiley & Sons Ltd.

This scene takes place, on average, almost once every minute in the United States. The tragedy is compounded by a lack of understanding by both the lay public and the medical profession as to the reason for these sudden deaths. Very often, sudden death is not caused by acute myocardial infarction or bradycardia, as is commonly claimed. Instead, likely the majority of the 400 000 sudden deaths that occur each year in the United States are due to ventricular tachycardia or ventricular fibrillation. To the extent that ventricular tachyarrhythmias can be adequately treated, many of these sudden cardiac deaths are potentially preventable.

During the past few decades, remarkable advances have been made in treating ventricular tachycardia and fibrillation, largely thanks to what has been learned in the electrophysiology laboratory. It was the recognition that the great majority of lethal arrhythmias are due to the mechanism of reentry, and that they therefore lend themselves nicely to study in the electrophysiology laboratory, that catalyzed the rapid expansion of electrophysiology centers during the 1980s. The original "Holy Grail" for electrophysiologists was to solve the problem of sudden cardiac death.

This goal was pursued for years through the careful study of ventricular tachyarrhythmias in the electrophysiology laboratory. For almost 20 years, electrophysiologists spent much of their time inducing and terminating ventricular arrhythmias and, most especially, trying to identify effective therapy for those arrhythmias by the serial testing of antiarrhythmic drugs – often requiring the repeated induction of ventricular tachyarrhythmias over the course of several days. Thankfully, serial drug testing for ventricular arrhythmias has become almost entirely obsolete.

In this chapter, we will review the current management of ventricular tachyarrhythmias, and outline the role that electrophysiologic testing plays in their evaluation and treatment. Details on the ablation of ventricular arrhythmias in the electrophysiology laboratory are presented in Chapter 10.

The evaluation of ventricular tachyarrhythmias

The mechanisms of ventricular arrhythmias

The appropriate evaluation and treatment of ventricular arrhythmias largely depends on the mechanism of those arrhythmias. Table 7.1 lists

Table 7.1 Mechanisms of ventricular arrhythmias

Automatic ventricular arrhythmias
- Premature ventricular complexes
- Ventricular tachycardia and fibrillation associated with acute medical conditions:
  - Acute myocardial infarction or ischemia
  - Electrolyte and acid–base disturbances, hypoxemia
  - Increased sympathetic tone

Reentrant ventricular arrhythmias
- Premature ventricular complexes
- Ventricular tachycardia and fibrillation associated with chronic heart disease:
  - Previous myocardial infarction
  - Cardiomyopathy (including bundle branch reentry and ventricular arrhythmias associated with arrhythmogenic right ventricular cardiomyopathy)

Triggered activity
- Pause-dependent triggered activity
- Catechol-dependent triggered activity

Miscellaneous ventricular arrhythmias
- Idiopathic left ventricular tachycardia
- Outflow tract ventricular tachycardia (repetitive monomorphic ventricular tachycardia)
- Brugada syndrome
- Catecholaminergic polymorphic ventricular tachycardia

---

the most common ventricular arrhythmias according to their mechanisms. Figuring out which mechanism is responsible when faced with a ventricular arrhythmia depends to a great extent on the clinical setting in which the arrhythmia occurs – and sometimes on its characteristics in the electrophysiology laboratory.

We will discuss these arrhythmias in the order of their clinical frequency, beginning with reentrant ventricular arrhythmias.

Reentrant ventricular arrhythmias

Reentry accounts for the majority of ventricular arrhythmias. Reentrant ventricular arrhythmias are most often associated with chronic underlying heart disease. Reentrant circuits within the ventricles usually do not appear until patients develop some form of heart disease which causes scarring in the ventricular myocardium. Such scarring mainly occurs with ischemic heart disease and the various cardiomy-opathies. In ischemic heart disease, reentrant circuits arise during the healing and ventricular remodeling that follow an acute myocardial infarction – usually, the reentrant circuits form in the border zone between the scar tissue and the normal myocardium. In contrast to automatic arrhythmias, in which the typical substrate (such as acute ischemia) is temporary in nature and most often reversible, in the case of reentrant arrhythmias the substrate (i.e., the reentrant circuit) is not temporary but fixed.

Once a reentrant circuit is formed, it is always present and can generate a reentrant ventricular tachyarrhythmia at any time and without warning. Thus, the "late" sudden deaths that occur in patients with myocardial infarction (i.e., sudden death occurring at a time between roughly 24 hours and months or even years after the acute infarction) are usually due to reentrant arrhythmias. Reentrant arrhythmias, then, are commonly seen in patients who have a history of cardiac disease but are not acutely ill at the time of the arrhythmia. The vast majority of sudden cardiac deaths in the United States are due to reentrant ventricular tachyarrhythmias.

Risk factors for reentrant ventricular arrhythmias

It is relatively straightforward to predict which patients are at risk for reentrant ventricular tachyarrhythmias (and, therefore, at risk for sudden cardiac death), as long as one has an understanding of the pathophysiology of reentrant arrhythmias. A reentrant arrhythmia requires both an anatomic circuit with electrophysiologic properties appropriate for sustaining a reentrant impulse and an appropriately timed premature impulse to trigger the reentrant arrhythmia.

Because reentrant circuits are common only in the setting of myocardial disease, the major risk factor for ventricular reentry is the presence of underlying cardiac disease. As noted, myocardial infarctions and cardiomyopathic diseases are the most common disorders associated with reentrant ventricular arrhythmias. Nonetheless, any cardiac condition that causes even a small amount of ventricular fibrosis can give rise to reentrant circuits. Such conditions include myocardial trauma, a myocardial infarction that has been "aborted" by reperfusion therapy, subclinical infarctions associated with bypass surgery, subclinical viral myocarditis, and infiltrative diseases such as sarcoidosis or amyloidosis.

In general, the more extensive the myocardial fibrosis, the higher the likelihood of developing a reentrant circuit. With disease states that cause large fibrotic patches (such as a myocardial infarction), reentrant circuits are reasonably likely to develop. In disease states that cause only microscopic fibrosis, however, the likelihood of reentrant arrhythmias is proportional to the degree of myocardial involvement in the underlying disease process.

Once an anatomic circuit exists whose electrophysiologic properties are appropriate for sustaining reentry, an appropriately timed premature impulse is required to trigger the reentrant arrhythmia. Thus, another risk factor for developing reentrant ventricular arrhythmias is ventricular ectopy. Complex ventricular ectopy is generally considered to be present if, on 24-hour Holter monitoring, there are more than 10 premature ventricular complexes (PVCs) per hour, or repetitive forms such as couplets, triplets, or runs of nonsustained ventricular tachycardia. Patients with underlying cardiac disease who have complex ventricular ectopy have a higher risk of sudden death than patients who have the same underlying disease without complex ectopy. Frequent ectopic beats are not, however, a requirement for developing reentrant arrhythmias, since a single PVC (or even a premature atrial complex [PAC]) has the potential to trigger a reentrant ventricular tachyarrhythmia, given the right reentrant circuit. Indeed, a substantial proportion of patients resuscitated from lethal arrhythmias have only negligible ventricular ectopy.

It should also be noted that complex ventricular ectopy in patients with normal heart muscles (who are therefore extremely unlikely to have a reentrant circuit within their ventricles) has not been shown to increase the risk of sudden death.

The role of ejection fraction

An individual's risk for sudden cardiac death from a reentrant tachycardia, therefore, is most directly dependent on the presence or absence of underlying myocardial disease and on the extent of that disease. In general, since lower ejection fractions imply more extensive scarring and therefore indicate a higher likelihood that a reentrant circuit is present, the lower the ejection fraction, the higher the probability of sudden death. The risk of a fatal arrhythmia correlates strongly, though not perfectly, with declining ejection fraction.

As we have noted, some degree of ectopy must also be present to trigger the reentrant arrhythmia, but that ectopy does not necessarily have to be very frequent for an arrhythmia to occur. The probability that a reentrant circuit will generate an arrhythmia is much more dependent on the characteristics of the circuit itself (e.g., the tachycardia zone of the circuit) than on the frequency of ectopic beats.

Many studies have attempted to quantify an individual's risk of sudden death, and most have focused on three risk factors: the presence of a prior myocardial infarction, the presence of a depressed left ventricular ejection fraction (arbitrarily, less than 40%), and the presence of complex ventricular ectopy.

At the risk of greatly oversimplifying the vast body of literature examining this issue, let us make the following generalizations.

- First, the presence of underlying heart disease is more important in determining risk than the presence of complex ectopy, because underlying heart disease alone increases one's risk for sudden death, whereas complex ectopy alone does not.
- Second, having one of these risk factors alone (except for complex ectopy) yields a 1-year risk of sudden death that can be grossly estimated at approximately 5%.
- Third, the risk entailed by the presence of more than one of these risk factors appears to be roughly additive (Table 7.2).

Table 7.2 Risk factors and probabilities of sudden cardiac death

Risk factors	One-year risk of sudden death
Moderate-risk group	
Previous MI or LV EF <40%	5%
Previous MI + LV EF <40% or previous MI + complex ectopy or LV EF <40% + complex ectopy	10%
Previous MI + LV EF <40% + complex ectopy	15%
High-risk group	
Sudden-death survivor	30–50%
VT with syncope	30–50%
VT with minimal symptoms	20–30%

LV EF, left ventricular ejection fraction; MI, myocardial infarction; VT, ventricular tachycardia.

Values on this table are loosely derived from data reported by the Multicenter Postinfarction Research Group (Bigger JT et al., Circulation 1984;69:250) and the Multicenter Investigation of the Limitation of Infarction Size (Mukharji J et al., Am J Cardiol 1984;54:31).

Thus, the presence of either a previous myocardial infarction or a depressed ejection fraction gives a 1-year risk of about 5%. The presence of any two risk factors gives a risk of about 10%, and the presence of all three factors gives a risk of about 15%. Obviously, these values represent only a gross estimate derived from the available literature.

The severity of each risk factor is also important. For instance, a large myocardial infarction yields a higher risk than a small infarction, an ejection fraction of 15% yields a higher risk than an ejection fraction of 35%, and the presence of nonsustained ventricular tachycardia yields a higher risk than a single PVC. Thus, a patient with a previous large myocardial infarction with severely depressed ventricular function and long runs of nonsustained ventricular tachycardia will have a 1-year risk substantially higher than 15%.

An old indicator that was sometimes used to estimate risk of reentrant ventricular arrhythmias is the signal-averaged surface electrocardiogram (ECG). We discuss this test here mainly because of its educational value, though it can still be helpful clinically under some conditions.

The signal-averaging process digitizes and processes a series of QRS complexes (usually several hundred) recorded from the body surface. The result is a clean, high-fidelity average QRS complex in which small (low-amplitude) details can be seen, which are not visible on a normal ECG. In many patients at risk for lethal arrhythmias, low-amplitude afterpotentials can be seen immediately following the QRS complex (Figure 7.1). In theory, these afterpotentials may represent electrical

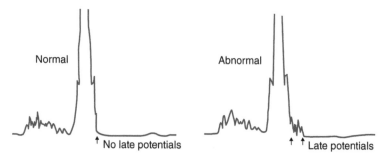

Figure 7.1 Signal-averaged ECG. The first panel shows a normal signal-averaged ECG, in which no late potentials are present. The second panel shows an abnormal signal-averaged ECG. The late potentials may indicate areas of slow conduction within the ventricular myocardium, suggesting the presence of a reentrant circuit.

activity caused by localized slow conduction in one or more reentrant circuits.

The predictive value of the signal-averaged ECG has not proven to be reliable enough to use in risk stratification in patients with coronary artery disease or heart failure. But the notion that an abnormal QRS complex can be a marker of a substrate capable of reentry is still important.

The signal-averaged ECG could be considered a fancy way to assess fragmentation of the QRS, which can often be found on a 12-lead ECG. Fragmented QRS complexes in the absence of bundle branch block (such as an R' wave or notching of a prominent S wave) suggest the presence of scar tissue capable of causing reentry, and have been correlated with an increased risk of life-threatening ventricular arrhythmias (Figure 7.2.)

In summary, patients who have survived a myocardial infarction or who have a depressed left ventricular ejection fraction from any cause are at increased risk for sudden death from reentrant ventricular tachyarrhythmias. The risk increases when the underlying cardiac disease is accompanied by complex ventricular ectopy or abnormal ventricular substrate. Considering only the fact that each year between 500 000 and 1 000 000 people in the United States suffer myocardial infarctions, the pool of patients at risk for sudden cardiac death is seen to be huge.

Clinical characteristics of reentrant ventricular tachyarrhythmias

The reentrant ventricular tachyarrhythmias take two major forms – ventricular tachycardia and ventricular fibrillation – and result in three major symptom complexes: sudden cardiac death, syncope, or minimal symptoms such as dizziness and palpitations.

Ventricular tachycardia (Figure 7.3) is a relatively organized tachyarrhythmia with discrete QRS complexes. It can be either sustained or nonsustained and can be monomorphic or polymorphic – polymorphic ventricular tachycardias tend to be faster and less stable than monomorphic tachycardias. The rate of ventricular tachycardia can be from 100 to more than 300 beats/min. At slower rates, ventricular tachycardia often does not cause significant hemodynamic compromise and may be relatively asymptomatic. The symptoms produced by ventricular tachycardia also depend on the morphology of the tachycardia, the severity of the underlying heart disease, the vascular tone, the geometry of ventricular contraction

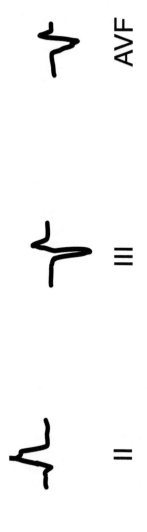

II   III   AVF

Figure 7.2 Fragmented QRS complex. QRS complexes from the inferior leads in a patient with prior inferior myocardial infarction show notching. Such QRS fragmentation in the distribution of a major coronary artery suggests the presence of scar tissue, even if Q waves are not present, and indicates an increased risk of ventricular arrhythmias.

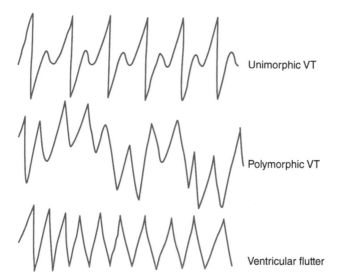

Unimorphic VT

Polymorphic VT

Ventricular flutter

Figure 7.3 Ventricular tachycardia. In monomorphic ventricular tachycardia, all QRS complexes are similar in morphology. In polymorphic ventricular tachycardia, the QRS complexes have constantly changing morphologies. In ventricular flutter, the ventricular rate is so rapid that the QRS complexes cannot be readily distinguished from T waves.

during the tachycardia, and whether the patient is upright or supine. At faster rates (usually 220 beats/min or faster), the tachycardia is so rapid that it may be impossible to distinguish the QRS complex from the T waves. This type of ventricular tachycardia is often referred to as ventricular flutter.

Ventricular fibrillation (Figure 7.4) is a completely disorganized tachyarrhythmia without discrete QRS complexes. This arrhythmia causes instant hemodynamic collapse and rapid loss of consciousness, because the heart immediately ceases to contract meaningfully. When ventricular fibrillation begins, it is associated with a coarse electrical pattern. As the heart becomes less viable (over a period of a few minutes), the amplitude of fibrillation waves seen on the ECG becomes finer and finer. Finally, all electrical activity ceases (flatline).

Recordings from patients who wore ambulatory monitors at the time of sudden cardiac death have often displayed the following progression of arrhythmias (Figure 7.5): an episode of ventricular tachycardia suddenly occurs (sometimes preceded by a brief period

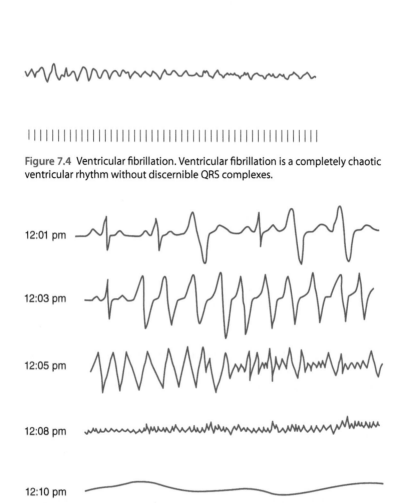

Figure 7.4 Ventricular fibrillation. Ventricular fibrillation is a completely chaotic ventricular rhythm without discernible QRS complexes.

Figure 7.5 A typical sequence of events in sudden death. This figure shows tracings from a Holter recording made in a patient who experienced sudden death. At 12.01 p.m. the patient is in sinus rhythm with PVCs. At 12.03 p.m. ventricular tachycardia occurs, which degenerates to ventricular fibrillation at 12.05 p.m. By 12.08 p.m., fine ventricular fibrillation is present. All electrical activity has ceased by 12.10 p.m.

of increased ventricular ectopy), which degenerates within seconds to minutes to coarse and then to fine ventricular fibrillation. After another 5–7 minutes, there is no electrical activity at all. Patients who are successfully resuscitated during such an episode (electrophysiologists have called them, oxymoronically, "sudden-death survivors") are often labeled as having had primary ventricular fibrillation, because that is the rhythm commonly seen by the time rescuers arrive. If the rescuers are a little too late, they see the flatline pattern of the dead heart. This has led to the popular misconception that sudden bradycardia is responsible for a large proportion of sudden deaths. The 1-year risk of arrhythmia recurrence for sudden death survivors is between 30% and 50%. Most recurrences are fatal.

When syncope occurs in a patient with a history of previous myocardial infarction or cardiomyopathy (especially if complex ventricular ectopy is present), a spontaneously terminating ventricular tachyarrhythmia must be high on the list of differential diagnoses. Such patients have up to a 50% chance of having inducible ventricular tachycardia during electrophysiologic testing, and those who have inducible arrhythmias subsequently have a high risk of sudden death (nearly as high as in sudden-death survivors). It is unlikely that a patient will survive multiple episodes of hemodynamically unstable (i.e., syncope-producing) ventricular arrhythmias. Indeed, patients with underlying heart disease who present with a single syncopal episode actually have a worse prognosis than patients who present with multiple syncopal episodes (in these latter patients, there is likely to be some other cause for the syncope).

Despite the fact that reentrant ventricular tachyarrhythmias are responsible for hundreds of thousands of sudden deaths each year in the United States, it is not unusual for sustained reentrant ventricular tachycardia to present with relatively minimal symptoms (minimal symptoms being palpitations, dizziness, lightheadedness, and other symptoms that are less severe than loss of consciousness). Sustained ventricular tachycardia that produces only minimal symptoms almost invariably presents as a monomorphic wide-complex tachycardia whose rate is less than 200 beats/min. Patients who present with these minimally symptomatic arrhythmias have a lower risk of sudden death than patients who have lost consciousness with their presenting arrhythmias – but their risk is still far higher than normal.

Owing to the lack of severe symptoms, a major problem that occurs with these patients is that physicians often mistake their relatively

Table 7.3 Clues for distinguishing ventricular tachycardia from supraventricular tachycardia with aberrancy

	Ventricular tachycardia	Supraventricular tachycardia with aberrancy
AV dissociation present	50%	Never
QRS duration	Often >0.14 seconds	Often <0.14 seconds
Precordial concordance	Often present	Usually not present
If RBBB configuration:		
Lead V₁	Initial R taller (Rsr)	Second R taller (rsR)
Lead V₆	Monophasic QRS common	Triphasic QRS common
	Axis commonly <−30°	Axis usually >−30°
If LBBB configuration:		
Lead V₁	Wide R wave, >0.04 seconds	Narrow R wave

Concordance, either all QRS complexes are positive or all are negative.
AV, atrioventricular; LBBB, left bundle branch block; RBBB, right bundle branch block.

well-tolerated ventricular tachycardia for supraventricular tachycardia with aberrancy. At some time in their careers, all physicians memorize a list of clues that helps them to distinguish ventricular tachycardia from supraventricular tachycardia with aberrancy in patients presenting with wide-complex tachycardia. Such a list of clues is presented in Table 7.3.

Unfortunately, within 15 minutes of taking the examination for which they memorized those clues, most physicians forget all of them. Instead, they often substitute the following simple rule (because it is easy to remember): "Ventricular tachycardia always causes loss of consciousness." *This tenet is patently false and often leads to mistaking sustained ventricular tachycardia for paroxysmal atrial tachycardia (PAT) with aberrancy.* Patients thus misdiagnosed may then be sent out of the emergency room without appropriate treatment. Because their reentrant ventricular tachycardia is not recognized, the opportunity to intervene to reduce their long-term risk of sudden death is missed.

Intravenous adenosine has come into common usage for termination of supraventricular tachycardias and thus is often administered to patients with wide-QRS complex tachycardia. When adenosine is administered, useful clues can often be seen that can lead one to a diagnosis of ventricular tachycardia. When supraventricular tachycardia of any type is treated with adenosine, careful observation usually reveals *some* transient change in the rhythm, even if the supraventricular tachycardia is not terminated. For instance, patients with atrial flutter or atrial tachycardia most commonly will have transient second- or third-degree atrioventricular (AV) block following IV adenosine, thus revealing the underlying mechanism of the arrhythmia. In contrast (unless the patient has one of the rare forms of ventricular tachycardia that responds to verapamil and adenosine), when adenosine is administered to a patient with ventricular tachycardia, *nothing happens.* Thus, when a patient with wide-complex tachycardia has no response at all to adenosine, ventricular tachycardia should immediately become the leading diagnosis.

Because the clues listed in Table 7.3 are difficult to remember, the authors propose an alternative simple rule.

> When patients with previous myocardial infarction or cardiomyopathy present with wide-complex tachycardia, it is ALWAYS ventricular tachycardia until proven otherwise, regardless of symptoms.

This rule will lead to the correct diagnosis in more than 95% of patients with underlying cardiac disease who present with wide-complex tachycardia. If such patients are referred for a more aggressive evaluation, the few who do have supraventricular arrhythmias will be diagnosed during electrophysiologic testing.

We would also propose another simple concept: Ventricular tachycardia (VT) starts in the ventricle. Unless the source is close to the Purkinje system, the QRS morphology will not look like a typical right bundle branch block (RBBB) or left bundle branch block (LBBB). VT is almost always broad in the initial portion of the QRS. The morphology of VT and its axis often suggests an origin in ventricular muscle. Supraventricular tachycardia (SVT) with aberration almost always starts with a sharp narrow deflection and looks similar to a RBBB or LBBB.

The electrophysiologic study in the evaluation of reentrant ventricular tachyarrhythmias

The electrophysiology study has revolutionized our understanding and management of lethal ventricular arrhythmias. Through the electrophysiology study, we have come to learn that most patients with ventricular tachyarrhythmias have reentrant foci as the source of their arrhythmias, that the arrhythmias can be reproduced safely in the laboratory, and that some reentrant circuits can be successfully ablated using transcatheter techniques.

The reasons for performing electrophysiology studies in patients known or suspected to have sustained ventricular tachyarrhythmias include:

- diagnosing the presence of a reentrant circuit that can cause a ventricular tachyarrhythmia
- assessing the feasibility of mapping and ablating a reentrant circuit; and
- optimizing the programming of an antitachycardia device.

Inducing ventricular arrhythmias

In considering the techniques used for inducing ventricular arrhythmias, we should begin by reviewing the prerequisites for reentry. First, an appropriate anatomic circuit should be present (see Figure 2.6). Second, the electrophysiologic characteristics of the circuit should be such that an appropriately timed premature impulse can block down one pathway (pathway B) and conduct down the other (pathway A) to establish a continuously circulating impulse. Third, the initiating premature impulse must reach the circuit at a critical instant in time (i.e., when pathway B is refractory and pathway A has recovered).

The successful induction of ventricular tachycardia in the EP laboratory depends on the first two prerequisites being in place: an anatomic circuit with appropriate electrophysiologic characteristics must be present. The only prerequisite for reentry supplied by the electrophysiologist is the critically timed premature impulse. By programmed stimulation, the electrophysiologist attempts to deliver a premature impulse to the reentrant circuit at just the right moment to induce ventricular tachycardia.

Delivering a premature impulse to a reentrant circuit at just the right moment is sometimes not easy. As noted in Chapter 4, the distance between the pacing electrode and the reentrant circuit, as well as the refractory characteristics and conduction velocity (i.e., the functional refractory period [FRP]) of the intervening tissue, determine whether it is possible for a paced impulse to reach the reentrant circuit early enough to initiate an arrhythmia. Unfortunately, the precise location of the suspected reentrant circuit is almost always unknown, and the FRP of the tissue between the pacing electrode and the reentrant circuit cannot be measured. Thus, the measures used to optimize conditions to allow premature paced impulses to arrive at the reentrant circuit early enough to initiate reentry are necessarily empiric.

As we have seen, pacing at faster rates (i.e., at shorter cycle lengths) decreases the refractory periods and increases the conduction velocity in ventricular myocardium, thus decreasing the FRP. Shorter FRPs will allow premature impulses to arrive at the reentrant circuit earlier and will increase the chances of initiating reentry. Stimulation protocols use two basic techniques to minimize the FRP of the ventricular myocardium: coupling multiple premature impulses together (typically up to three programmed extrastimuli) and pacing incrementally at rapid rates.

In addition, most stimulation protocols call for pacing from more than one catheter location, on the simple premise that one location may be closer to a reentrant circuit than another. Typically, pacing is performed initially from the right ventricular apex, and if no arrhythmias are induced, the electrode catheter is moved to the right ventricular outflow tract and pacing is repeated. Some electrophysiologists will also pace from the left ventricle (LV). The experience of most, however, is that LV stimulation is unlikely to induce an arrhythmia if no arrhythmias have been inducible from two right ventricular sites.

Finally, the inducibility of a reentrant ventricular arrhythmia can occasionally be improved by infusing isoproterenol. Presumably, in some patients, catecholamines act on potentially reentrant circuits to optimize the electrophysiologic characteristics for reentry.

Programmed stimulation protocols vary somewhat from institution to institution. The basic organization of stimulation protocols is to use progressively more aggressive pacing techniques, until either the desired arrhythmia is induced or the protocol is finished (in which case the patient is declared to be "noninducible").

A typical stimulation protocol is outlined in Table 7.4. The electrode catheter is initially positioned in the right ventricular apex. Following a drive train of eight incrementally paced beats (S1 beats) at a cycle length of 600 ms, a single programmed extrastimulus (S2) is introduced at a coupling interval of 500 ms (Figure 7.6a). If no arrhythmia is induced, the pacing sequence is repeated. With each pacing sequence, the coupling interval between the last S1 stimulus and the S2 stimulus is decreased by 10–20 ms, until the S2 no longer captures (i.e., the effective refractory period [ERP] for the S2 is reached). This procedure

Table 7.4 A typical stimulation protocol

Endpoints for the electrophysiology study

- >10 beats of reproducibly inducible ventricular tachycardia (positive study)[a]
- Completing protocol without inducing ventricular tachycardia (negative study)

The following pacing sequences are introduced from the right ventricular apex

- Step 1: single extrastimulus brought in to ventricular refractoriness at three drive cycle lengths
- Step 2: double extrastimuli brought in to ventricular refractoriness at three drive cycle lengths
- Step 3: triple extrastimuli brought in to ventricular refractoriness at three drive cycle lengths
- Step 4 : 8–12 incrementally paced beats brought in to ventricular refractoriness

If ventricular tachycardia is not induced, these steps are repeated from the right ventricular outflow tract

If ventricular tachycardia is still not induced, isoproterenol is infused and pacing is repeated

---

[a] Many authorities require 30 seconds of induced ventricular tachycardia to consider a test positive.

is then repeated, with S1 drive train cycle lengths of 500 then 400 ms. If no VT is induced with single extrastimuli at any of the three drive cycle lengths, the S2 stimulus is "parked" at a coupling interval approximately 20 ms longer than its ERP and a second extrastimulus (an S3) is added (Figure 7.6b). At drive cycle lengths of 600, 500, and 400 ms, the S1–S2–S3 coupling intervals are brought in as closely as possible. If double extrastimuli also fail to induce the arrhythmia, a third extrastimulus is added (S4; Figure 7.6c). At drive trains of 600, 500, and 400 ms, the S1–S2–S3–S4 intervals are brought in as tightly as possible.

If no VT is induced with single, double, or triple extrastimuli at any of the three drive cycle lengths, incremental pacing is performed. Incremental trains consisting of 8–12 stimuli are introduced with progressively shorter cycle lengths, beginning at a cycle length of 350 ms and decreasing to ventricular refractoriness (Figure 7.6d). If no VT is induced from the right ventricular apex, the electrode catheter is repositioned to the right ventricular outflow tract and the entire

(a)

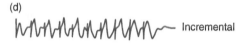 Single extrastimulus

S_1 S_1 S_1 S_1 S_1 S_1 S_1 S_1 S_2

(b)

Double extrastimuli

S_1 S_1 S_1 S_1 S_1 S_1 S_1 S_1 S_2 S_3

(c)

Triple extrastimuli

S_1 S_1 S_1 S_1 S_1 S_1 S_1 S_1 S_2 S_3 S_4

(d)

Incremental

Figure 7.6 Typical stimulation protocol for inducing ventricular tachycardia. Right ventricular pacing is illustrated. (a) Pacing begins with the introduction of a single extrastimulus (S2) following drive trains of incrementally paced beats (S1). (b) If ventricular tachycardia is not induced, two extrastimuli are used (S3). (c) If ventricular tachycardia is not induced with two extrastimuli, three extrastimuli are used (S4). (d) If ventricular tachycardia is still not induced, incremental bursts are used.

stimulation sequence is repeated. If VT is not induced, an iso-proterenol infusion is begun (to produce sinus tachycardia of 110–140 beats/min), and the entire stimulation sequence is repeated.

If no ventricular tachycardia has been induced with any of these measures, the patient is deemed to be "noninducible."

The meaning of "inducibility" and "noninducibility"

We touch here on the endearing notion that the EP study defines the patient definitively as being in one of two states: inducible or noninducible. While this conceptualization is fundamentally flawed, it is still clinically useful in many cases.

For instance, the EP study is often performed for diagnostic purposes. The whole point of doing the study here is to see whether an arrhythmia is inducible or not. If it is, the patient is presumed to have a high probability of developing spontaneous ventricular tachyarrhythmias; if it is not, that probability is presumed to be low. The best example of such a diagnostic study is the use of EP testing for syncope of unknown origin. (The evaluation of syncope will be covered in Chapter 15.) Obviously, in such diagnostic tests, one wants the stimulation protocol to have a very high chance of inducing arrhythmias that are clinically relevant, but a very low chance of inducing arrhythmias that are artifacts of an aggressive stimulation protocol, and that are never likely to become clinically manifest.

Electrophysiologists have yet to agree on the "best" stimulation protocol or on the correct definition of "inducibility." Although ideally one wishes to minimize both false positives and false negatives, in reality, when the electrophysiologist selects a stimulation protocol and a definition of inducibility, he or she is deciding whether to err on the side of producing more false positives (inducing non-clinical arrhythmias, which can lead to inappropriately aggressive therapy) or more false negatives (failing to induce truly clinical arrhythmias, leading to undertreatment). The aggressive stimulation protocol outlined in Table 7.4 errs on the side of producing more false positives.

Studies in apparently normal patients suggest that in a substantial minority (20–30%), more than 10 beats of polymorphic VT can be induced when triple extrastimuli are used, but that virtually none have inducible arrhythmias when only double extrastimuli are used. Thus, stimulation protocols using triple extrastimuli are likely to produce some false-positive studies. On the other hand, many patients who have had documented sustained ventricular tachyarrhythmias require triple extrastimuli to induce the clinical arrhythmias. Thus, stimulation protocols using less than three extrastimuli will tend to eliminate false positives but will miss some of the true positives.

Any definition chosen for "inducibility" necessarily takes into account the morphology and duration of the induced arrhythmia. The morphology of the induced arrhythmia is an issue because the studies in "normals" mentioned earlier suggest that when a false-positive VT is induced, the arrhythmia is almost always polymorphic. Thus, an induced arrhythmia that is polymorphic tends to be nonspecific. Some institutions accordingly attempt to limit their false-positive studies by stipulating that for a study to be considered positive, inducible VT must be monomorphic. However, although induced polymorphic tachycardia is a relatively nonspecific result, patients do, in fact, develop spontaneous polymorphic ventricular tachycardias. Insisting on a monomorphic arrhythmia will thus cause one to ignore some true-positive studies.

Regarding the duration of the induced tachycardia, most electrophysiologists recognize that in a substantial minority of patients presenting with sustained arrhythmias, only a nonsustained tachycardia will be inducible in the EP laboratory. Therefore, most laboratories will accept nonsustained tachycardia (if it is of sufficient duration) as a positive study. The determination of how many beats in duration that nonsustained tachycardia should be is completely empiric. In many laboratories, an inducible arrhythmia is defined by the ability to reproducibly induce at least 10 beats of VT (Figure 7.7). The number 10 is chosen arbitrarily. Some electrophysiologists consider anywhere from 3 to 15 beats of induced tachycardia to represent a positive study. Others require at least 30 seconds of VT before an arrhythmia is considered inducible.

One must be mindful of Bayes' theorem when deciding on an appropriate stimulation protocol and definition of inducibility. This theorem states that the specificity of any test is determined largely by the true incidence of the condition for which the test is being performed in the population being tested. In EP studies in patients who present with spontaneous sustained ventricular tachyarrhythmias, it is appropriate

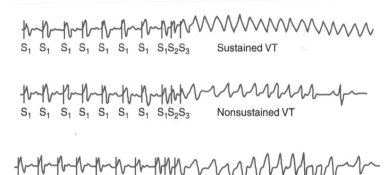

S_1 S_1 S_1 S_1 S_1 S_1 S_1 $S_1S_2S_3$ Sustained VT

S_1 S_1 S_1 S_1 S_1 S_1 S_1 $S_1S_2S_3$ Nonsustained VT

Polymorphic nonsustained VT

Figure 7.7 Types of inducible ventricular tachycardia. When inducing ventricular tachycardia in the electrophysiology laboratory, the goal is to induce sustained monomorphic ventricular tachycardia (shown in the top panel). This response is considered to be specific. The middle and bottom panels display two induced arrhythmias (nonsustained monomorphic ventricular tachycardia and polymorphic ventricular tachycardia) whose interpretation is controversial.

to use a more aggressive stimulation protocol and a more liberal definition of "inducibility." In such patients, positive tests are statistically less
likely to be falsely positive than in the general population, and are more
likely to be truly positive. If programmed stimulation is to be used in
patients who are in lower-risk groups (such as patients with syncope of
unknown origin), it might be reasonable to use a less aggressive pacing
protocol and a stricter definition of "inducibility," because the odds of
a positive study being falsely positive are higher in such patients.

Electrophysiologists have perhaps done too much hand-wringing
because they cannot agree on standardized pacing protocols and
definitions of "inducibility." They worry that the many differences
between centers render the electrophysiologic literature impossible to
interpret. The authors' opinion is that, on the contrary, the different
approaches being used are not particularly harmful and may, in
fact, be beneficial. An appraisal of the literature suggests that the
clinical results achieved with EP testing in patients who present with
sustained ventricular arrhythmias actually have been quite similar
among different centers. This suggests that in high-yield patient
populations, the variations in methodology have not been significant.
Further, as noted previously, different approaches will probably be of
benefit when the EP study is applied to different patient populations.
It may be harmful to be locked into a standardized protocol that errs
too much on the side of either false-positive or false-negative studies
when studying new populations.

In recent years, the advent of advanced imaging has aided in the
inducible vs noninducible tension. Magnetic resonance imaging
(MRI), for instance, can identify even small areas of scar. In such a
patient, a 10–20-second run of polymorphic VT may be considered
"positive" but if an MRI scan is normal, one may feel more confident
calling the same nonsustained VT a "nonspecific" finding.

Table 7.5 summarizes the factors that must be considered when estimating the specificity of the electrophysiology study.

Terminating ventricular arrhythmias

Termination of induced ventricular tachyarrhythmias is accomplished
by one of two methods: programmed stimulation (possible only with
VT, not with ventricular fibrillation) or direct current (DC) cardiover-
sion/defibrillation.

Terminating a reentrant arrhythmia with programmed stimulation
requires that a premature impulse encounters the reentrant circuit at

Table 7.5 Estimating the specificity of a positive electrophysiology study

Factors increasing specificity of a positive study
- Induced arrhythmia is monomorphic ventricular tachycardia
- Induced ventricular tachycardia is sustained
- Tachycardia is induced with single or double extrastimuli
- Patient studied is in a high-risk group

Factors decreasing specificity of a positive study
- Induced arrhythmia is polymorphic ventricular tachycardia or ventricular fibrillation
- Induced arrhythmia is nonsustained
- Arrhythmia is induced with triple extrastimuli or incremental pacing
- Patient studied is not in a high-risk group

a critical time. In this way, initiating and terminating reentry are similar, and the considerations for inducing arrhythmias discussed earlier (i.e., the distance between the electrode catheter and the reentrant circuit on one hand, and the FRP of the intervening tissue on the other) also pertain to termination of the tachycardia. Thus, techniques for pace-termination of VT are similar to techniques for pace-induction.

Several methods for pace-termination of VT have been proposed, but they essentially boil down to the incremental and extrastimulus techniques that we have seen before (Figure 7.8). The incremental method is used most commonly. Generally, incremental pacing to terminate VT begins with 8–12 beats at a cycle length 10–20 ms faster than the cycle length of the tachycardia. If this is unsuccessful, pacing is repeated at faster rates. When the extrastimulus technique is used to terminate VT, the extrastimuli are generally coupled to the intrinsic tachycardia beats rather than to a train of incrementally paced beats.

Whichever pacing method is used to terminate VT, there is a real risk of accelerating the tachycardia or causing it to degenerate to ventricular fibrillation (Figure 7.9). This poor result tends to occur more frequently with more aggressive pace-termination measures (such as rapid incremental pacing or triple extrastimuli), but these more aggressive pacing measures are also the most efficacious at terminating the tachycardia. If degeneration of the rhythm results from efforts at pace-termination, the patient usually needs to be rescued with a DC shock.

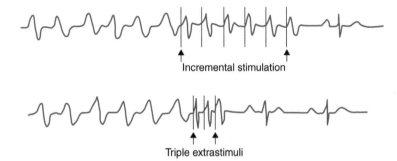

Incremental stimulation

Triple extrastimuli

Figure 7.8 Pace-termination of ventricular tachycardia. The top panel shows termination of ventricular tachycardia using a six-beat burst of incremental stimuli. The bottom panel shows termination of ventricular tachycardia using three programmed extrastimuli.

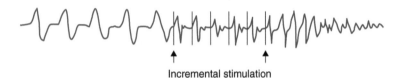

Incremental stimulation

Figure 7.9 Degeneration of ventricular tachycardia with pacing. This figure shows one of the inherent hazards in attempting to pace-terminate ventricular tachycardia. In this example, a six-beat burst of incremental stimuli degenerates the ventricular tachycardia into ventricular fibrillation.

Successful pace-termination of VT is easier to accomplish with arrhythmias that are relatively slow and monomorphic. The faster and less organized the arrhythmia, the harder it is to pace-terminate.

The choice of the timing and method of terminating the induced arrhythmia depends on several factors, including the rate and morphology of the induced arrhythmia, the duration of the arrhythmia, and the patient's blood pressure, symptoms, and level of consciousness. In most laboratories, if the patient is tolerating the induced VT, no attempt will be made to terminate the arrhythmia for 30 seconds (both in order to assess the patient's tolerance of the arrhythmia and to see if the arrhythmia will terminate spontaneously). If the patient is awake but is uncomfortable (experiencing lightheadedness, severe palpitations, or angina) or severely hypotensive, the electrophysiologist immediately attempts to pace-terminate the arrhythmia. If at any time the patient becomes unconscious, a DC shock is delivered. In most laboratories, once attempts to terminate the arrhythmia are begun, patients remain in VT for an average of 10–15 seconds. Deaths from inducing ventricular arrhythmias in the EP laboratory are extremely rare (<0.01%), and even the need for full cardiopulmonary resuscitation is very uncommon (<0.10%).

Testing the effect of drugs on the reentrant circuit
From the early 1980s until the mid-1990s, serial drug testing was the major reason for studying patients with reentrant ventricular tachyarrhythmias. This practice has largely fallen away for two reasons. First, large studies showed that pharmacologic therapy based on serial drug testing was not nearly as effective as had previously been thought. Second, results obtained with the implantable cardioverter-defibrillator (ICD) were far better than those obtained with serial drug testing – or with any other treatment. Today, serial drug testing is done only rarely, and is generally limited to patients who refuse therapy with the ICD or for whom the intention is to reduce the frequency of recurrent arrhythmias in the presence of an ICD.

The principle behind drug testing for ventricular tachyarrhythmias is simple. As discussed in Chapter 3, antiarrhythmic drugs work by changing the shape of the cardiac action potential, thus altering the conduction velocity or refractoriness of cardiac tissue. By so doing, these drugs are capable of altering the electrophysiologic properties of a reentrant circuit to make a reentrant arrhythmia less (or more) likely to occur. If a ventricular arrhythmia that was inducible during baseline (drug-free) testing is no longer inducible after administering a drug, then that drug has probably had a favorable effect on the reentrant circuit (Figure 7.10). For years, it was thought that treatment with a drug that rendered a previously inducible arrhythmia noninducible would protect against recurrent arrhythmias. As it turns out, a drug defined as being "successful" during serial drug testing probably delays the onset of an arrhythmia, but may not substantially reduce the patient's long-term risk of sudden death.

We leave this section in the chapter mostly for historical and physiologic reasons.

The electrophysiology study in the treatment of reentrant ventricular tachyarrhythmias

The EP study is useful in managing ventricular arrhythmias in at least two ways. First, it plays an essential role in the transcatheter ablation

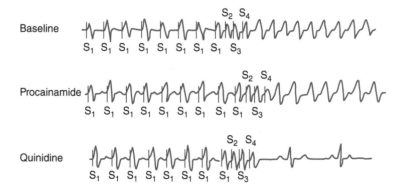

Figure 7.10 Successful serial drug testing for ventricular tachycardia. At baseline (top) and after administration of procainamide (middle), sustained ventricular tachycardia is inducible. After administration of quinidine (bottom), however, no ventricular tachycardia is inducible. Quinidine would appear to have a favorable effect on the reentrant circuit in this patient.

of ventricular arrhythmias. This technique will be discussed in Chapter 10. Second, electrophysiologic testing is potentially useful in in programming ICDs to optimize therapy for recurrent arrhythmias.

Preoperative electrophysiologic testing for ICDs

Appropriately programming ICDs often requires several complex decisions. One such decision is whether and how to use antitachycardia pacing (ATP) to terminate recurrent VT. In programming ATP, the physician sets a rate zone in which ATP is to be attempted. For instance, one might choose to attempt ATP for arrhythmias whose rate is between 150 and 190 beats/min. If a VT of more than 190 beats/min was to occur, ATP would not be used – a DC shock would be administered instead. A shock would also be given if a preselected number of ATP attempts failed to stop an episode of VT, or if the arrhythmia were to accelerate with an ATP attempt.

Programming ATP inappropriately can lead to serious problems. Because ATP is a potentially "kinder, gentler" therapy, the physician might be tempted to try it even for rapid, hemodynamically unstable tachycardias that would otherwise be treated immediately with high-energy shocks. Because rapid tachycardias are (most electrophysiologists agree) more difficult to terminate with ATP than slower tachycardias, prolonged attempts at ATP could conceivably allow prolonged hemodynamic compromise before "definitive" therapy was finally administered.

Conversely, the availability of ATP might tempt physicians to use implantable devices to treat slow, relatively well-tolerated tachycardias that might be better treated by other means. In such cases, the ICD might be programmed to deliver therapy at slower heart rates which are often reached when the patient develops sinus tachycardia or atrial fibrillation, thus potentially triggering inappropriate ATP attempts. Not only would such inappropriate ATP sequences fail to stop the supraventricular tachycardia, but they might also induce the very ventricular tachycardias that they were supposed to terminate.

This is problematic because in most cases, once an ICD begins delivering therapy, it does not stop until the heart rate falls below the programmed rate cut-off. Thus, unless the supraventricular arrhythmia terminates spontaneously, the device gradually, inexorably, and inappropriately escalates therapy until a series of high-energy shocks are delivered.

The exception to this rule is that newer generation ICDs have the ability to program a "slow VT" zone in which only ATP would be allowed. The number of patients for whom this is a viable option is limited. Far more typical is that an electrophysiologist targets slower VTs with catheter ablation.

Some electrophysiologists feel that pre-ICD testing is extremely useful, and they do it routinely. In recent years, however, most electrophysiologists point out that the characteristics of a patient's induced VT are often quite different from those of their spontaneous tachycardia, and that the odds of successfully pace-terminating a patient's induced arrhythmia frequently vary from day to day – and thus that the usefulness of preoperative testing is questionable. Further, this species of electrophysiologist feels that one achieves adequate (and even equivalent) success rates simply by programming ATP empirically. The authors, having done scores of preoperative EP studies and observed the results, now tend to agree with the latter group. That being said, some electrophysiologists swear by preoperative testing, which therefore remains a somewhat common and legitimate indication for electrophysiologic testing. A pre-ICD electrophysiology test may also detect another arrhythmia, such as paroxysmal supraventricular tachycardia (PSVT), which could be ablated and hence reduce the probability of inappropriate shocks.

Automatic ventricular arrhythmias

Abnormal automaticity accounts for a minority of lethal ventricular tachyarrhythmias. In distinction to reentrant ventricular arrhythmias, which are almost always associated with chronic, underlying disease of the myocardium, automatic ventricular arrhythmias tend to be associated with acute, reversible medical conditions, such as acute myocardial ischemia, hypoxemia, acid–base disturbances, electrolyte abnormalities (especially hypokalemia and hypomagnesemia), and high adrenergic tone. Thus, automatic ventricular arrhythmias tend to be seen in two general clinical settings: in patients who are acutely ill (e.g., in the intensive care setting) and in those who are having acute myocardial ischemia or infarction. It can be argued that patients who are desperately ill in the intensive care unit are not candidates for truly "sudden" death and, indeed, these patients are not included in most of the statistics on sudden death. On the other hand, lethal arrhythmias secondary to acute myocardial ischemia or infarction can and do occur "suddenly."

The automatic ventricular arrhythmias that occur during the first 24–48 hours after an acute myocardial infarction are thought to account for about 20% of the sudden cardiac deaths in the United States. The automatic arrhythmias seen during the first day or two after an acute myocardial infarction are probably related to the residual ischemia seen acutely in the zone of infarction. Once the infarction heals, the substrate for these early arrhythmias disappears. Therefore, the automatic ventricular arrhythmias that occur early during an acute myocardial infarction are thought to have little long-term prognostic significance (provided, of course, that the patient survives them).

Because automatic arrhythmias generally occur secondarily to metabolic abnormalities, treatment should be aimed at identifying and reversing the underlying cause whenever possible. In many instances, intravenous antiarrhythmic drugs (particularly lidocaine and amiodarone) can be helpful in temporarily suppressing automaticity while the primary problem is being addressed.

Automatic ventricular arrhythmias are not inducible in the EP laboratory and the EP study is not useful in their evaluation or treatment.

The authors note here that in many cases of VT, clinicians recommend coronary angiography to exclude new ischemic disease as the cause. The presence of a new ischemic lesion as a cause of ventricular arrhythmia is much more likely when the VT is polymorphic or when there are other symptoms (angina) or signs (ECG changes such as ST depression or elevated troponins) of ischemia. It is uncommon for new monomorphic VT to be caused by an acute ischemic lesion. Slower monomorphic VTs are almost always due to long-standing scar. Coronary angiography in these situations often acts merely to delay definitive therapy.

Triggered activity

As noted in Chapter 2, triggered activity is a mechanism for ventricular arrhythmias that has features of both automaticity and reentry. In recent years, the clinical features of arrhythmias mediated by triggered activity have been better characterized. Although triggered activity is a relatively uncommon cause of ventricular arrhythmias, the clinician must be alert to such arrhythmias for two reasons. First, like any ventricular tachyarrhythmia, these arrhythmias are life-threatening. Second, the successful treatment of arrhythmias mediated by triggered activity can be uniquely different from treatment used for other forms of ventricular arrhythmia.

Two fairly distinct clinical syndromes have been identified involving triggered activity: pause-dependent arrhythmias and catechol-dependent arrhythmias. In each syndrome, patients typically develop the polymorphic ventricular tachycardias that have been called torsades de pointes. Although these arrhythmias tend to occur in relatively short bursts and are usually accompanied by lightheadedness or syncope, the arrhythmias can persist long enough to cause sudden death.

Pause-dependent triggered activity

Pause-dependent triggered activity is caused by afterdepolarizations that occur during phase 3 of the cardiac action potential; hence they are called *early* afterdepolarizations (EADs; Figures 7.11 and 7.12). If the afterdepolarization reaches the threshold potential of the cardiac cell, another action potential can be generated (Figure 7.12b). Pause-dependent triggered activity is almost always related to conditions that prolong the duration of the cardiac action potential, such as electrolyte abnormalities (hypokalemia and hypomagnesemia) or the use of class Ia or III antiarrhythmic agents.

One way to think about pause-dependent torsades de pointes is akin to a plane crash: it is almost never due to one thing. Rather, there are

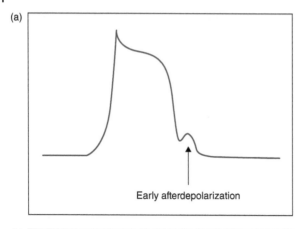

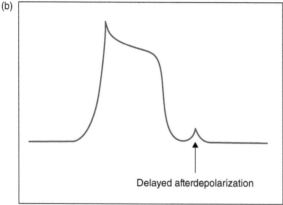

Figure 7.11 Afterdepolarizations. (a) An early afterdepolarization (EAD), the type of afterdepolarization associated with pause-dependent triggered activity. EADs occur during phase 3 of the action potential. (b) A delayed afterdepolarization (DAD), the type associated with catechol-dependent triggered activity. DADs occur after the end of phase 3.

numerous causes: a patient on a QT-prolonging drug who gets diarrhea and low potassium or a person on a QT-prolonging drug who is then put on a QT-prolonging antibiotic.

Repolarization reserve
Individuals who develop triggered arrhythmias when their QT intervals are prolonged most likely have an inborn subclinical abnormality

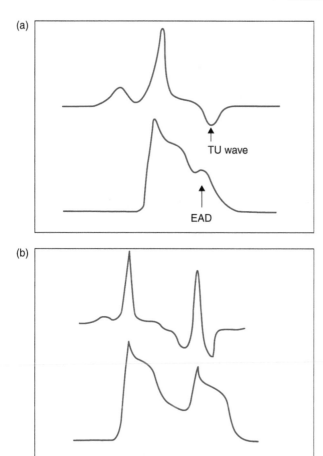

Figure 7.12 The relationship between early afterdepolarizations (EADs), TU wave abnormalities, and premature ventricular complexes. (a) The temporal association between EADs and the TU abnormalities as seen on the surface ECG. The TU wave is most likely the surface manifestation of the EADs themselves. (b) If an EAD is of sufficient magnitude to reach threshold potential, a premature complex results. Note that the timing of the premature complex is such that it occurs precisely on the TU wave of the previous beat.

of the cardiac cell membrane, which becomes manifest only when their action potential durations are increased.

This concept is increasingly recognized as the amount of repolarization reserve a person has. Some patients can tolerate large doses of

QT-prolonging drugs or very low potassium levels with little budging of the QT interval. Others, on the other hand, cannot tolerate any amount of QT-prolonging drug. The amount of reserve is largely genetically determined and is the reason why electrophysiologists often start QT-prolonging drugs (sotalol and dofetilide) in the hospital.

Future generations of clinicians may be able to identify repolarization reserve with advanced genetic testing. For now, we have to use trial and error type testing of QT-prolonging drugs.

The ventricular arrhythmias themselves are typically polymorphic and tend to occur in short bursts. The ECG, while in sinus rhythm, usually shows prolongation of the QT interval and distortion of the T wave; often, a distinct U wave occurs. Studies using the monophasic action potential have shown that the U waves are the ECG manifestation of the EADs themselves. When a burst of VT occurs, the first beat of tachycardia is invariably superimposed onto the U wave (or the distorted T wave), suggesting that the EAD (represented by that U wave) has reached the transmembrane potential for generating an action potential (Figure 7.12).

The TU wave abnormalities in this condition are usually dynamic. They tend to wax and wane, depending largely on the previous cycle length; the longer the previous cycle length, the more exaggerated the TU wave aberration of the following complex – hence, the condition is "pause dependent." Once a burst of VT has been initiated, it tends to repeat in a pattern of "ventricular tachycardia bigeminy" – the burst of VT causes a compensatory pause, and that pause causes the following sinus beat to develop marked U-wave abnormalities (i.e., a pronounced EAD occurs). Thus, another burst of tachycardia is generated after that first sinus beat. Pause-dependent triggered activity should be strongly suspected when this ECG pattern occurs either in the setting of QT interval prolongation or in the setting of conditions that predispose to QT interval prolongation, even if overt QT prolongation is not present (Figure 7.13).

The treatment of pause-dependent triggered activity is aimed at reducing the duration of the action potential. Drugs that prolong the QT interval should be discontinued and avoided – specifically, antiarrhythmic drugs that prolong action potential duration should not be used (some commonly used drugs that cause this type of triggered activity are listed in Table 3.3). Electrolyte abnormalities should be rapidly corrected. Intravenous magnesium sulfate often

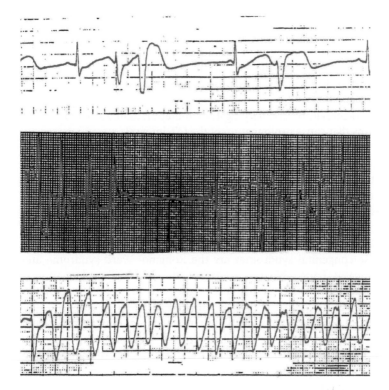

Figure 7.13 Ventricular arrhythmias caused by pause-dependent triggered activity (torsades de pointes). Features of pause-dependent ventricular arrhythmias are shown in a patient with QT prolongation caused by quinidine. In the top panel, "late" premature ventricular complexes (coincident with the onset of the U wave) arise immediately after a relatively long interval (i.e., a "pause") between QRS complexes. In patients prone to developing these arrhythmias, the pause itself induces afterdepolarizations (see text), thus triggering ectopic complexes. The bigeminal pattern seen here is typical, because each ectopic complex tends to produce a compensatory pause which, in turn, produces another ectopic complex. In the middle panel, the ectopy has become more sustained. Compensatory pauses still follow each burst of ventricular tachycardia, so that the patient now displays "ventricular tachycardia bigeminy." In the bottom panel, the arrhythmia has become even more prolonged and now displays a more typical "torsades de pointes" morphology. The key to recognizing torsades de pointes is to recognize the pause-dependent nature of the arrhythmia; the key to treating these arrhythmias is to eliminate the pauses. Thus, overdrive pacing reliably suppresses these arrhythmias.

ameliorates these arrhythmias, even when the serum magnesium level is not depressed. The mainstay of emergent treatment of these arrhythmias, however, is to eliminate pauses; that is, to increase the heart rate. This is usually accomplished either by atrial or ventricular pacing or by beginning an isoproterenol infusion.

Because the conditions that lead to pause-dependent triggered activity are generally reversible, long-term therapy is aimed at avoiding conditions that cause prolongation of the QT interval.

Catechol-dependent triggered activity

Catechol-dependent triggered activity is caused by afterdepolarizations that occur during phase 4 of the cardiac action potential. Thus, they are called *delayed* afterdepolarizations (DADs). DADs occur in the setting of digitalis toxicity, in cardiac ischemia, and in some patients who have congenital QT interval prolongation. These congenital syndromes are the Romano–Ward syndrome and the Jervell–Lange–Nielsen syndrome (in which QT prolongation is accompanied by neural deafness). Patients with catechol-dependent triggered activity have been postulated to have an imbalance in sympathetic innervation of the heart, with predominant input from the left stellate ganglion, stimulation of which can reproduce DADs.

Catechol-dependent triggered activity generally is not dependent on pauses (although pause-dependent features are seen in some patients). Instead, it is brought out in conditions of high sympathetic tone. Thus, patients experience VT (manifested by syncope or cardiac arrest) during times of exercise or emotional stress. Often, the QT interval is normal at rest. During stress testing, QT prolongation occurs, and often VT is seen. Left stellate sympathectomy has eliminated arrhythmias in some patients.

Treatment of catechol-dependent triggered activity usually consists of β-blockers and, because DADs are thought to be mediated by calcium-dependent channels, calcium channel blockers. In addition, more and more clinicians are using ICDs in these patients.

Miscellaneous types of ventricular arrhythmia

Clinical syndromes involving unusual ventricular arrhythmias have been described in which the arrhythmias do not fit clearly into any of the categories described so far. In many cases, these arrhythmias occur in the setting of a structurally normal heart, and in most cases, their mechanisms are not well understood. The literature is confusing regarding their classification and nomenclature, which is merely a reflection of our incomplete understanding of these arrhythmias. The following is a brief description of these syndromes.

Idiopathic left ventricular tachycardia

This arrhythmia tends to occur in younger patients without structural heart disease. The arrhythmia has a RBBB morphology often with a left, superior axis. It is inducible with programmed stimulation, and each QRS complex is preceded by a distinct His spike. The arrhythmic focus maps to the inferior aspect of the septum, and in several patients it has been successfully ablated. It tends to respond to therapy with β-blockers and calcium channel blockers. Both reentry and triggered activity have been advanced as the mechanism of this arrhythmia.

Outflow tract ventricular tachycardia

This arrhythmia, which has also been termed "repetitive monomorphic ventricular tachycardia," originates in the right or left ventricular outflow tract. It manifests as a nonsustained LBBB tachycardia with an inferior axis and is often provoked by exercise. Although the arrhythmia is often not inducible with programmed extrastimuli, pacing the heart at a rapid rate or instituting an isoproterenol infusion (i.e., simulating the heart rate response with exercise) can often induce it. It is usually seen in younger patients without structural heart disease. The arrhythmia tends to be responsive to therapy with β-blockers and calcium channel blockers, but the treatment of choice is usually transcatheter ablation, which has a high success rate in completely eliminating the arrhythmia. Whether this arrhythmia represents automaticity or triggered activity is unknown.

In recent years, electrophysiologists are increasingly seeing patients with frequent PVCs – often from the outflow tract area. Whether the increased volume of patients with outflow area PVCs is a true increase or simply more recognition that this arrhythmia can be ablated is unknown. The indications to ablate these PVCs are mostly twofold: symptoms and worsening LV function.

Symptoms due to PVCs can be severe and not reduced by medications. In these patients, electrophysiologists may recommend ablation. Another reason for ablation would be if the PVCs were more than 20k per day and associated with worsening of LV systolic function.

We discuss ablation of PVCs further in Chapter 11.

Arrhythmogenic right ventricular cardiomyopathy

Arrhythmogenic right ventricular cardiomyopathy (ARVC) is a rare condition, usually seen in younger patients, in which a variable amount of right ventricular myocardium is replaced by fatty and fibrous tissue. This condition appears to be genetic in origin; several genetic mutations have been identified that account for at least 30% of cases. The VT seen in right ventricular cardiomyopathy usually has a LBB morphology, and is almost invariably inducible with programmed stimulation. The treatment of this arrhythmia is similar to treatment for the reentrant ventricular tachycardias seen in the setting of coronary artery disease. Catheter ablation often requires epicardial access as the scar can extend to the epicardial surface. Surgery to cause electrical isolation of the dysplastic areas of the right ventricle has been tried, and although it has been successful in controlling the arrhythmia, right ventricular failure commonly follows. In general, patients with this condition who have had episodes of sustained VT or ventricular fibrillation should be offered an ICD.

A major new finding in ARVC syndromes has been the importance of curtailing endurance exercise. Patients with this syndrome have gene defects of the myocardial connection proteins and clinical studies have found that persistent endurance exercise can exacerbate the condition. In other words, exercise can worsen the phenotype of this genetic condition. Another recent development in ARVC is that the signal-averaged ECG – a rapid, noninvasive, readily repeatable test – can be useful in identifying family members of patients with this condition who also may be at risk for arrhythmias.

Bundle branch reentry

Bundle branch reentry is a distinct form of VT seen rarely in patients with idiopathic cardiomyopathy who also have intraventricular conduction disturbances. Most of these patients present with rapid monomorphic ventricular tachycardia that has an LBBB morphology. The reentrant circuit uses the right bundle branch in the downward direction and the left bundle branch in the upward direction. Its significance lies in the fact that it can be cured with transcatheter ablation of the right bundle branch. The ablation of bundle branch reentrant ventricular tachycardia is discussed in Chapter 10.

Brugada syndrome and sudden unexpected nocturnal death syndrome

Brugada syndrome was first recognized as a clinical complex consisting of ventricular tachyarrhythmias – often presenting as sudden death, cardiac arrest, or syncope – in patients who have unusual baseline ECGs displaying nonischemic ST segment elevation in leads V1–V3, as well as pseudo-RBBB. These patients are now thought to have genetic abnormalities involving the cardiac sodium channel (the channel that is mostly responsible for depolarization – phase 0 – of the cardiac action potential). Brugada syndrome affects males far more often than females, and the arrhythmias seen with it frequently occur during sleep. This condition appears to be the cause of the sudden unexpected nocturnal death syndrome (SUNDS) that has been described in apparently healthy Asian males.

There are several variants of the Brugada syndrome, probably reflecting various mutations in the cardiac sodium channel gene. In some patients, baseline ST changes are transient, in which case the characteristic ST changes can often be brought out by administering class I antiarrhythmic drugs (the drugs that operate on the sodium channel) or by pacing or vagal maneuvers. The arrhythmias associated with this syndrome are often inducible with programmed pacing, so a diagnostic EP study may be useful if Brugada syndrome is suspected. A history of prior cardiac arrest or syncope or a family history of sudden death greatly increases the risk of sudden death in a patient with Brugada syndrome.

The only treatment demonstrated to reduce the risk of sudden death in patients with Brugada syndrome is the ICD. β-blockers and amiodarone have not been shown to protect these patients. The generally accepted approach to treatment is to use clinical parameters to assess the patient's risk of sudden death and, if the risk is deemed to be relatively high, to insert an ICD. Fever has been shown to exacerbate the condition and patients with Brugada syndrome should be educated to take fever-reducing drugs in the event of infection.

Catecholaminergic polymorphic ventricular tachycardia

Catecholaminergic polymorphic ventricular tachycardia is a congenital disorder manifesting as rapid, polymorphic ventricular tachycardia or ventricular fibrillation, which is triggered by exercise or emotional stress. This condition presents as stress-induced sudden death or stress-induced syncope, usually in children or teenagers. There is often a family history of similar events. Notably, there is no prolongation of the QT interval in this condition.

Catecholaminergic polymorphic ventricular tachycardia has been associated with two specific genetic mutations (the cardiac ryanodine receptor and calsequestrin 2). These mutations are often inherited but can occur spontaneously. The mechanism of the polymorphic arrhythmia itself is not clear, but generally the arrhythmia is not inducible during electrophysiologic testing.

The polymorphic arrhythmias in this condition are often reduced in frequency by the use of β-blockers and flecainide. Patients who have survived cardiac arrest, or who have had a recurrence of symptoms on β-blockers, should be offered an ICD.

Ventricular tachyarrhythmias associated with mitral valve prolapse

Ventricular tachyarrhythmia associated with mitral valve prolapse is mentioned only to point out its minimal significance. Although there are many case reports in the medical literature that attribute sudden death to mitral valve prolapse, there is no epidemiologic study showing that patients with prolapse are any more susceptible to ventricular tachyarrhythmias than the general population. The purported association between sudden death and prolapse is probably related to the fact that between 5% and 10% of the general population have mitral valve prolapse, so that 5–10% of patients with unexplained sudden death are found to have prolapse on autopsy.

An overview of the treatment of ventricular arrhythmias

The optimal treatment of ventricular arrhythmias has changed radically since the first edition of this book was published in 1990. Today, thanks to advances in technology and the new knowledge gained from large randomized clinical trials, thousands of patients are being offered therapies they could not have received in earlier decades, and are being kept alive as a result. The progress has been remarkable.

The following discussion offers an overview of what we have learned over the last few decades on the treatment of ventricular arrhythmias, as well as a perspective on what the future might hold.

Four general truths we have learned about treating ventricular arrhythmias

Suppression of ventricular ectopy with antiarrhythmic drugs does not reduce risk

As noted previously, in the setting of underlying cardiac disease, complex ventricular ectopy is one of the risk factors for sudden death. For years, it was assumed that antiarrhythmic drugs aimed at suppressing such ectopy would reduce the risk. The medical community was finally disabused of this benign view of ectopy suppression in 1989, with the results of the Cardiac Arrhythmia Suppression Trial (CAST; Echt DS et al., N Engl J Med 1991;324:781). CAST was designed to study whether suppressing ventricular ectopy in patients with recent myocardial infarctions reduced the risk of death. What it showed instead was that the successful suppression of ectopy with two of the three drugs studied (encainide and flecainide) actually *doubled* or *tripled* the risk of death or cardiac arrest, while successful suppression of ectopy with the third drug (moricizine) provided no survival benefit. There were plenty of other reasons at the time to suspect that using antiarrhythmic drugs to suppress ectopy was risky but CAST drove home the point – suppression of ambient ventricular ectopy with antiarrhythmic drugs does not lead to a reduction in mortality and in fact may increase mortality.

CAST highlights the trouble with surrogate markers of disease. PVCs and ventricular ectopy are known to correlate with increased risk of cardiac arrest. Rhythm drugs reliably suppress the ectopy. But this did not lead to lower mortality. Ventricular ectopy therefore is a poor surrogate for cardiac arrest and overall mortality.

While antiarrhythmic drugs chosen by serial electrophysiologic testing allowed clinicians to avoid most of the proarrhythmic effects of these drugs, the overall survival of patients whose lethal ventricular arrhythmias were treated in this way proved to be very disappointing.

The bottom line is that the use of antiarrhythmic drugs, whether the therapy is aimed at suppressing ventricular ectopy or at inhibiting the induction of ventricular tachyarrhythmias in the EP laboratory, is not an effective method of reducing the risk of sudden death.

Yet antiarrhythmic drugs can have a role – especially in patients with backup ICDs – for the suppression of ventricular arrhythmias that cause symptoms, such as palpitations, tachycardia, or ICD shocks.

In recent years, many patients who have frequent, symptomatic or potentially dangerous PVCs have been treated with ablation therapy. Chapter 10 discusses this in detail.

Empiric treatment with amiodarone does not sufficiently reduce risk

Amiodarone is a uniquely effective antiarrhythmic drug and, in addition, has the virtue of not causing very much proarrhythmia. On the negative side, it has complex pharmacokinetic properties (its half-life is between 30 and 100 days, and it does not achieve its peak efficacy until it has been loaded for several weeks) and it has to be used carefully with close attention for side-effects or organ toxicity (refer to Table 3.4). Because amiodarone must be administered for weeks before it becomes fully effective, and because, when it is discontinued, measurable amounts of amiodarone will be present in a patient's serum for a very long time, the drug is most often used empirically – that is, without any form of formal testing of its effectiveness in a given patient. Still, despite these drawbacks, its relative efficacy leads electrophysiologists to use amiodarone fairly often.

Several randomized clinical trials have now tested the hypothesis that empiric treatment with amiodarone is an adequate method of reducing the risk of sudden death in high-risk patients. Some of the more important studies that have examined this issue are listed in Table 7.6. The bottom line is that, while amiodarone may improve mortality in some subsets of patients (a conclusion that has by no means been firmly established), it is not nearly as effective as the ICD. The use of amiodarone in high-risk patients should generally be limited to those who are not eligible for (or refuse) the ICD, or to adjunctive therapy to an ICD in order to reduce the frequency of recurrent arrhythmias.

Ablation of reentrant foci is an effective way of treating some patients with ventricular tachycardia

Because ablation can eliminate the reentrant substrate for ventricular arrhythmias, for patients whose VT is suitable, ablation should be strongly considered as a treatment option. Due to the risk of complications from ablation, patient selection and procedure

Table 7.6 Major clinical trials using amiodarone empirically in different groups of patients at increased risk for sudden death from ventricular arrhythmias

Study	Patient population	Randomization	Results
GESICA[a]	516 pts, NYHA class II/IV, cardiac enlargement	Amiodarone vs placebo	Significant survival benefit with amiodarone at 13 months (33.5% vs 41.4%)
CHF-STAT[b]	674 pts, LVEF <0.4, complex ectopy, cardiac enlargement	Amiodarone vs placebo	No significant survival benefit, but pts with nonischemic cardiomyopathy showed a trend toward amiodarone benefit
CAMIAT[c]	1202 MI survivors, complex ectopy	Amiodarone vs placebo	No significant survival benefit
EMIAT[d]	1500 MI survivors, LVEF <0.4	Amiodarone vs placebo	No significant survival benefit
SCD-HeFT[e]	2521 pts, LVEF ≤0.35, NYHA class II/III	ICD vs amiodarone vs conventional therapy	No reduction in mortality with amiodarone, but survival benefit with ICD

There is no evidence of a survival benefit with amiodarone in patients with ischemic heart disease. While two earlier trials (GESICA and CHF-STAT) showed a trend toward benefit in patients with nonischemic cardiomyopathy, the much larger SCD-HeFT trial subsequently revealed no such trend.

GESICA, Study Group on Survival of Heart Failure in Argentina; CHF-STAT, Survival Trial of Antiarrhythmic Therapy in Congestive Heart Failure; CAMIAT, Canadian Amiodarone Myocardial Infarction Trial; EMIAT, European Myocardial Infarction Trial; SCD-HeFT, Sudden Cardiac Death in Heart Failure Trial; ICD, implantable cardioverter-defibrillator; LVEF, left ventricular ejection fraction; MI, myocardial infarction; NYHA, New York Heart Association Functional Class; pts., patients.

[a]Doval HC et al. Lancet 1994;344:493.
[b]Singh SN et al. N Engl J Med 1995;333:77.
[c]Cairns JA et al. Lancet 1997;349:675.
[d]Julian DG et al. Lancet 1997;349:667.
[e]Bardy GH et al. N Engl J Med 2005;352:225.

planning is vital. Transcatheter ablation of VT will be discussed in Chapter 10.

In the majority of high-risk patients, the ICD is the only treatment that reliably reduces the risk of death from ventricular arrhythmias

The ICD automatically and reliably terminates the ventricular tach-yarrhythmias responsible for sudden death. Except for those cases in which ablation is a good option, in patients at high risk for lethal ventricular arrhythmias no other therapy approaches the level of efficacy achieved with the ICD.

A brief overview of the ICD

Like a pacemaker, an ICD employs a pulse generator, electrodes for sensing and pacing, and electrodes for defibrillation. With most ICDs, which we can call transvenous ICDs, intracardiac electrodes are used, although completely subcutaneous ICDs are now available (see below). For transvenous ICDs, the defibrillation electrodes and ventricular sensing/pacing electrodes are incorporated into one lead, which is placed into the right ventricle. If dual-chamber pacing is to be used, a second sensing/pacing lead is placed in the right atrium. Some ICDs also incorporate cardiac resynchronization therapy (CRT – see Chapter 14), in which case a third lead is placed into the coronary sinus for sensing and pacing the left ventricle.

The pulse generator contains circuitry for pacing, sensing and therapy, as well as separate large-voltage batteries and capacitors for defibrillation. Most contemporary ICDs will last for 6–12 years before battery depletion.

ICDs employ detection algorithms that are generally able to distinguish between ventricular arrhythmias that require therapy and other arrhythmias that do not. They are able to treat ventricular arrhythmias either with pacing therapy or with a shock, and can be programmed to do either or both, based on the "rate zone" of the ventricular arrhythmia being treated.

Programming ICDs

Programming ICDs for optimal behavior can quickly become an exercise in complexity. Many electrophysiologists try to tailor ICD therapy to treat the arrhythmias they are able to induce in the laboratory. With tailored therapy, in general the treatment employed is "tiered," the aggressiveness of treatment being escalated according to the rate of the arrhythmia being treated. The purpose of this approach is to attempt to treat as many arrhythmias as possible with pacing therapy instead of shock therapy. In most cases, however, tailored therapy is no more effective at preventing shocks than using an empiric approach.

With an empiric approach to ICD therapy, in general the ICD is programmed to administer treatment only for high-rate arrhythmias, after a relatively long delay. The MADIT-RIT trial (Moss et al., NEJM, 2012;367:2275–2283) compared "conventional" rapid therapy (2.5-second delay for rates 170–199 BPM, 1-second delay for rates of 200 BPM or higher) to either delayed therapy (60-second delay for rates of 170–199 BPM; 12-second delay for rates of 200 BPM or higher) or high-rate therapy (no therapy for rates <200 BPM, 2.5-second delay for rates of 200 BPM or higher). The authors reported surprising findings in that programming of ICD therapies for tachyarrhythmias of 200 beats/min or higher or with a prolonged delay in therapy at 170 beats/min or higher, compared with conventional programming, was associated with reductions in inappropriate therapy and all-cause mortality during long-term follow-up.

Based on this study, most electrophysiologists now program ICDs empirically, except in patients known to have recurrent, monomorphic ventricular tachycardias that respond well to ATP.

Complications of ICDs

Most complications of ICDs are related to the implantation procedure, and include infection, pocket bleeding and hematoma, lead dislodgment, and pneumothorax. Because ICD infections involve intravascular foreign bodies (i.e., the leads), treating them effectively usually requires removing the entire ICD system – an often difficult and potentially risky procedure if the ICD leads have been in for more than a few months.

Many late ICD complications are related to the intracardiac leads, including lead dislodgment, lead fracture, and insulation defects. Other late complications include skin erosion, skin necrosis, or pulse generator migration at the pocket site. Premature battery depletion and pulse generator malfunction are uncommon but can have serious consequences.

Inappropriate shocks are not uncommon but fortunately have declined with smarter ICD programming. These are usually due to treating supraventricular tachycardias, including sinus tachycardia, but can also be seen with lead or pulse generator problems that cause electrical noise or other forms of inappropriate sensing. Inappropriate shocks can occur in clusters (especially if due to sinus tachycardia or electrical noise), and can have a devastating psychological impact.

Subcutaneous ICDs

ICDs are now available that are entirely subcutaneous. That is, the leads are located under the skin instead of being intravascular – and this is the chief advantage of a subcutaneous ICD. Subcutaneous leads have several potential advantages over intravascular leads. The most difficult-to-manage complications of the standard ICD system usually involve the leads. With a subcutaneous system, if a lead complication occurs – and in particular, if an infected system occurs – it is less difficult to remove and replace the entire ICD system. The chief disadvantage is that the subcutaneous ICD is a shock-only device and is incapable of prolonged pacing, either for bradycardia support or for terminating VT. In addition, inappropriate shocks are more likely to occur with subcutaneous ICDs, and can be more difficult to manage than with transvenous ICDs.

Most electrophysiologists consider using subcutaneous ICDs in younger patients who need ICDs, in order to avoid problems associated with very long-term intravascular leads, and for patients who are at high risk for infection (such as patients on dialysis). Subcutaneous ICDs are still in their early iterations, and the optimal indications for their usage are still evolving.

Wireless monitoring of ICDs

Most modern ICDs have the capacity to store and wirelessly transmit data about the function of the devices themselves, and about the patient's heart rhythms and the response to any therapy that has been administered. This data can be transmitted remotely according to a fixed schedule, or at any time the doctor would like to see it. The remote monitoring capability has made it much simpler to troubleshoot and avoid device problems, and to detect and manage inappropriate shocks. Observational studies have found associations between remote monitoring and improved outcomes, though the possibility remains that healthier patients with better socioeconomic outcomes have higher adherence to remote monitoring. This is a form of selection bias.

The Evidence-based approach to using the ICD

ICDs – and the physicians who use them – have come under significant scrutiny, and clinicians are best advised to apply this therapy under close adherence to formal, approved guidelines. Because the guidelines for using ICDs are changeable, and because the variable emphasis which payers give to certain aspects of those guidelines may occasionally appear at least somewhat arbitrary, the authors will not attempt to reproduce formal ICD guidelines here, or to prescribe how a clinician ought to behave in light of them. Rather, it would be more useful to briefly review the current state of clinical evidence regarding ICDs, as derived from the randomized clinical trials that form the basis for those guidelines.

The randomized clinical trials assessing the benefits of ICDs can be divided into two general categories: the secondary prevention trials (in which ICDs were studied in patients who had already experienced life-threatening ventricular arrhythmias) and the primary prevention trials (which studied patients judged to be at elevated risk but who had not yet experienced life-threatening arrhythmias). Because the secondary prevention trials were the first to be conducted, we will begin with those.

Secondary prevention trials

Results from at least three randomized clinical trials have now demonstrated that therapy with the ICD can significantly prolong the survival of patients presenting with sustained ventricular tachyarrhythmias, compared to other therapies (most specifically, amiodarone) (Table 7.7). The designs of these studies were relatively straightforward, and so are the subsequent ICD indications they support. The ICD is now generally recognized as the treatment of choice for most patients presenting with sustained ventricular tachyarrhythmias. Caveats include patients who have severe life-limiting comorbid conditions, such as cancer, dementia, or frailty.

Table 7.7 The three major randomized clinical trials conducted with the ICD in patients presenting with sustained ventricular tachyarrhythmias (i.e., the secondary prevention trials)

Study	Patient population	Randomization	Results
AVID[a]	1016 pts with life-threatening sustained VT/VF	ICD vs amiodarone or sotalol	Survival benefit with ICD
CASH[b]	288 survivors of cardiac arrest	ICD vs one of three drug treatment arms	Survival benefit with ICD
CIDS[c]	659 pts with sustained VT/VF	ICD vs amiodarone	Trend toward survival benefit with ICD

These trials confirmed the effectiveness of the ICD in patients presenting with life-threatening, sustained ventricular tachyarrhythmias.

AVID, Antiarrhythmics vs Implantable Defibrillators; CASH, Cardiac Arrest Study Hamburg; CIDS, Canadian Implantable Defibrillator Study; ICD, implantable cardioverter–defibrillator; pts, patients; VT/VF, ventricular tachycardia or ventricular fibrillation.

[a] Antiarrhythmics versus Implantable Defibrillators (AVID) Investigators. N Engl J Med 1997;337:1576.

[b] Kuck KH et al. Circulation 2000;102:748.

[c] Connolly SJ et al. Circulation 2000;101:1297.

Primary prevention trials

While the secondary prevention trials with the ICD were aimed at confirming the correctness of ICD usage in patients with manifest ventricular arrhythmias, the primary prevention trials have been aimed instead at testing the ICD in high-risk patients who have not yet had sustained ventricular arrhythmias. As one might predict, the designs of these studies (and therefore resulting ICD indications) are much less straightforward than those of the secondary prevention trials. Table 7.8 lists the major primary prevention trials that have affected indications for the ICD and their most relevant design features.

MADIT I (Multicenter Automatic Defibrillation Implantation Trial) was the first primary prevention trial to be completed. In this study, patients with prior myocardial infarctions, left ventricular ejection fractions of less than 0.35, spontaneous nonsustained ventricular tachycardia, and inducible sustained ventricular tachycardia that was not suppressed with drug testing in the EP lab were randomized to

Table 7.8 The major randomized clinical trials conducted with the ICD in patients with an increased risk of sudden death but who had never experienced sustained ventricular tachyarrhythmias (i.e., the primary prevention trials)

Study	Patient population	Randomization	Results
MADIT I[a]	196 MI survivors, NSVT, LVEF <0.35, inducible VT, failed drug trial	ICD vs drug (mainly amiodarone)	Survival benefit with ICD
MUSTT[b]	704 MI survivors, NSVT, LVEF ≤0.4, inducible VT	No therapy vs EP-guided therapy	Survival benefit in EP-guided therapy pts who received ICD
MADIT II[c]	1232 MI survivors, LVEF ≤0.3	ICD vs conventional therapy	Survival benefit with ICD
SCD-HeFT[d]	2521 pts, LVEF ≤0.35, NYHA class II/III	ICD vs amiodarone vs conventional therapy	Survival benefit with ICD; none with amiodarone
DINAMIT[e]	674 pts, recent acute MI, LVEF ≤0.35, sympathetic overdrive	ICD vs conventional therapy	Reduced arrhythmic deaths with ICD, but no overall survival benefit

Table 7.8 (Continued)

Study	Patient population	Randomization	Results
IRIS[f]	898 pts, recent acute MI, LVEF ≤0.4, sympathetic overdrive	ICD vs conventional therapy	Reduced arrhythmic deaths with ICD, but no overall survival benefits
DANISH[g]	1116 pts, nonischemic CM, LVEF ≤0.35	ICD vs optimal med therapy including CRT where indicated	No survival benefit with ICD for whole group; improved survival in subgroup under 59 years old

Each of these trials except DINAMIT showed a survival benefit with the ICD. Owing to the varied subsets of patients entered into these trials, the resulting indications for the ICD are also somewhat complicated (see text).

MADIT, Multicenter Automatic Defibrillator Implantation Trial; MUSTT, Multicenter Unsustained Tachycardia Trial; SCD-HeFT, Sudden Cardiac Death in Heart Failure Trial; DINAMIT, Defibrillator in Acute Myocardial Infarction Trial; IRIS, Immediate Risk Stratification Improves Survival; DANISH, Defibrillator Implantation in Patients with Nonischemic Systolic Heart Failure; CM, cardiomyopathy; EP, electrophysiology study; ICD, implantable cardioverter–defibrillator; LVEF, left ventricular ejection fraction; MI, myocardial infarction; NSVT, nonsustained ventricular tachycardia; NYHA, New York Heart Association Functional Class; VT, ventricular tachycardia.

[a]Moss AJ et al. N Engl J Med 1996;335:1933.
[b]Buxton AE et al. N Engl J Med 1999;341:1882.
[c]Moss AJ et al. N Engl J Med 2002;346:877.
[d]Bardy GH et al. N Engl J Med 2005;352:225.
[e]Hohnloser SH et al. N Engl J Med 2004;351:2481.
[f]Steinbeck G et al. N Engl J Med 2009;361:1427.
[g]Kober L et al. N Engl J Med 2016;375:1221.

receive either the ICD or the "best" antiarrhythmic drug therapy (in most cases, amiodarone). At the end of the trial, patients randomized to the ICD had significantly improved overall survival. Subsequently, ICD indications were expanded to include patients who met *all* the MADIT I requirements (including electrophysiologic testing and at least one drug trial).

MUSTT (Multicenter Unsustained Tachycardia Trial) was even more complex in design than MADIT I, and it was in fact not specifically designed as an ICD trial at all. But for our purposes, this trial can be thought of as being similar to MADIT I, except that it was more liberal in terms of its ejection fraction entrance criterion (patients were allowed into MUSTT with ejection fractions of ≤ 0.4). In this trial, the ICD again significantly improved survival.

MADIT II randomized patients with prior myocardial infarctions and left ventricular ejection fractions of ≤ 0.3 to either ICDs or conventional medical therapy. The requirements for nonsustained VT and electrophysiologic testing were dropped in this trial. The results of MADIT II showed the group receiving ICDs as having significantly improved survival.

SCD-HeFT (Sudden Cardiac Death in Heart Failure Trial) enrolled patients with heart failure due to either prior myocardial infarction or nonischemic cardiomyopathy (this is the first primary prevention trial to include nonischemic patients). Enrollees were required to have left ventricular ejection fractions of ≤ 0.35 and NYHA class II or III heart failure. They were randomized to ICD implantation, empiric amiodarone, or placebo. At the end of the trial, the ICD produced a significant reduction in overall mortality compared to either amiodarone or placebo, while amiodarone itself offered no survival benefit compared to placebo.

DINAMIT (Defibrillator in Acute Myocardial Infarction Trial) randomized patients to receive either an ICD or conventional medical therapy an average of 18 days after an acute myocardial infarction. All patients had left ventricular ejection fractions of ≤ 0.35 and evidence of sympathetic overstimulation (either reduced heart rate variability or an increased resting heart rate) but no overt congestive heart failure. The ICD reduced arrhythmic death by 50% but did not reduce overall mortality. The "excess" in nonsudden deaths in the ICD group – deaths that cancelled out the reduction in arrhythmic deaths – was due to pump failure and mainly occurred in patients who earlier had been rescued from arrhythmic death by their ICDs.

The *IRIS* (Immediate Risk Stratification Improves Survival) trial, like DINAMIT, also enrolled patients within a month of an acute myocardial infarction and randomized them to ICD versus medical therapy. IRIS patients all had left ventricular ejection fractions of 40% or less, and also had episodes of nonsustained ventricular tachycardia. Further, they all had heart rates at rest of at least 90 beats\min. After a mean follow-up of about 3 years, there was no difference in overall mortality. The ICD group had a lower risk of sudden death but a higher risk of nonsudden cardiac death.

The conclusion generally drawn from the DINAMIT and IRIS trials is that any decision on implanting an ICD should be delayed for 4–6 weeks following an acute myocardial infarction, since ICD implantation during this interval has not been shown to be of benefit. It is noteworthy, however, that all patients enrolled in these two studies had evidence of impending heart failure, manifested by elevated resting heart rates or reduced heart rate variability. Given that a rapid resting heart rate is, prognostically, the worst heart rhythm one can have after a heart attack, it is likely that these two trials selected patients who had a particularly high risk of developing pump failure as their hearts remodeled. Patients who were similar but had normal resting heart rates might well have enjoyed an overall survival benefit with the ICD – but neither of these studies enrolled any such patients. And since they were not studied, subsequent guidelines have not allowed for ICD implantation in such patients.

The all-important DANISH trial

Finally, the DANISH trial (Køber L et al., N Engl J Med 2016;375:1221–1230) has to at least some extent called into question the use of the ICD in patients with nonischemic cardiomyopathy. In this study, 1116 patients with nonischemic cardiomyopathy and ejection fractions ≤0.35 were randomized to receive an ICD plus optimal medical therapy or optimal medical therapy alone. Optimal background therapy in the Danish study (in contrast to the older studies examining the use of ICDs for primary prevention) included CRT therapy in 58% of patients in both groups. The impressive nature of the background therapy was a key feature of DANISH.

After a median follow-up of 5.8 years, there was no significant difference in total mortality between the two groups (21.6% in the ICD group vs 23.4% in the non-ICD group).

DANISH had an important twist. A subgroup analysis found a heterogeneous effect based on age. Patients younger than 59 years had a statistically significant 49% relative reduction in death vs no significant reduction in death for those between 59 and 68 years and the group older than 68 years. While the statistical test for an interaction based on age was significant, the interpretation of subgroups in trials where the overall average effect was not significant is controversial. We believe a conservative take of DANISH is that implantation of ICDs in older patients with nonischemic cardiomyopathy is unlikely to reduce death rates.

Evidence-based indications for the ICD

Based on the evidence from randomized clinical trials, current indications for using an ICD can be summarized as follows.

- Patients who have had a cardiac arrest from a ventricular tachyarrhythmia, or who have had an episode of sustained, hemodynamically unstable VT, in whom no reversible cause is identified, and in whom the arrhythmia did not occur within the first 48 hours after a myocardial infarction.
- Patients with ejection fractions ≤0.35 who have not had an acute myocardial infarction in the last 4–6 weeks, and have NYHA class II/III heart failure after at least 3 months of optimal medical therapy. Since publication of the DANISH trial, this indication is less solid than previously believed, especially for older patients.
- Patients with ejection fraction less ≤0.30 despite maximally tolerated medical therapy who have distant myocardial infarction but have not had revascularization with either percutaneous coronary intervention or coronary artery bypass surgery within 90 days
- Patients with a prior myocardial infarction more than 4–6 weeks ago, and an ejection fraction that remains ≤0.3 with optimal medical therapy.
- Patients who meet CMS requirements for CRT and are NYHA class IV can receive a CRT device that also provides defibrillation therapy. This is the only group of patients in NYHA class IV that currently has an indication for implantable defibrillation therapy; the rationale here is that class IV patients who receive CRT therapy often experience a significant improvement in their functional class – and would thus find themselves eligible for an ICD a few weeks or months after receiving a CRT-only device. CRT devices are discussed in Chapter 13.

- High-risk patients with hypertrophic cardiomyopathy, arrhythmogenic right ventricular cardiomyopathy, congenital long QT syndrome with recurrent arrhythmias despite medical therapy, catecholaminergic polymorphic ventricular tachycardia, or other congenital forms of potentially lethal ventricular arrhythmias.
- ICD therapy should not be used in patients who have no reasonable expectation of survival for at least 1 year even if sudden death can be prevented, including those with refractory class IV heart failure who are ineligible for cardiac transplantation or CRT.
- ICDs should also not be used for patients with reversible forms of ventricular arrhythmias, or those with ventricular arrhythmias that are likely to be treatable with ablation therapy.

Despite its life-saving properties, we strongly feel that due to the potential for harm from the ICD, it remains a preference-sensitive decision. Patients considered for an ICD should undergo thorough shared decision making, preferably with a decision support tool. In fact, it is now mandated that US patients insured by Medicare have a shared decision-making session using a decision support tool. Decision support tools have been shown to improve knowledge, enhance risk perception, and increase patient participation in decision making.

8

Transcatheter Ablation: Therapeutic Electrophysiology

Over the past few decades, the most important advance in the field of electrophysiology has been the rapid transformation of the electrophysiology study from a largely diagnostic procedure to a largely therapeutic one. Many cardiac arrhythmias that formerly required the use of potentially toxic drugs or cardiac surgery can now be routinely cured (or at least palliated) in the electrophysiology laboratory by means of transcatheter ablation techniques.

The basic idea behind transcatheter ablation is to position a catheter at a critical area within the heart, and to apply damaging energy through the catheter in order to create a precisely localized scar. Strategically placed scar tissue, being electrically inert, can disrupt the pathways necessary for pathologic tachyarrhythmias. In this chapter, we will briefly review the technologies used to ablate cardiac arrhythmias in the electrophysiology laboratory. Later chapters will describe the specific techniques used, and specific considerations that must be taken into account, when ablating supraventricular tachycardia, atrial fibrillation, atrial flutter, premature ventricular complexes (PVCs), and ventricular tachycardia.

The technology of transcatheter ablation

Successful transcatheter ablation requires three things. First, it requires a thorough understanding of the arrhythmia being treated – specifically, the precise location and physiology of the electrical pathways involved must be carefully defined. Second, it requires an understanding of the cardiac anatomy associated with those arrhythmias. Finally, the technology must be available to

Fogoros' Electrophysiologic Testing, Seventh Edition. Richard N. Fogoros and John M. Mandrola.
© 2023 John Wiley & Sons Ltd. Published 2023 by John Wiley & Sons Ltd.

precisely position the ablation catheter, and to create the right kind of lesion at a critical location that will disrupt the arrhythmia. The rapid advance of transcatheter ablation as a therapeutic technique has hinged on steady progression in all three of these requirements.

Direct-current shocks

The use of direct-current (DC) shocks for transcatheter ablation is now of historical interest only, as DC energy has been entirely supplanted for this use by radiofrequency (RF) energy and cryothermal energy. From the first successful ablation in a human in 1982 until approximately 1989, however, DC shocks were the most commonly used energy source for the performance of transcatheter ablation.

To ablate with DC energy, a standard electrode catheter was connected to a conventional defibrillator and shocks were delivered to the distal electrode of the catheter, using a surface electrode as the energy sink. DC shocks delivered in this way required general anesthesia, and tended to produce significant complications. The relatively few electrophysiologists who used this technique did, however, demonstrate that appropriately placed intracardiac lesions could successfully treat certain cardiac arrhythmias. This proof of concept led researchers to develop alternative means of creating intracardiac lesions that would be less dangerous and more effective.

Radiofrequency (RF) energy

As it turned out, such a means was readily available. RF energy had been used for many years in operating rooms (in the form of Bovie machines) to cauterize small bleeding vessels within the surgical wound. It was not long before electrophysiologists recognized that attaching an RF generator to an electrode catheter would permit the creation of a discrete, well-demarcated intracardiac lesion.

The RF energy provided by the Bovie machine consists of alternating current (AC) with a frequency range of 100 kHz to 1.5 MHz. In the electrophysiology lab, relatively low frequencies are used in order to avoid the sparking seen with the higher frequencies used in the operating suite. The RF current flow causes localized heating at the tip of the catheter and leads to desiccation and coagulation necrosis of the underlying tissue. The voltage created during RF ablation is relatively low (40–60 V), thus avoiding the barotrauma (i.e., the explosion) seen with DC shocks.

Today, the RF energy used for ablation during electrophysiology procedures is generated by equipment specifically designed for this application. These specialized RF generators allow for instantaneously monitoring the energy being delivered to the cardiac tissue. The voltage, current, wattage, impedance, and contact force can be tracked, permitting the operator to carefully titrate the applied energy. In addition, most ablation systems allow monitoring of the temperature at the catheter tip, thus allowing the operator to more easily avoid coagulation of blood (temperatures in excess of 100 °C are associated with formation of a coagulum at the catheter tip, thus dramatically decreasing the energy delivered to the target tissue).

Special catheters have also been developed for use during RF ablation procedures. These come in a variety of shapes and sizes, and allow the operator to apply variable amounts of "bend" to the distal end, in order to facilitate accurate manipulation of the tip of the catheter. Ablation catheters also come equipped with enlarged tip electrodes (4 and 8 mm, instead of the "standard" electrode size of 1 mm). The enlarged surface area provides for a more efficient application of RF energy.

More recently, saline irrigation of the catheter tip and force sensing have been added to the standard RF catheter. Saline irrigation helps to prevent coagulum formation and force sensing helps the operator confirm adequate tissue tip contact.

RF energy has several advantages for intracardiac ablation. It can be applied, in judicious amounts, to thin-walled structures such as the coronary sinus and cardiac veins without producing rupture. RF energy produces very little stimulation of muscle or nerve, so it can be applied without using general anesthesia. It can be easily titrated, so graded amounts can be delivered to cause partial tissue damage. Finally, RF energy produces small, homogeneous, discrete lesions, which tend not to be arrhythmogenic.

There are also two disadvantages to the use of RF energy. First, the lesions it produces are small (4–5 mm in diameter and approximately 3 mm in depth). Extremely precise mapping is thus required in order to damage the target area sufficiently, and target tissue that is relatively broad or deep (e.g. a bypass tract located epicardially) might not be readily amenable to RF ablation. Further, the delivery of RF energy is not instantaneous. This means that stable contact between the catheter tip and the tissue must be maintained while RF energy is being applied. Monitoring of the impedance and contact force in the ablation system during the application of energy is helpful in ensuring adequate tissue contact.

Other energy sources

Another common source of thermal energy used for catheter ablation is cryothermal energy (i.e., freezing). There are two main types of cryoablation: freezing via a catheter tip and freezing via a balloon.

Electrophysiologists often use catheter-based cryoablation in areas where permanent damage can be problematic, such as areas close to the atrioventricular (AV) node. The advantage of cryoablation in these areas is that tissue can be partially frozen to assess for success or damage to the AV node. If the partial freeze successfully ablates the aberrant pathways without causing heart block, a complete freeze can be performed. Pediatric electrophysiologists sometimes use cryothermal catheter ablation in the region of the AV node.

Cryoablation has also been developed in balloon systems for use in single-shot isolation of the pulmonary veins for AF ablation (see Chapter 11). A randomized controlled trial called Fire and Ice compared cryoballoon to RF energy for the ablation of AF and the results were similar in both efficacy and safety (Kuck K-H et al., N Engl J Med 2016;374:2235). The main advantage of cryoballoon ablation, which has led to its widespread adoption in many electrophysiology programs, is its shorter learning curve.

Several other kinds of energy are being developed for ablation. One especially promising form of energy is called pulse field ablation or PFA – which harks back to the DC current ablation days. PFA is actually a nonthermal energy that uses super-short pulses of DC energy. Another name for it is electroporation, and it works by producing irreversible pores in cell membranes. The key advantages of PFA are its speed and cardiac selectivity. It ablates cardiac cells but does not affect adjacent structures such as phrenic nerves or the esophagus. At the time of this writing, PFA has been shown, in preliminary studies, to successfully ablate left atrial tissue. PFA is promising and worth noting in this text, but widespread adoption will depend on larger studies that are currently ongoing.

Electroanatomic mapping systems

The past several years have seen the advent of practical computer-based systems for mapping and ablating cardiac arrhythmias. This new type of mapping – which is often called "electroanatomic mapping" – has revolutionized ablation therapy.

As long as the electrophysiologist had to rely on whatever electro-physiological data could be synthesized from a few (or even many) intracardiac electrograms, and on whatever limited anatomic data could be discerned from fluoroscopic images, ablation procedures generally had to be limited to treating the simpler arrhythmias, such as AV nodal reentry or arrhythmias mediated by AV bypass tracts.

Electroanatomic mapping breaks both informational barriers – the electrophysiologic and the anatomic – to successful ablation. These new mapping systems allow detailed, three-dimensional maps to be constructed for an entire cardiac chamber (or chambers), which can show how the electrical impulse propagates across the heart and where there might be areas of ectopic origin, slow conduction, and low voltage (such as in areas of scar tissue). The 3-D display delineates both electrical activation and critical anatomic landmarks (such as blood vessels and valves). The 3-D maps are usually detailed enough that, once they are constructed, any further catheter maneuvering within the mapped cardiac chamber can mostly be accomplished without fluoroscopy.

Electroanatomic mapping permits the electrophysiologist to see the details of complex reentrant arrhythmias and identify specific anatomic areas – such as regions of slow conduction or scarring – which may be good targets for ablating reentrant arrhythmias. The origin of ectopic arrhythmias can be readily identified and pinpointed. Some systems allow for detailed mapping even when arrhythmias are nonsustained, very rapid, or otherwise unsuitable for typical mapping procedures.

These new mapping systems are especially helpful for mapping and ablating those "nonsimple" arrhythmias that are difficult or impossible with more traditional ablation procedures. Chief among these are atrial fibrillation and any complex reentrant arrhythmia involving abnormal areas of conduction.

Successful ablation of atrial fibrillation usually requires producing complete electrical isolation of the pulmonary veins, and in some cases also the ablation of ectopic foci. Because left atrial anatomy is so variable (with frequent variations in the number and sites of pulmonary veins, and numerous unexpected pits and ridges), it is difficult to effectively isolate the pulmonary veins without a detailed anatomic map of the left atrium. By providing the electrophysiologist with detailed anatomy and the means to maneuver within it, and providing a mechanism for mapping any remaining atrial ectopic foci, electroanatomic mapping makes the ablation of atrial fibrillation feasible in many more patients than it has ever been before.

Several electroanatomic mapping systems are now available. None are without limitations. We will briefly discuss the three systems which are in broadest use, and compare their relative advantages and disadvantages.

There is one major caveat: although these systems and their mapping algorithms are innovative tools with impressive displays, it has to be recognized that these powerful algorithms work best when there is accurate data collection with thoughtful and skillful mapping. The impressive colorful propagation arrhythmia maps are graphic aids to guide the operator and hence have to be cross-checked with other tools such as properties of local electrograms and entrainment maneuvers.

Magnetic field mapping (CARTO® mapping system, Biosense Webster)

A magnetic field can be used to create a 3-D, color-coded image of the cardiac chambers. With the CARTO system, the necessary magnetic field is generated from a three-coil location pad mounted beneath the catheterization table. The specialized catheters used with the CARTO system, which are now available as both ablation catheters and multipolar mapping catheters, contain a magnet at the distal tip, which can sense the field strength from each of the three magnetic coils. The precise location of the ablation catheter (and also other mapping catheters) can then be triangulated in real time, and the position of these catheters within the 3-D image of the relevant cardiac chamber can be continuously displayed.

Because the maps made with the CARTO system are dependent on the patient's location, they can become inaccurate if the patient moves. To mitigate this issue, a special set of patches are placed directly on the patient's back to serve as a location reference. The mapping system records the original location of these patches as a reference, so that if the patient moves (or the electrode is displaced), the original position can be found again.

When mapping tachycardias, it is also important to establish a timing reference, to use as "time zero" for gating the electrical signal from the mapping catheter. Typically, for ablating supraventricular arrhythmias the coronary sinus electrogram is used as a reference; for ventricular arrhythmias, the peak upstroke or downstroke of a surface QRS is used.

Once everything is in place, the mapping catheter is advanced to the cardiac chamber of interest and an electroanatomic map is generated. This is accomplished by slowly moving the mapping catheter across the endocardial surface and acquiring and processing both anatomic and electrical data from multiple points. The software has become so advanced that maps of thousands of points can be acquired in minutes. In the resultant map (which is continuously updated as the point-to-point mapping proceeds), the electrical data are superimposed on the anatomic map, in a color-coded fashion. These electrical data can be displayed in multiple ways – as an activation map, a dynamic propagation map, or a voltage map. Important anatomic features (such as valve rings, blood vessels, and the His bundle) can be labeled on the map. The maps can be viewed in virtually any projection.

Recent iterations of the system allow much easier creation of both the anatomy and the electrical properties of the chamber of interest. Activation and voltage maps can be made simultaneously.

Care must be taken in generating the map, so that all the key landmarks of the chamber of interest are identified. For instance, in mapping the right atrium, the operator usually begins by advancing the mapping catheter to the superior vena cava under fluoroscopy and, while directing the tip along the lateral wall, withdrawing it to the junction of the superior vena cava and the high right atrium. No longer is it necessary to take single points. The catheters do this automatically. Some operators can use this system to do zero to ultra-low fluoroscopy. All four cardiac chambers can be mapped in this way.

In many cases, it will be important to create the electroanatomic map after inducing the arrhythmia of interest, so that cardiac activation can be observed during the arrhythmia. When superimposed on the anatomic image, activation maps acquired during the arrhythmia should allow the confirmation of the mechanism of the arrhythmia and the identification of targets for ablation. But for scar-related arrhythmias, such as left atrial flutter or ischemic ventricular tachycardia, it is useful to identify low-voltage scar areas before tachycardia induction. See the following chapters for details.

In ablating atrial fibrillation, on the other hand, the emphasis is on the anatomy and not as much on electrical activation. Because the anatomy of the left atrium is so variable, a very detailed anatomic image is sometimes necessary in order to adequately isolate the pulmonary veins. To assist in producing this detailed anatomy, the CARTO system allows integration of the electroanatomic map with an image of the heart previously obtained using CT scanning or MRI. The CARTO system also makes available a module that superimposes the electroanatomic map on to an image derived from intracardiac echocardiography. With such anatomic tools, placement of lesions to isolate the pulmonary veins can often be carried out with remarkable precision.

The chief disadvantage of the CARTO system is that it requires the use of an expensive, proprietary, single-use mapping/ablation catheter.

Electrical field mapping (EnSite Precision® mapping system, Abbott)

Since the last edition of this chapter, the two major mapping systems (CARTO and EnSite) have become more similar.

The EnSite system consists of both hardware and disposables. The current systems have a field frame mounted underneath the patient bed, which generates a low-powered magnetic field within which the position of an electromagnetic sensor catheter is detected. The hardware connects catheters, patient reference sensors, and the field frame and relays the information to the EnSite amplifier via a fiberoptic connection.

The disposable kit consists of a system reference surface electrode and six surface electrodes placed on the patient in pairs, which send low-power currents through the patient's chest in three orthogonal (x, y, z) directions to form a 3-D transthoracic electrical field with the heart at the center. As standard catheter electrodes (from diagnostic and ablation catheters) are maneuvered within the chambers, each catheter electrode senses the corresponding levels of impedance derived from the measured voltage and a unique point is registered.

The original Ensite systems used only impedance technology for localization. The most recent versions incorporate magnetic field. Either impedance or magnetic mapping environment can be tailored to the specifics of the patient and procedure type.

During geometry creation, the operator assigns points based on local electrogram characteristics and anatomic location based on fluoroscopy or echo (e.g., tricuspid or mitral annular points, appendage, pulmonary veins, etc.), usually gated to ECG to prevent variation with the cardiac cycle.

Unlike CARTO, with Ensite, the chamber geometry and tachycardia mapping can be determined with any nonproprietary diagnostic or ablation catheter, which is timed against a fiducial point on the reference catheter.

If needed, image integration functionalities (like CARTO) allow images from a preacquired CT/MRI scan on the real-time electroanatomic image of the cardiac chamber to facilitate anatomical accuracy, which may be particularly helpful for complex ablation of atrial fibrillation, adult congenital heart disease, etc. See Table 8.1.

Table 8.1 Comparison between CARTO and EnSite systems.

	CARTO	EnSite
External magnet reference	Essential	Optional in newer systems
Catheter visualization	Any catheter (max. 3)	Any catheter (no limit)
Geometry creation	Only magnetic tip proprietary catheter	Any catheter
Arrhythmia mapping	Only magnetic tip proprietary catheter	Any catheter
Disposable patches	Less expensive	More expensive
Visualization of catheters	Only limited to thorax	Pelvis to thorax
Intracardiac reference for geometry creation	Not required	Required (if not using system reference)
Pacing from ablation catheter during RF	Not possible	Possible
Noncontact mapping	Not possible	Possible with ESI array
Image integration with CT and MRI	Possible	Possible
Image integration with ICE	Possible	Not possible
Catheter localization in sheath	Possible	Not possible

CT, computed tomography; ESI, Endocardial Solutions, Inc.; ICE, intracardiac echocardiography; MRI, magnetic resonance imaging; RF, radiofrequency.

Complications of ablation

RF ablation carries the same risks as a standard electrophysiology study (discussed in Chapter 4), plus the added risks related to performing the RF ablation itself.

The two most common of these are the risk of creating inadvertent, complete heart block (usually when ablating in proximity to the normal conducting system) and the risk of causing cardiac perforation and tamponade (usually when ablating from the atria, the right ventricle, or within the coronary sinus or other cardiac veins). These complications each occur in less than 2% of patients treated with RF ablation.

Even rarer complications include the creation of arrhythmogenic foci (uncommon, since RF energy tends to create homogeneous lesions); production of mitral or tricuspid regurgitation (when ablating at or near the valvular apparatus); systemic embolization (when mapping and ablating in the left heart); and the creation of fixed lesions within the coronary arteries. In addition, in complicated or difficult cases, the patient's exposure to radiation may be substantial.

AF ablation has specific complications related to left atrial ablation: first, the transseptal procedure can lead to perforation or inadvertent aortic puncture; thrombus in the left atrium (LA) may lead to stroke, and one of the more feared complications is esophageal fistula formation from ablation on the LA posterior wall. Cryoballoon pulmonary vein (PV) isolation has all of these potential complications plus phrenic nerve injury during freezes of the right pulmonary veins.

Overall, the risk associated with RF ablation is low. For arrhythmias that are life-threatening or significantly symptomatic, and that have a high probability of being successfully treated with RF ablation, this is an extremely attractive option. In addition, if a patient has an arrhythmia that is readily amenable to RF ablation, then ablation should be strongly considered whenever daily antiarrhythmic drug therapy would otherwise be required.

Acknowledgment

The authors thank Dr Shanta Chakrabarti for his kind assistance with this section.

9

Ablation of Supraventricular Tachycardias

This chapter discusses the general approach to ablating supraventricular tachycardias, except for atrial fibrillation (AF) and atrial flutter. Those two arrhythmias present special challenges and will be discussed in separate chapters.

Ablation of the AV junction

While not strictly an ablation procedure for supraventricular tachycardia, ablation of the atrioventricular (AV) junction is performed almost exclusively in patients with persistent supraventricular tachycardias – almost always AF or atrial flutter. In fact, the original indication for transcatheter ablation was to produce complete heart block in patients with chronic atrial fibrillation and persistently rapid ventricular rates. Ablation of the AV junction is aimed at producing complete heart block at the level of the AV node. While insertion of a permanent pacemaker is always required after this procedure, in some cases the patient is left with a relatively stable escape rhythm after AV nodal ablation.

To perform ablation of the AV junction, a temporary pacemaker is first placed into the right ventricle. In some cases, a permanent pacer has already been placed. The ablation catheter is then used to map the His bundle. Once the largest His deflection is carefully localized, the catheter is gradually withdrawn, while recording from the distal (ablating) electrode, until the His and ventricular deflections become relatively small and the atrial deflection becomes relatively large. This position indicates that the catheter tip is in the region of the compact AV node. Excellent contact of the catheter tip with the

Fogoros' Electrophysiologic Testing, Seventh Edition. Richard N. Fogoros and John M. Mandrola.
© 2023 John Wiley & Sons Ltd. Published 2023 by John Wiley & Sons Ltd.

cardiac tissue must be maintained, and the catheter position must be entirely stable. When optimal positioning has been confirmed, radiofrequency (RF) energy is applied to the tip electrode (usually 20–35 W for 30–60 seconds). Successful AV nodal ablation is often heralded by the development of an accelerated junctional tachycardia during application of the RF energy (hence, junctional tachycardia during RF application is a "good sign"). If the attempt is unsuccessful, the catheter is repositioned and RF ablation is repeated. In the hands of an experienced operator, successful RF ablation of the AV junction is possible in over 98% of cases, although in 5–10% of cases a second procedure is required to assure permanent block.

Occasionally, ablations of the AV junction using this technique will be unsuccessful, and in these cases ablation from the left ventricle may be required. Ablating the AV junction from the left ventricle is accomplished by positioning the ablation catheter just inferior to the aortic valve along the septal wall of the left ventricle. The intracardiac electrogram during left-sided ablation should show a His bundle deflection at least 35–50 ms earlier than the ventricular deflection (a closer spacing between the His deflection and the ventricular deflection means that the catheter is not actually recording the His bundle, but instead is recording the left bundle branch).

A few cases of sudden death have been reported within several days of ablation of the AV junction. It is thought that these deaths are likely due to torsades de pointes, most probably provoked in susceptible patients by a sudden, relative bradycardia. The risk for this event appears to be transient, and can be avoided by pacing patients relatively rapidly (i.e., 80–100 beats/min) for a few days to a few weeks after AV junction ablation.

Though it is permanent and results in pacer dependence, ablation of the AV node has become a more prevalent procedure in recent years. One reason is that modern medical care has led to increasing numbers of older people who present with comorbid conditions that preclude drug or ablation therapy for AF. Another reason is that this procedure can be combined with cardiac resynchronization devices that not only pace but also resynchronize left and right ventricle contraction.

Ablation of AV nodal reentrant tachycardia

RF ablation is now the treatment of choice for AV nodal reentrant tachycardia (AVNRT).

Successfully ablating AV nodal reentrant tachycardia has required a change in the way electrophysiologists visualize the AV node. In the past, most electrophysiologists thought of the AV node simply as a compact, button-like structure, as depicted in Figure 9.1a. It has now become apparent that the AV node behaves more as depicted in Figure 9.1b. The AV node does indeed appear to have a compact distal component (i.e., the part of the node that gives rise to the His bundle), but the more proximal portion of the AV node appears to be "diffuse."

To visualize what this means, it is helpful to imagine the course of the electrical impulse as it approaches the AV node from the atria. We have seen that the electrical impulse arises in the sinus node and then travels across the atria in a radial fashion. Recent findings suggest that as this electrical impulse approaches the AV node, it is gathered into bands of conducting fibers, which coalesce into "tracts," which in turn coalesce to form the compact AV node. At some point, the cellular electrophysiology of these coalescing tracts changes (in what is referred to as a "transition zone") from behaving like typical atrial tissue to behaving like typical AV nodal tissue. Thus, the point at which the AV node "begins" is inherently indistinct and diffuse, and probably varies from patient to patient.

The tracts of atrial fibers that coalesce to form the AV node are ill defined, and until recently were completely theoretical. It now appears, however, that (at least in patients with AV nodal reentrant tachycardia, and probably in all individuals) two distinct tracts can be localized anatomically – the anterior tract (which corresponds to the fast AV nodal pathway) and the posterior tract (which corresponds to the slow AV nodal pathway).

The "classic" way of visualizing the two pathways involved in AV nodal reentrant tachycardia is shown in Figure 6.11, in which the two tracts are seen as a functional division within the button-like AV node. To visualize the dual AV nodal pathways as currently conceptualized, one must be familiar with the anatomy of Koch's triangle (Figure 9.2).

The three sides of Koch's triangle are defined by the tricuspid annulus (the portion of the annulus adjacent to the septal leaflet of the tricuspid valve), the tendon of Todaro, and the os of the coronary sinus. The His bundle is located at the apex of Koch's triangle. Therefore, the major landmarks that define Koch's triangle (the tricuspid valve, the os of the coronary sinus, and the His bundle) are readily identifiable during electrophysiologic testing.

(a)

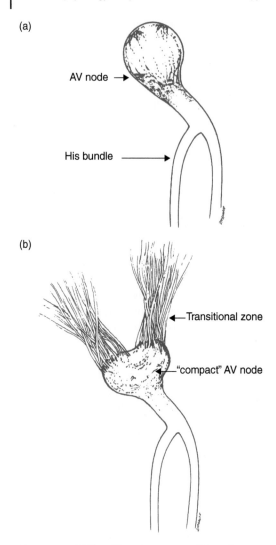

(b)

Figure 9.1 "Old" and "new" concepts of AV node anatomy and physiology. (a) The AV node as it commonly used to be conceived, namely as a compact "button" of specialized tissue. (b) The AV node as it is currently conceptualized by electrophysiologists. In this "new" model, tracts of conducting fibers coalesce to form the compact AV node. The transition from atrial electrophysiology to AV nodal electrophysiology probably occurs proximal to the compact node. Anatomists have been describing this for years but until ablationists arrived on the scene, there seemed to be no good reason to believe them.

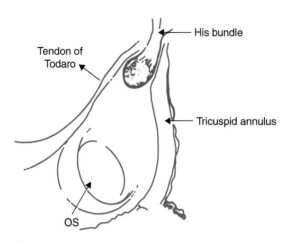

Figure 9.2 The triangle of Koch. Long described by anatomists and long ignored by electrophysiologists, Koch's triangle has become vitally important in performing transcatheter ablations. Koch's triangle is defined posteriorly by the os of the coronary sinus. The apex of the triangle is defined anteriorly by the His bundle. The tendon of Todaro and the tricuspid valve annulus compose the other two sides of the triangle. In the electrophysiology laboratory, the landmarks of Koch's triangle are identified by one catheter recording the His deflection and another placed in the os of the coronary sinus. Koch's triangle lies between these two catheters.

It is important to recognize that the apex of Koch's triangle (i.e., the angle where the AV node and His bundle reside) is an *anterior* structure – in fact, the apex of Koch's triangle defines the anterior aspect of the atrial septum. In contrast, the os of the coronary sinus is a *posterior* structure and defines the posterior portion of the atrial septum.

In patients with AV nodal reentrant tachycardia, the fast and slow pathways can be visualized as two tracts of atrial fibers that coalesce to form the compact AV node (Figure 9.3). The fast pathway is an *anterior* and *superior* tract of fibers, located along the tendon of Todaro. The slow pathway is a *posterior* and *inferior* tract of fibers, located along the tricuspid annulus near the os of the coronary sinus. Thus, the anatomic correlates of the "functional" dual AV nodal pathways have now been identified. Because the two pathways can be discretely localized, they can be discretely ablated.

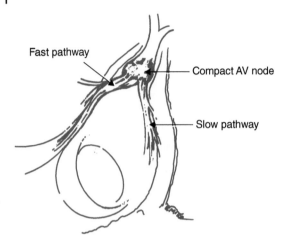

Figure 9.3 The fast and slow pathways in patients with AV nodal reentrant tachycardia, relating to Koch's triangle. The dual AV nodal pathways seen in patients with AV nodal reentrant tachycardia have classically been considered to lie within a button-like AV node. Electrophysiologists performing RF transcatheter ablation, however, have now clearly shown that the fast and slow pathways are readily discernible and can be distinctly localized within Koch's triangle. Both pathways appear to be located proximally to the compact AV node. The fast pathway is an anterior and superior structure and lies near the compact AV node along the tendon of Todaro. The slow pathway is a posterior and inferior structure and can usually be identified along the tricuspid annulus near the os of the coronary sinus. Because the slow pathway is farther away from the AV node than the fast pathway, the slow pathway can usually be selectively ablated without causing complete heart block.

When the anatomy of dual AV nodal pathways was first recognized, most attempts at curing AV nodal reentry focused on ablating the fast pathway. These attempts were generally successful, but unfortunately they yielded a relatively high incidence of complete heart block (up to 20%). The heart block most likely resulted from the fact that the fast pathway and the compact AV node are in close proximity (i.e., both structures are anterior).

The ablation of AV nodal reentry in recent years has been generally accomplished by ablating the slow pathway. Since the slow pathway is posterior, it is relatively distant from the AV node, and thus ablation of this structure yields a low incidence of complete heart block (generally less than 1%).

In general, two approaches are commonly used for ablation of the slow AV nodal pathway – the "mapping" approach and the anatomic approach. Both approaches begin by first identifying the anatomic limits of Koch's triangle, by placing one catheter in the His position and another in the os of the coronary sinus. The ablation catheter is then advanced from the femoral vein to the tricuspid annulus, near the os of the coronary sinus. Although 3-D mapping is not necessary for slow pathway ablation, it does help sort out the important structures, including the location of the His spike, coronary sinus ostium, and tricuspid valve annulus.

With the "mapping" approach, the ablation catheter is carefully manipulated along the tricuspid annulus, searching for discrete "slow potentials" that presumably represent depolarization of the slow pathway itself (Figure 9.4). These slow potentials are located between

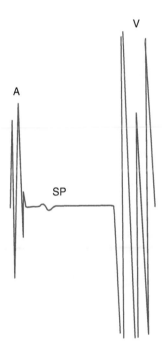

Figure 9.4 Slow AV nodal pathway potential. Mapping of the slow pathway in patients with AV nodal reentrant tachycardia is accomplished by seeking the slow potential (SP) along the tricuspid annulus within Koch's triangle. See text for details. A, atrial deflection; V, ventricular deflection.

the atrial and ventricular deflections in the intracardiac electrogram. Mapping of AV nodal reentrant tachycardia is thus best accomplished during sinus rhythm and not during tachycardia, so that the atrial and ventricular deflections during mapping remain separate and distinct. When the slow potentials are identified, an RF lesion applied at their location almost always ablates the slow pathway.

With the anatomic approach to slow pathway ablation, no attempt is made to map the slow potentials. Instead, ablation sites are identified by fluoroscopic and 3-D electroanatomic means. Generally, the length of the tricuspid annulus between the os of the coronary sinus and the His bundle is visually divided into three equal sections – posterior (closest to the os of the coronary sinus), middle, and anterior (closest to the His bundle). The ablation catheter is positioned across the tricuspid valve in the posterior section and gradually withdrawn until both atrial and ventricular deflections are recorded, with the ventricular deflection being larger than the atrial deflection. An RF lesion is made, and if the slow pathway has not been successfully ablated, the catheter is moved further anteriorly and the procedure is repeated. Lesions are placed in each of the three sections serially, from posterior to anterior, until the slow pathway has been ablated.

Many electrophysiologists have evolved an integrated approach which begins with ablations posteriorly and moving anteriorly (as with the anatomic approach), but which adds at least a brief search for slow pathway potentials within that anatomic zone prior to applying RF energy.

Accelerated junctional tachycardia occurs during RF application in virtually 100% of successful slow pathway ablations. Therefore, if no tachycardia occurs after 10–15 seconds of RF application, the RF should be terminated and the catheter repositioned. If tachycardia does occur, 30–60 seconds of RF energy should be applied – with the caveat described in the next paragraph. Successful ablation is documented by confirming that the physiology of dual AV nodal pathways is either no longer present or significantly modified so as not to maintain AVNRT (see Chapter 6).

The accelerated junctional tachycardia that occurs with this ablation must be intensely monitored for signs of ventricle to atrium (VA) or AV block. In particular, all junctional beats should be associated with an atrial and ventricular signal. If VA Wenckebach or VA block is noted, it means that permanent AV block is being created and the operator must terminate ablation immediately – as in, less than 1 second.

One clue to impending VA or AV block of the junctional tachycardia is rapid acceleration of the rate. This often heralds block and it is wise to terminate ablation if the junctional beats accelerate. Successful ablation of the slow pathway often requires numerous short applications of energy.

AV block as a result of inadvertent injury to the compact AV node can be avoided with carefully monitored ablation. One trick for operators is to use a foot pedal to deliver RF. This technique allows RF to be terminated without telling another person to terminate RF. One rule of thumb of ablation reigns supreme in ablating AVNRT: *you can always burn more, but you cannot take away a burn.*

When one or both of these techniques for slow pathway ablation is used, successful treatment of AV nodal reentrant tachycardia can be achieved in over 98% of patients, with a very low risk of producing complete heart block.

Ablation of bypass tracts

In the late 1980s, RF ablation of bypass tracts was considered a difficult and somewhat mystical technique performed by only a few adventurous shamans. During the 1990s, however, it evolved into a widely available and highly effective procedure. For most patients with significantly symptomatic or life-threatening bypass tracts, RF ablation is now the therapy of choice.

Characteristics of bypass tracts

As noted in Chapter 6, bypass tracts are tiny bands of myocardial tissue that form a bridge across the AV junction, connecting atrial tissue to ventricular tissue. They can occur anywhere along the AV groove, except along the portion directly between the mitral and aortic valves. Because they are composed of bands of myocardial tissue, bypass tracts tend to exhibit the electrophysiologic features of myocardial tissue instead of AV nodal tissue; that is, their refractory periods tend to shorten instead of lengthen with decreases in cycle length, and they tend to develop second-degree block in a Mobitz II pattern instead of a Mobitz I pattern.

Localization of bypass tracts begins by studying the surface electrocardiogram (ECG) and continues with intracardiac mapping.

ECG localization of bypass tracts

Bypass tracts are divided into five general categories according to their location (Figure 9.5). These categories are left free wall, right free wall, posterior septal, anterior septal, and mid-septal. The general approach to mapping in the EP laboratory is different for each of these categories, so it is important to have some idea as to the location of a bypass tract before the ablation procedure begins. In most cases, the surface ECG fortunately gives a very good indication of where the bypass tract is located.

Table 9.1 lists the ECG criteria for grossly localizing bypass tracts. The "key" is to look for the leads with the negative delta wave, because the negative delta wave "points" to the bypass tract (Figure 9.6).

Consider the delta waves in ECG lead I, which is a "left-sided" lead. Delta waves in lead I are negative for left free-wall tracts, are biphasic (or isoelectric) for left posterior to right posterior tracts, and are positive for right free-wall tracts.

The delta waves in lead V_1 (a right-sided lead) are positive for left free-wall and posterior septal tracts and negative for right free-wall tracts. They are biphasic (or isoelectric) for anteroseptal tracts.

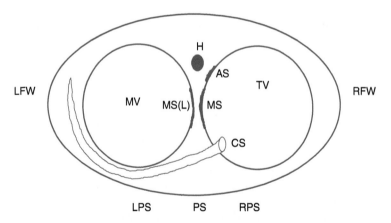

Figure 9.5 Location of bypass tracts. The anatomic structures shown in this figure are the mitral valve (MV), the tricuspid valve (TV), the coronary sinus (CS), and the His bundle (H). AS, anteroseptal tracts; LFW, left free-wall tracts; LPS, left paraseptal tracts; MS, midseptal tracts; MS(L), left-sided midseptal tracts; PS, posteroseptal tracts; RPS, right paraseptal tracts; RFW, right free-wall tracts. See text for details.

Table 9.1 Electrocardiographic localization of bypass tracts.

Location of tract	Characteristics of preexcited QRS
Left free wall	Negative delta wave in AVL and often in lead I. Positive delta wave in inferior and precordial leads. Normal QRS axis
Right free wall	Negative delta wave in leads III and AVF. Positive delta waves in leads I and II. Normal QRS axis
Posteroseptal	Negative delta waves in inferior leads. Positive delta waves in leads I and AVL. R/S ratio in V_1 <1; left superior axis
Anteroseptal	Negative delta wave in leads V_1 and V_2. Positive delta wave in leads I and II. Normal QRS axis
Midseptal	ECG similar to anteroseptal, except that in inferior leads, delta waves are not positive

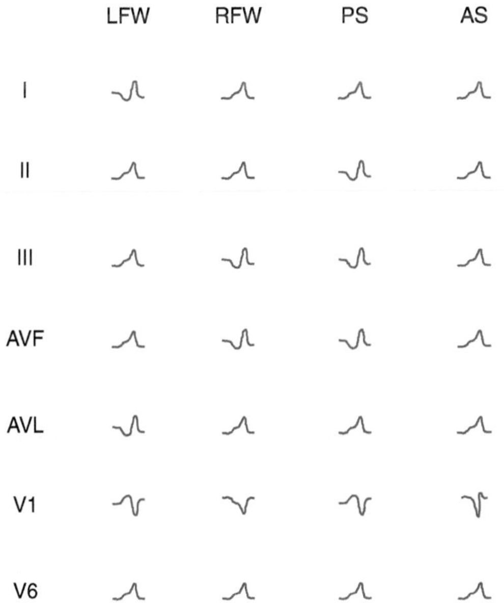

Figure 9.6 Electrocardiographic manifestations of the major categories of bypass tract. Typical electrocardiographic patterns are shown for left free-wall tracts (LFW), right free-wall tracts (RFW), posteroseptal tracts (PS), and anteroseptal tracts (AS). See text and Table 9.1 for details.

The delta waves in leads II, III, and AVF (inferior leads) are negative for posterior septal tracts and become positive as the tracts move anteriorly toward the anteroseptal regions.

Based on this general concept, and on the more specific criteria listed in Table 9.1, a very good idea of the location of a bypass tract can be ascertained before the electrophysiologic procedure is begun, allowing an accurate preliminary action plan.

Considerations for successfully mapping and ablating bypass tracts

Before outlining specific approaches to various types of bypass tract, let us review some general considerations for successfully mapping and ablating these tracts.

1. Mapping can be conducted on either the atrial or ventricular aspect of the AV groove. In general, when mapping on the ventricular aspect, antegrade conduction over the bypass tract (i.e., the delta wave) is mapped. Maximal preexcitation is helpful in mapping the delta wave. This can be accomplished by pacing the atrium at a rate that maximizes preexcitation, or by administering drugs (such as verapamil) that increase refractory periods in the normal conducting system. When mapping on the atrial aspect of the AV groove, or when mapping concealed bypass tracts, retrograde conduction over the bypass tract is studied. This is best accomplished during orthodromic macroreentrant tachycardia (i.e., tachycardia that uses the bypass tract for retrograde conduction and the normal conducting system for antegrade conduction) or with ventricular pacing at a rate that optimizes retrograde conduction via the bypass tract.

2. When the mapping catheter is located near the bypass tract (whether on the atrial or ventricular aspect of the AV groove), the interval between the atrial and ventricular depolarizations (assuming that either antegrade or retrograde conduction of impulses is occurring across the bypass tract) will be short. Generally, the localized AV interval is no more than 60 ms, and sometimes the atrial and ventricular depolarizations are virtually continuous (Figure 9.7).

3. When the mapping catheter is near the bypass tract and preexcitation is occurring, the local ventricular depolarization should be earlier than the earliest ventricular depolarization seen on any surface ECG lead.

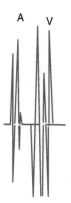

Figure 9.7 Depiction of the narrow AV interval seen when the mapping catheter is in proximity to the bypass tract. Compare this to the more "usual" AV interval shown in Figure 9.4. When mapping bypass tracts, the optimal localized AV interval is generally less than 60 ms.

4. Loss of preexcitation (i.e., disappearance of the delta wave) when pressure is applied with the tip of the mapping catheter is an excellent indication that the site of the bypass tract has been localized. 3-D mapping systems can help mark these "bump" locations.
5. In many patients, a localized potential from the bypass tract itself can be recorded (Figure 9.8). These bypass tract potentials tend to be relatively low in amplitude, but have discrete, sharp onsets. They generally resemble His bundle electrograms more than they do the

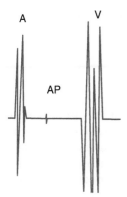

Figure 9.8 Recording of a bypass tract potential. Often, a localized potential from the bypass tract itself (AP, "accessory pathway" potential) can be recorded from a well-positioned mapping catheter.

slow pathway potentials seen when mapping the slow AV nodal pathways. Sometimes it can be difficult to differentiate between a bypass tract potential and a part of the atrial or ventricular depolarizations. Pacing techniques can often be used to demonstrate that the bypass tract potentials are distinct from either the atrial or the ventricular potentials. A clear-cut bypass tract potential is an excellent indication that RF ablation at that site will be successful.

6. Unipolar recordings from the tip of the mapping catheter can be extremely helpful in localizing the bypass tract, as these recordings give information about the direction of the cardiac impulse being recorded (a positive deflection means the impulse is moving toward the unipolar electrode, while a negative deflection means it is moving away). When the QRS complex is preexcited, the unipolar ventricular electrogram should be predominantly negative (i.e., a QS complex should be recorded). A negative unipolar ventricular electrogram indicates that the electrical impulse during ventricular depolarization is always moving away from the catheter tip – which is possible only if the catheter tip is located at the site of earliest ventricular activation. A negative ventricular deflection on the unipolar electrogram is entirely analogous to a negative delta wave seen on the corresponding surface ECG leads.

7. Finally, once the bypass tract has been carefully mapped and it is time to perform the ablation, catheter stability is critical since RF energy must be continuously applied to the target tissue for a sustained period of time (often 60 seconds or longer). The catheter is considered to be sufficiently stable when the ratio of the amplitudes of atrial to ventricular deflections on the local intracardiac electrogram varies by less than 10%.

The approach to bypass tracts according to location

Left free-wall bypass tracts

More than 50% of bypass tracts referred for RF ablation are located in the left free wall. These tracts cross the AV groove along the anterolateral, lateral, posterolateral, or posterior aspects of the mitral valve annulus. The coronary sinus also courses along the same portion of the mitral annulus, and thus provides a convenient means of mapping the annulus in patients with left free-wall pathways.

Standard electrode catheters are placed in the high right atrium, His position, and right ventricular apex. A multipolar electrode catheter is placed into the coronary sinus (often a 10-lead catheter is used) and multiple bipolar recordings are established along its length.

After the earliest sites of antegrade and retrograde preexcitation are approximated using the electrodes within the coronary sinus, the mapping and ablation catheter is inserted.

There are two general approaches for ablating left free-wall pathways: the retrograde approach and the transseptal approach.

In the past, the retrograde approach was the most commonly used technique, but in the era of AF ablation, many more electrophysiologists are comfortable with transseptal puncture. With the retrograde approach, the mapping catheter is inserted through a femoral artery and advanced across the aortic valve into the left ventricle. The catheter tip is then maneuvered into the AV groove beneath the mitral valve leaflets and the bypass tract is localized. One advantage of the retrograde approach is good tissue–catheter contact, usually on the ventricular side of the mitral annulus.

With the transseptal approach, the mapping catheter is inserted through a femoral vein and advanced across the intraatrial septum into the left atrium. In most cases, crossing the intraatrial septum requires that a puncture be made through the septal wall, using a catheter-based tool designed specifically for that purpose. When the transseptal approach is used, the atrial aspect of the mitral annulus is mapped. An advantage of this approach is that it allows the catheter to be moved along the annulus with relative ease. But this is also its disadvantage, since catheter stability can become a problem. Deflectable sheaths are often used to stabilize the ablation catheter on the annulus.

With either approach, the multipolar coronary sinus catheter is used as a stable reference for guiding mapping maneuvers. Also with either approach, successful ablation of left free-wall bypass tracts can be achieved in more than 95% of cases.

Right free-wall bypass tracts

Right free-wall tracts are seen in approximately 10% of patients with bypass tracts referred for ablation. These tracts are more difficult to map and ablate than left free-wall tracts, because a stable catheter position is more difficult to attain and there is no anatomic structure analogous to the coronary sinus to aid in mapping.

Standard electrode catheters are placed in the high right atrium, His position, right ventricular apex, and coronary sinus. The mapping

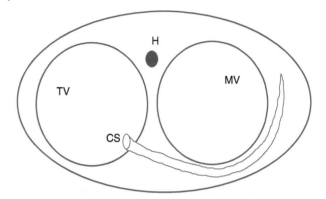

Figure 9.9 Orientation of the tricuspid annulus (TV) in the left anterior oblique (LAO) projection. In the LAO projection, the tricuspid annulus can be visualized as the face of a clock, with the His bundle (H) in the 1 o'clock position and the os of the coronary sinus (CS) in the 5 o'clock position. MV, mitral valve annulus.

and ablation catheter is usually inserted via a femoral vein, advanced across the tricuspid valve, and then withdrawn so that the mapping electrodes are positioned along the tricuspid annulus in such a way that both atrial and ventricular deflections are recorded. Mapping is often conducted using the left anterior oblique (LAO) projection, which allows the tricuspid annulus to be visualized as the face of a clock (Figure 9.9). In this projection, the His bundle is located at approximately 1 o'clock, and the os of the coronary sinus at approximately 5 o'clock. If the bypass tract proves to be difficult to map or if catheter stability is a problem, alternative approaches can be tried. Introducing the mapping catheter via the superior instead of the inferior vena cava is sometimes helpful. Long intravascular sheaths with preformed geometry are extremely helpful in lending stability to the mapping catheter. Catheter stability and gaining adequate contact are the chief barriers to right-sided accessory pathway ablations.

In experienced hands, right free-wall pathways can be successfully ablated in over 90% of cases.

Mahaim bypass tracts

Mahaim bypass tracts, as originally described, supposedly connect the AV node to either the right bundle branch (nodofascicular fibers) or ventricular muscle (nodoventricular fibers). Recently, it has been determined with careful mapping that Mahaim tracts actually do not arise within the AV node itself but rather within atrial muscle. Thus, these bypass tracts actually form connections between atrial muscle and the right bundle branch (atriofascicular fibers) or ventricular muscle (AV fibers).

The original confusion as to their site of atrial insertion arose from the fact that atriofascicular and AV tracts display the same sort of decremental conduction usually associated with AV nodal tissue; that is, with atrial pacing, faster pacing rates *increase* the stimulus–delta wave interval, unlike in a more typical bypass tract, where faster pacing rates *decrease* the stimulus–delta wave interval. Further, Mahaim bypass tracts tend to respond to adenosine similarly to AV nodal tissue. For practical purposes, therefore, while Mahaim fibers turn out to be anatomically distinct from the AV node, they are electrophysiologically similar to it. Conceptually, Mahaim fibers can be visualized as strands of slow AV nodal fibers (i.e., the fibers that course along the tricuspid annulus within Koch's triangle) that abnormally veer off, bypassing the AV node and connecting directly to the right bundle branch or right ventricular myocardium.

The electrophysiologic characteristics of atriofascicular tracts are as follows. These tracts tend to display relatively little preexcitation during sinus rhythm but yield left bundle branch block (LBBB) (since they connect to the right bundle branch) with atrial pacing or during tachycardia. As noted, these tracts display decremental conduction and responsiveness to adenosine. Retrograde conduction is absent in atriofascicular fibers. The tachycardias mediated by these tracts, therefore, always use the bypass tract in the antegrade direction (and are thus manifested by an LBBB configuration) and the AV node (or a second bypass tract) in the retrograde direction. During preexcitation, the earliest ventricular activation is seen in the apex of the right ventricle, since it is the right bundle branch that is being preexcited.

AV Mahaim fibers display the same electrophysiologic characteristics, except that the right ventricular apex is *not* the site of earliest ventricular activation during preexcitation, since it is the ventricular muscle adjacent to the tricuspid valve that is being preexcited and not the right bundle branch.

Mapping and ablation of atriofascicular and AV fibers is performed in a manner similar to that described for other right-sided bypass tracts, except that antegrade mapping must always be performed, since these tracts do not display retrograde conduction. This generally requires mapping either during tachycardia or at an atrial pacing rate that maximizes preexcitation. Mapping is conducted along the tricuspid annulus between the His bundle and the os of the coronary sinus. 3-D mapping has made this easier because it reduces the need for fluoroscopy and allows for anatomic marking of the Mahaim potential.

Posterior septal (and paraseptal) bypass tracts

Posterior septal and paraseptal bypass tracts account for over 20% of bypass tracts referred for ablation (Figure 9.10).

Posterior septal tracts cross the AV groove near the os of the coronary sinus, where the right atrium and left ventricle are in proximity. Thus, the atrial insertion of a posterior septal tract is in the *right atrium,* while the ventricular insertion is in the *left ventricle.* In contrast, right paraseptal bypass tracts cross the AV groove just to the right of this region and connect the right atrium with the right ventricle. Left paraseptal bypass tracts cross the AV groove just to the left of this region and connect the left atrium with the left ventricle.

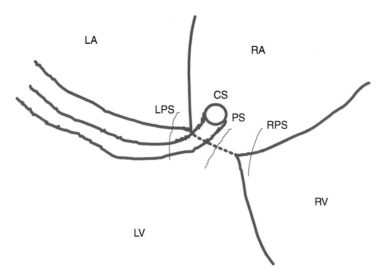

Figure 9.10 Insertions for bypass tracts located in the posterior septal region. The anatomic structures shown are the left atrium (LA), right atrium (RA), left ventricle (LV), right ventricle (RV), and coronary sinus (CS). Posterior septal tracts (PS) connect the right atrium with the left ventricle. Right paraseptal tracts (RPS) connect the right atrium with the right ventricle. Left paraseptal tracts (LPS) connect the left atrium with the left ventricle. See text for details.

Because the connections of posterior septal, left paraseptal, and right paraseptal tracts are all different from one another, the response to bundle branch block that occurs during macroreentrant tachycardia can be useful in differentiating among these three types of posterior bypass tract. Recall that when bundle branch block occurs during macroreentrant tachycardia and the block is on the same side as a bypass tract, the cycle length of tachycardia increases (see Figure 6.10). Accordingly, with left paraseptal bypass tracts, the onset of LBBB will increase the cycle length of the tachycardia whereas for right paraseptal tracts, only right bundle branch block (RBBB) will increase the cycle length. Finally, with posterior septal tracts (which connect the left ventricle with the right atrium), LBBB will prolong the cycle length but RBBB will not.

When ablating posterior septal or paraseptal tracts, the mapping catheter is inserted first into the right atrium. Mapping is begun anteriorly in Koch's triangle, along the tricuspid annulus near the bundle of His. Gradually, the mapping progresses posteriorly to the os of the coronary sinus. Then the right posterior paraseptal region is explored (posterior to the os of the coronary sinus along the tricuspid annulus), and finally mapping is performed within the os of the coronary sinus.

Posterior septal tracts are associated with anomalies of the coronary sinus in more than 15% of cases; often, a coronary sinus diverticulum is present and, if so, the bypass tract is almost invariably located in the neck of the diverticulum. An injection of dye into the coronary sinus may be necessary to visualize the anatomy. Ablating within the coronary sinus or other cardiac veins is feasible in these cases, and is usually successful. This procedure does carry the risk of perforation, which can lead to cardiac tamponade. In addition, it has been recognized that when ablating within the coronary sinus (especially if a diverticulum exists or if ablation is necessary in the middle cardiac vein), significant chronic lesions can be produced in the posterior descending coronary artery. Saline-irrigated catheters have improved the safety of ablation within the coronary sinus.

If the bypass tract cannot be localized using these maneuvers, mapping of the left posterior paraseptal region may be necessary; this requires insertion of a mapping catheter retrogradely across the aortic valve. Generally, at least one attempt at ablating the "earliest" site on the right side is made before moving to the left side.

Successful ablation of posterior septal and paraseptal tracts can be achieved in 85–90% of patients.

Anteroseptal and midseptal bypass tracts

In the preablation era, anteroseptal and midseptal pathways were lumped together as "anteroseptal bypass tracts" owing to their similar electrocardiographic manifestations. These tracts are now known to be quite distinct. They require different approaches during ablation procedures, so their differentiation is important. Bypass tracts arising in the region anterior and superior to the His bundle are termed *anteroseptal tracts*. Bypass tracts arising in the area between the His bundle and the os of the coronary sinus (i.e., in the triangle of Koch) are termed *midseptal pathways* (see Figure 9.5).

On the surface ECG, anteroseptal pathways display positive delta waves in leads I, II, III, and AVF; normal QRS axis; biphasic or positive delta waves in lead V_1; and positive delta waves in V_2–V_6 (see Figure 9.6).

The electrocardiographic manifestations of midseptal pathways are similar to those of anteroseptal pathways, with the following exceptions: for midseptal tracts close to the AV node, the delta wave is isoelectric (instead of positive) in leads III and AVF; for midseptal tracts closer to the coronary sinus, the delta wave is predominantly negative in leads III and AVF, and isoelectric in lead V_1 (Figure 9.11).

The techniques used in ablating anteroseptal and midseptal tracts are similar to those used for any other bypass tract. In either case, reference electrodes are placed in the right atrium, His position, coronary sinus, and right ventricular apex. The mapping and ablation catheter is inserted from the jugular or subclavian vein (for anteroseptal tracts) or from the femoral vein (for either anteroseptal or midseptal tracts).

For anteroseptal bypass tracts, mapping can be accomplished from either the atrial or ventricular aspect of the tricuspid valve. In general, a careful attempt should be made to record the anteroseptal bypass tract potential itself, and to carefully differentiate it from the His potential (since anteroseptal tracts are often in close proximity to the His bundle). To differentiate the bypass tract from the His bundle, mapping during macroreentrant tachycardia is often very helpful since during tachycardia, the bypass tract is depolarized retrogradely and the His bundle antegradely. Administering adenosine to selectively block AV conduction via the normal conducting system is also helpful in differentiating between the two.

Ablating anteroseptal pathways can be tricky due to the proximity to the compact AV node and His bundle. During sinus rhythm

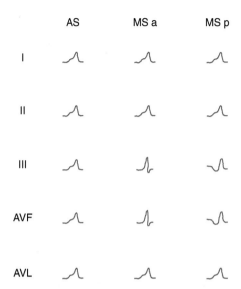

Figure 9.11 Electrocardiographic differentiation between anteroseptal and midseptal bypass tracts. Midseptal tracts are more posterior than anteroseptal tracts, and thus tend to have some of the electrocardiographic manifestations of posterior septal tracts. The more posterior the midseptal tracts, the more negative the delta waves in the inferior ECG leads (i.e., leads II, III, and AVF) (see text). AS, anteroseptal; MS a, midseptal tracts located relatively anteriorly; MS p, midseptal tracts located relatively posteriorly.

and manifest preexcitation, the preexcitation may obscure the His deflection. One trick is to ablate during orthodromic tachycardia. This ensures that the ablation catheter does not have a His deflection on it. For concealed anteroseptal pathways, the earliest site of retrograde conduction can be mapped during ventricular pacing (or tachycardia) but ablation should not be performed during ventricular pacing as it would be impossible to assess for AV block. Ablation can be performed during tachycardia or empirically during sinus rhythm. Some authors have reported successful ablation of anteroseptal pathways from the noncoronary cusp of the aortic valve, as this sits in close proximity to the region.

The procedure for ablating midseptal pathways is similar to that for performing slow pathway ablation in AV nodal reentrant tachycardia. Mapping is performed on the tricuspid annulus, between the His bundle and the os of the coronary sinus. If ablation cannot be accomplished from the right side, left-sided mapping (along the mitral annulus between the His bundle and the os of the coronary sinus) may be required.

In general, successful ablation of these bypass tracts can be accomplished in more than 90% of patients. The incidence of inadvertent, complete heart block is generally reported as being less than 5%, but RBBB has occurred in up to 40% of patients who have ablation of anteroseptal tracts.

Ablation of focal atrial tachycardias

Focal atrial tachycardias can be paroxysmal or incessant and, depending on their frequency, duration, and rate, can produce symptoms that are anywhere from mild to severe. These arrhythmias can be caused by automatic foci, foci of triggered activity, or microreentrant circuits.

Because they are focal, atrial tachycardias can often be mapped and are thus amenable to RF ablation. The site of atrial tachycardia is often associated with particular anatomic structures, most commonly the crista terminalis in the right atrium (see Chapter 12), the ostia of the pulmonary veins in the left atrium, the os of the coronary sinus, and the tricuspid annulus.

Ablating atrial tachycardia is usually performed with activation mapping – the earliest atrial deflection is sought that precedes the P wave on the surface electrogram. Electroanatomic mapping can also be helpful. Activation mapping depends on the ability to induce atrial tachycardia during the ablation procedure, or in the presence of incessant or very frequent tachycardia. Application of RF energy should also be performed during the tachycardia.

10

Ablation of PVCs and Ventricular Tachycardia

Modern treatment of PVCs

One of the newest targets for the modern electrophysiologist is the premature ventricular complex or PVC. Although PVCs can occur in up to 75% of the general population, these are usually infrequent and only minimally symptomatic. Most often, patients with PVCs who have no structural heart disease can be reassured, given time and the problem will resolve itself.

The four most common situations when treatment, including ablation, of PVCs could be considered are:

- frequent PVCs (usually greater than 20 k per day) believed to be causing or worsening left ventricle (LV) dysfunction
- frequent PVCs that cause life-altering symptoms
- PVCs that initiate ventricular tachycardia (VT) or ventricular fibrillation (VF)
- PVCs frequent enough to reduce pacing from cardiac resynchronization therapy (CRT).

Drug therapy of PVCs is often ineffective or associated with side-effects. What is more, previous data from the Cardiac Arrhythmia Suppression Trial (CAST) has shown that type IC drugs used to treat PVCs in patients with previous myocardial infarction can increase mortality (see Chapter 7). Catheter ablation has emerged as an effective strategy for elimination of PVCs: a focal problem (aberrant focus) and a focal solution (ablation).

Fogoros' Electrophysiologic Testing, Seventh Edition. Richard N. Fogoros and John M. Mandrola.
© 2023 John Wiley & Sons Ltd. Published 2023 by John Wiley & Sons Ltd.

Once the electrophysiologist has decided to target the PVCs, the first step is to study the electrocardiogram (ECG). The ECG is an elegant mapping tool. Each of the 12 leads sees the ECG from a different point of view. Pattern recognition is key. The ECG gets the electrophysiologist in the right neighborhood of the heart. For instance, PVCs with a right bundle branch block (RBBB) pattern in lead V_1 originate in the left ventricle; PVCs with an inferiorly directed axis (large r waves in leads II, III, aVF) originate in the superior aspects of the heart. We will expand on using the ECG to estimate the site of the arrhythmia in the section of this chapter on VT ablation.

All 12 leads of the ECG are important, but lead V_1 has special importance for localizing the site of outflow tract arrhythmias (Figure 10.1). A QS pattern in V_1 indicates the most anterior area – the right ventricular outflow tract (RVOT). As the focus moves posteriorly, the size of the r wave in lead V_1 increases gradually.

In the electrophysiology (EP) laboratory, two global strategies are used to locate and ablate PVCs.

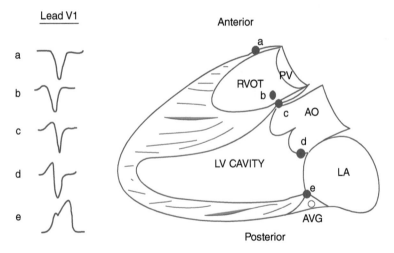

Figure 10.1 Site of origin of ventricular arrhythmias – lead V_1. This diagram shows typical lead V1 configurations for ventricular ectopic beats from five common sites of origin. **Site a** is the anterior right ventricular outflow tract. **Site b** is the posterior right ventricular outflow tract. **Site c** is from beneath the right coronary cusp of the aortic valve. **Site d** is from beneath the left coronary cusp of the aortic valve. **Site e** is from the upper posterior wall of the left ventricle near the AV groove. Ao, aorta; AVG, posterior AV groove; LA, left atrium; LV, left ventricle; PV, pulmonary valve; RVOT, right ventricular outflow tract.

Activation mapping

The operator places a mapping/ablation catheter at points in the vicinity of the PVC and measures the timing of the electrogram from the catheter tip. The earlier the electrogram relative to the initial QRS deflection on the surface leads, the closer the tip is to the PVC site (Figure 10.2). Successful ablation sites usually inscribe an electrogram

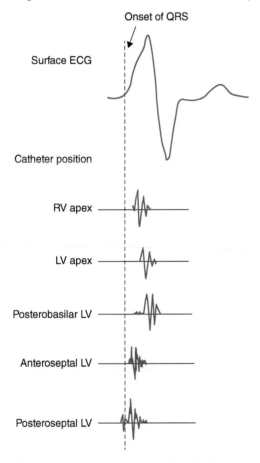

Figure 10.2 Activation mapping of ventricular ectopy. By recording intracardiac electrograms from multiple ventricular positions during a PVC, the earliest site of ventricular activation is sought (in this example, in the posteroseptal left ventricle). The site of earliest activation should be near the site of origin of the PVC. LV, left ventricle; RV, right ventricle.

at least 25 ms before the onset of the QRS and have a QS pattern on the unipolar electrogram (all forces away from the catheter tip). Activation mapping is usually combined with 3-D electroanatomic mapping where the timing is color coded. 3-D maps help localize the structure with less use of fluoroscopy. Activation mapping requires a sufficient burden of PVCs. Infrequent PVCs are often a major challenge when ablating PVCs.

Pace mapping

The ablation catheter tip can be used to pace the heart. As the operator approaches the site of the PVC, the paced QRS starts to look similar to the PVC. The closer to the site, the better the pace map. When the paced QRS matches the PVC in all 12 leads, the operator is likely on the successful site for ablation. Pace mapping can be an adjunct to activation mapping, or it can be used alone when the PVC burden is too low to use activation mapping. One caveat for pace mapping is that its use depends on a stable exit point of the PVC focus. PVCs arising from the region of the left ventricular outflow tract (LVOT), near the aortic cusps, can have variable exit points, which makes pace mapping less useful in that area.

Anatomic considerations of the outflow tract

Although a PVC can occur from any area of the heart, they tend to cluster in typical locations. We will discuss the most common of these regions.

The superior aspect of the heart, near the outflow tract of the right and left ventricle, including the valves and epicardial area, is the most likely site of PVCs, especially in patients without structural disease (Figure 10.1).

RV outflow tract (RVOT)

The RVOT is separated into three areas – the rightward aspect (free wall) anterior, leftward aspect (septal), and posterior. The RVOT courses anterior and leftward of the LVOT. The pulmonic valve is superior to the aortic valve. Importantly, myocardial sleeves can extend from a few millimeters to 2 cm into the pulmonary artery. And the inferior portion of the RVOT is continuous with the area of the His bundle, tricuspid valve annulus, and intraventricular septum.

LV outflow tract

Whereas the RVOT is muscular, the LVOT contains both muscular and fibrous elements. Ventricular muscle from the LVOT extends northward into and between the semilunar valve cusps. Remember, the pulmonic valve is superior to the aortic valve, so the muscular area of the RVOT sits at the same level as the right and left coronary cusps of the aortic valve. These two cusps of the aortic valve are the most common sites for LVOT PVCs. They reside immediately posterior to RVOT. The noncoronary cusp resides even more posteriorly, adjacent to the intraatrial septum, and is more often associated with septal atrial tachycardias than PVCs. The complex extensions of the myocardial sleeves in the outflow tract can cause ventricular arrhythmias originating there to have variable exit sites, and hence variable QRS morphology.

Epicardial and coronary sinus sites

A little less than 10% of idiopathic VT and outflow tract PVCs originate from epicardial sites. Typically, these occur from myocardium reachable from the distal coronary sinus. The coronary sinus courses through the AV groove, continuing on around the lateral mitral annulus as the great cardiac vein. The junction of the anterior intraventricular vein (AIV) and great cardiac vein is just lateral to the left coronary cusp of the aortic valve.

Left ventricular summit

The most northerly part of the left ventricle lies between the left anterior descending and left circumflex coronary arteries, near the junction of the great cardiac vein and AIV. This area is even superior to the aortic valve cusps.

Mitral annulus and papillary muscle

A smaller proportion of PVCs originate from the mitral annulus or papillary muscle. These areas tend to be approachable with an ablation catheter. The morphology of the QRS depends on the site of origin on the valve. A characteristic feature of these arrhythmias relates to the posterior location of the mitral valve relative to the pulmonic and AV valve. This means the forces are back to front and have positive deflections in V_1–V_3.

Ablation of outflow tract PVCs and ventricular tachycardia

When an outflow tract origin is suspected, it is best to begin mapping in the RVOT, preferably after generating a 3-D map to help define the anatomic structure. The ECG guides the mapping procedure. For instance, if the R waves are especially tall in the inferior leads, areas above the pulmonic valve should be explored. An attempt should be made to "bracket" the activation, exploring east, west, north, and south of the earliest point.

The three characteristics of a successful ablation site are activation that precedes the QRS by ≥25–30 ms, a pace map that matches the QRS in all 12 leads, and a QS pattern on the unipolar recording from the catheter tip.

If the earliest endocardial activation in the RVOT is not greater than 20 ms before the QRS, or if the pace map does not match in more than 10 or 11 leads, the focus is not likely to be in the right ventricle (RV). Sometimes ablation in the posterior RVOT can transiently suppress the PVCs. If so, the next step should be to map in the LVOT, in either the right or left coronary cusp, as these structures lie immediately behind the RVOT (Figure 10.3).

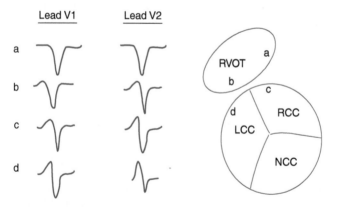

Figure 10.3 Relationship of locations in the RVOT and right and left coronary cusps. In the figure, locations a, b, c, and d represent common locations of origin for ventricular arrhythmias, and their correlating ECG characteristics. Note the close proximity of these sites. These areas of origin are the same as depicted in Figure 10.1. LCC, left coronary cusp; NCC, noncoronary cusp; RCC, right coronary cusp; RVOT, right ventricular outflow tract.

Mapping in the LVOT should begin above the valve. It helps to display the RVOT area on the 3-D map. Many operators will use intracardiac echocardiography (ICE) imaging to define the coronary cusps. Fortunately, the focus of these arrhythmias is usually inferior to the origin of the left main coronary artery. Some operators routinely perform angiography before ablating in the region of the coronary cusps. Other operators visualize the left main origin on ICE images. (The proximity of these arrhythmias to major structures emphasizes the importance of informed consent and slow decision making before the procedure, especially when ablation is used for treatment of mild symptoms. See below on the complications of ventricular ablations.)

If the aortic cusp areas are not sufficiently early, mapping can then proceed to the LVOT under the aortic valve. Sometimes it is helpful to use a short curved catheter that can be fully deflected into the LV and pulled back so that the tip is pointing upward (Figure 10.4).

Another place to look for sites of origin near the left ventricular out-flow area is the epicardial region. Epicardial sites can be reached by advancing the ablation catheter into the coronary sinus and around the lateral mitral valve annulus in the great cardiac vein. The most

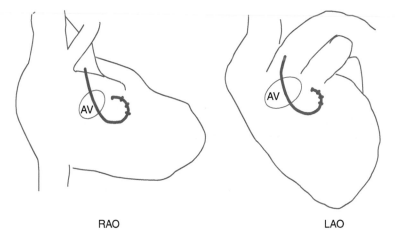

RAO   LAO

Figure 10.4 Mapping the left ventricular outflow area. A short-curved mapping catheter can be used to cross the aortic valve and, after fully deflecting the catheter, pulling it back so that the tip reaches the left ventricular outflow area. This diagram depicts RAO and LAO fluoroscopy projections.

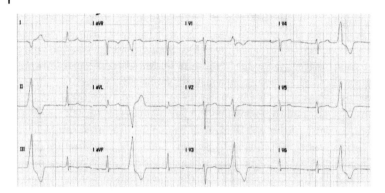

Figure 10.5 12-lead ECG of PVCs originating at the junction of the great cardiac vein and the anterior intraventricular vein. This is the most common epicardial site associated with frequent ventricular arrhythmias. The superior axis and early precordial transition are characteristic (see text).

common area of interest from within the coronary sinus is at the junction of the great cardiac vein and AIV. PVCs from the site usually have a marked inferior axis and very early transition in the precordial leads, often with a typically slurred upstroke in the initial upstroke of the QRS (Figure 10.5).

Mitral annular PVCs

The mitral valve is a posterior structure. This means arrhythmias coming from the area of the mitral valve move from back to front (posterior to anterior), and thus record positive deflections in all the precordial leads. Two characteristics confirm a mitral annular location: when mapped to the site of origin, the catheter tip is in the typical mitral annular location in the right anterior oblique (RAO) and left anterior oblique (LAO) projection (similar to ablation of left-sided accessory pathways), and both atrial and ventricular signals are recorded from the ablation catheter. When moving from lateral mitral annulus to septal annulus, the QRS narrows as the catheter approaches the conduction system.

Idiopathic left centricular PVCs and ventricular tachycardia

Idiopathic left ventricular tachycardia, also called left posteroseptal tachycardia, is a verapamil-sensitive arrhythmia originating in the posteroapical aspect of the left ventricular septum, in the region of the left posterior fascicle. It was first described by Belhassen and colleagues, so it also goes by the name Belhassen VT. The arrhythmia has a right bundle branch morphology with left axis deviation. It is also seen in patients who have otherwise normal hearts.

The most common mechanism for fascicular VT is macroreentry using the left posterior (less commonly, the anterior fascicle) as one limb and abnormal Purkinje fiber or adjacent myocardium as the other limb (Figure 10.6). The usual VT mechanism involves retrograde conduction over the left posterior fascicle and antegrade conduction over the abnormal myocardial or Purkinje fibers. The VT circuit likely includes the entire length of the fascicle.

In addition to this "classic" reentrant tachycardia, frequent PVCs also occasionally originate from this area, as well as automatic or triggered tachycardias. Some experts believe papillary muscle VT also arises from the distal Purkinje network. The ECG manifestations of left posterior fascicular VT include RBBB with a superior axis. Left anterior fascicular VT, in contrast, has a RBBB and an inferior axis. Importantly, there are subtle differences between fascicular VT and papillary muscle VT: VT from the papillary muscle typically has qR or a monophasic pattern in V_1 whereas fascicular VT has a typical rSR'

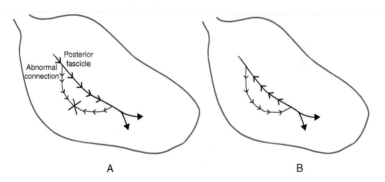

A   B

Figure 10.6 Idiopathic left ventricular tachycardia. This figure depicts idiopathic left ventricular tachycardia (Belhassen tachycardia), which utilizes one of the left ventricular fascicles (typically the posterior fascicle), along with an abnormal connection consisting of myocardial or Purkinje fibers, to form a reentrant circuit. Panel A shows the baseline state, with normal conduction down the left posterior fascicle, and into both ends of an abnormal connection. Panel B shows the most typical form of this arrhythmia, using the posterior fascicle in the retrograde direction and the abnormal connection in the antegrade direction (see text).

in V_1; papillary muscle VT is wider than fascicular VT; fascicular VT inscribes small q waves in leads 1 and aVL; finally, papillary muscle VT usually has large R waves that transition to an rS transition in leads V_4–V_6.

Ablation of posterior fascicular VT can be accomplished in two ways. One is to target the abnormal diastolic potentials that precede the QRS by up to 110 ms. These pathways form the antegrade limb of the circuit, so as one moves the mapping catheter apically, the diastolic potentials are seen later. Another way to ablate this tachycardia is to target the posterior fascicle itself by searching for the earliest fascicular potential, which is a sharp His-like spike just before the QRS. Ablation is ideally performed from the mid-base down to the apex, along the fascicle. It is best to avoid ablation in basal locations, which risks causing LBBB or complete AV block. Successful ablation can be performed in approximately 75–80% of patients with idiopathic left ventricular tachycardia.

Even when fascicular VT is not inducible, empiric ablation can still be successfully performed. The operator can either target the diastolic potentials which are seen after the QRS as late potentials, or linear ablation lesions can be created along the fascicle from mid-base to the apical inferior wall.

A recent observation from numerous centers shows that PVCs from the Purkinje network can be triggers of ventricular fibrillation. The characteristic VF-inducing PVC has a narrow QRS and is tightly coupled. These VF-inducing PVCs have been reported in patients without structural heart disease and in patients with cardiomyopathy.

Bundle branch reentrant tachycardia

Bundle branch reentrant tachycardia, as opposed to the other forms of readily ablatable ventricular tachycardia, does not occur in patients who have otherwise "normal" ventricles. Patients with sustained bundle branch reentry generally have underlying nonischemic dilated cardiomyopathy that is relatively severe, and also have intraventricular conduction defects on their ECGs. The arrhythmia is rapid, usually symptomatic (often presenting with syncope or cardiac arrest), and is most often of left bundle branch morphology.

The reentrant circuit uses one bundle branch (usually the right bundle branch) in the antegrade direction and the other bundle

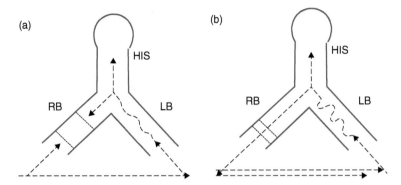

Figure 10.7 Bundle branch reentry. The His bundle and right and left bundle branches are depicted. Sustained bundle branch reentrant tachycardia requires intrinsic conduction delay in the bundle branches, most often manifested by an intraventricular conduction delay on the ECG. In (a), a premature ventricular impulse blocks retrogradely in the right bundle branch (RB), then conducts up the left bundle branch (LB), but finds the RB still refractory in the antegrade direction. Bundle branch reentry is thus not established. A more appropriately timed premature impulse (b) might encounter very slow retrograde conduction up the LB, so that antegrade penetration of the RB is now possible. A sustained reentrant arrhythmia using the RB antegradely and LB retrogradely is now established.

branch (usually the left) in the retrograde direction (Figure 10.7). Establishing a sustained bundle branch reentrant tachycardia requires a conduction delay within the bundle branches (and thus intrinsic conduction system disease). Thus, bundle branch reentry should be suspected in patients with nonischemic cardiomyopathy and intraventricular conduction delays on their 12-lead ECGs who present with ventricular tachycardia that has left bundle branch morphology.

During the electrophysiology study, each QRS complex of the tachycardia is preceded by a His bundle deflection. The HV interval during tachycardia may be the same as, slightly longer than, or slightly shorter than that during sinus rhythm, depending on the site of the recording catheter and the conduction velocity in the right bundle branch during the tachycardia. AV dissociation is usually present during bundle branch reentrant tachycardia.

During this tachycardia, the interval between the His deflection and the right bundle branch deflection is usually shorter than that during sinus rhythm. This finding helps to differentiate bundle branch reentry from supraventricular tachycardias with aberrancy (in which the His right bundle deflection is normal or prolonged). Further, any variations in the tachycardia cycle length during bundle branch reentry are preceded by variations in the HH interval; that is, by variations in the interval between His spikes in two successive beats of the tachycardia. This is in contradiction to what one would see in other forms of ventricular tachycardia, in which the retrograde activation of the His bundle occurs passively, following ventricular activation. The resultant ventricular tachycardia will have an LBBB configuration.

Once bundle branch reentry has been confirmed, ablation of the right bundle branch eliminates the reentrant circuit. Ablating the right bundle branch is accomplished by first manipulating the ablation catheter to record the His bundle electrogram and then slowly advancing the catheter into the right ventricle until a distinct right bundle branch deflection is seen.

Successful ablation of the right bundle branch can be achieved in more than 95% of patients with bundle branch reentrant tachycardia. Unfortunately, owing to the significant underlying cardiac disease that burdens these patients, their long-term prognosis – from both an arrhythmic and a hemodynamic standpoint – remains relatively poor. Many electrophysiologists often consider implanting defibrillators in these patients, even after "curing" their bundle branch reentry.

Ablation of reentrant VT in the presence of structural heart disease

As noted in Chapter 7, reentrant ventricular tachycardia is generally possible only when areas within the ventricular muscle become damaged. In patients with focal areas of scar due to previous myocardial infarction, nonischemic cardiomyopathies, such as arrhythmogenic right ventricular cardiomyopathy (ARVC), or sarcoidosis, ventricular tachycardia (usually) occurs because conduction proceeds through channels of surviving myocardium within and through the area of scar. Channels of surviving but damaged myocardium conduct slowly, while the scarred areas serve as anatomic boundaries. Unidirectional block, slow conduction, and the presence of multiple pathways set the stage for reentry.

The approach to ablation of scar-related ventricular tachycardia includes four steps.

Table 10.1 Using the ECG to locate the exit point of scar-related VT.

	Exit point
Right bundle branch block	Left ventricular exit
Left bundle branch block	Septal or RV exit
Superior axis (+aVR, AVL)	Inferior wall exit
Inferior axis	Anterior wall exit
Positive precordial concordance	Basal exit
Negative precordial concordance	Apical exit
QS in any lead	Wavefront moving away from that lead
The wider the QRS and more slurred the upstroke	The more likely an epicardial origin

Step 1

Use the ECG. Its 12 leads give 12 clues to the exit point of the circuit. Table 10.1 gives some rules of thumb that relate the ECG to likely critical locations within a ventricular reentrant circuit.

Step 2

The second step for scar-related VT is to create a 3-D map during sinus rhythm to identify the low-voltage areas of scar and late potentials. Figure 10.8 demonstrates typical late potentials. Mark these areas on the anatomic map. The later the potential during sinus rhythm, the more interesting this site may be during VT. Another way to get an idea of the exit points of the VT is to pace from areas that you think the VT is exiting. These are called pace maps, and they are a bit less useful for scar-related VT but can help identify a general area of interest. The time between the stimulus and the QRS can be a clue. If the S–QRS interval is long, it is possible you are within a scar area of interest (see below).

Step 3

The third step is to induce the clinical VT with programmed stimulation. A 12-lead ECG of the VT should be recorded, taking note of the cycle length of tachycardia and its morphology. Some operators use pressors to maintain an adequate blood pressure during this part of the test, but this needs to be done with extreme caution in patients with precarious cardiac function or severe coronary artery disease.

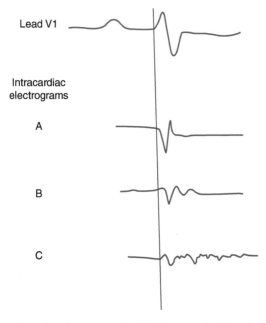

Figure 10.8 Late potentials. This figure depicts lead V_1 during normal sinus rhythm, and three locations near an area of scar recorded with a mapping catheter (intracardiac electrograms A, B, and C). Electrogram A is normal. Electrogram B shows some fractionation. Electrogram C shows a lot of fractionation in the electrical signal, along with electrical activity that persists for a long time – that is, late potentials (see text).

Hemodynamic compromise can occur very quickly. In rare cases, for instance, in patients with advanced heart failure, hemodynamic support devices can be used during mapping. Expert centers vary a lot in their use of these devices.

If the VT is clinically stable, find a reference electrode (often, a surface ECG lead with a reliable upstroke or downstroke on the QRS) and perform activation mapping. To perform activation mapping, it is helpful to have a conceptual idea of how scar-related ventricular tachycardia often behaves (Figure 10.9).

During reentrant ventricular tachycardia, the earliest portion of the QRS complex marks the exit point as it leaves the damaged area of slow conduction and begins depolarizing normal ventricular myocardium (sites X in Figure 10.10). By recording localized electrograms during ventricular tachycardia, the earliest site of ventricular activation can

(a)

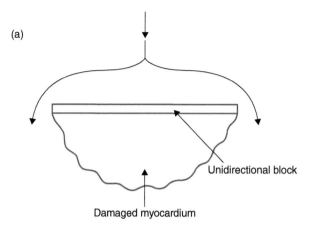

Unidirectional block

Damaged myocardium

(b)

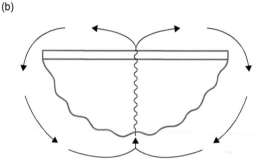

Figure 10.9 A model of scar-related ventricular tachycardia. Substantial evidence indicates that reentrant ventricular tachycardia operates according to this mechanism in many patients. (a) A patch of damaged myocardium that is protected in the antegrade direction by a line of unidirectional block. An electrical impulse encountering this line of block is forced around the periphery of the damaged area. (b) The completed reentrant circuit. The electrical impulse enters the damaged area from the retrograde direction. After conducting slowly through the damaged myocardium, it exits back into normal tissue, thus completing the circuit. This is sometimes called a figure-of-eight reentrant circuit.

be assumed to be near the "exit point" of the reentrant circuit. This technique is called "activation mapping." Most of these arrhythmias involve macroreentrant circuits, so there will be an "early-meets-late" spot on a 3-D map. It is important to note, however, that ablating at an exit point may not eliminate the reentrant circuit, as demonstrated in Figure 10.10.

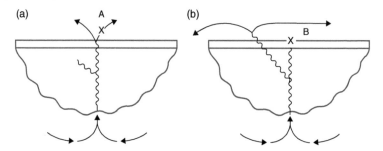

Figure 10.10 Why activation mapping may not lead to successful ablation of ventricular tachycardia. In this figure, activation mapping has successfully identified the point of "exit" from the area of damaged myocardium, and attempts at ablation are performed (ablation lesions are denoted by "X"). In (a) the lesion that has been created is extremely close to the exit point (lesion A), but yet has not been placed in an area critical to the reentrant circuit. In (b), the precise exit point has been ablated (lesion B). Although this lesion has successfully abolished the original reentrant pathway, a second exit point has now appeared, and ventricular tachycardia (probably with a somewhat different morphology) persists.

The reality is even more complex than this. Figure 10.11 shows a more detailed model of a scar-related VT. In this model, a classic figure-of-eight reentrant tachycardia is shown (outer loop, A). The pathway the reentrant circuit takes through the scar tissue, however, is complicated, and includes a potential inner loop (B), as well as two blind loop bystander pathways (D and E).

The key to successfully ablating this arrhythmia is to find a critical zone that will eliminate all reentry. Ablating at any sites along pathway A will fail, as will ablating at sites on the inner loop B or ablating channels D or E. Further, ablating at the exit point of the circuit (X) or the entrance point of the circuit (Y) will also fail. Only lesions placed at critical points (C) can be expected to reliably eliminate reentry through this circuit.

So the key is not merely to identify points on the reentrant circuit for ablation, but to identify *critical* points.

Step 4

The fourth step is to perform entrainment pace mapping in areas of interest – especially at exit points, scar border zones, and at areas of low-voltage fractionated potentials.

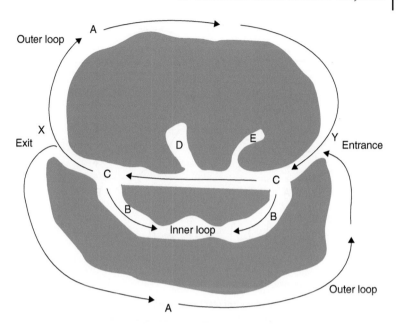

Figure 10.11 Complex model of scar-related ventricular reentry. See text for explanation. A, outer loop of reentry; B, inner loop; C, critical areas for ablation; D,E, blind alleys; X, exit for reentrant impulse; Y, entrance for reentrant impulse.

Entrainment mapping

Entrainment mapping, a variation of pace mapping, is a method of detecting critical areas within reentrant circuits (Figure 10.12). Entrainment is performed by pacing from various areas within the heart during reentrant tachycardia, at a cycle length slightly shorter (usually by 20–30 ms) than that of the tachycardia.

Classically, entrainment is supposed to be accompanied by fusion beats. This is because the paced impulse travels in both directions through the reentrant circuit, and in the backwards direction it "collides" with the impulse coming around from the previous cycle. (This collision is depicted in Figure 10.12, panel B.) Since at least part of the myocardium within the circuit is being depolarized from two different directions, fusion occurs.

With reentrant ventricular tachycardia, however, successful entrainment usually occurs within the area of slow conduction, as shown.

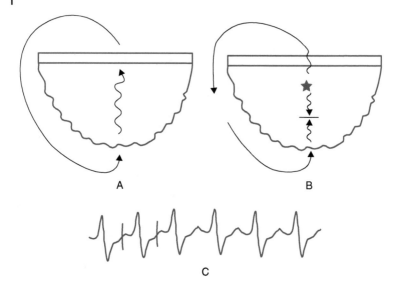

Figure 10.12 Entrainment of ventricular tachycardia. Panel A depicts reentrant ventricular tachycardia made possible by a zone of slow conduction, as shown in previous figures. Panel B depicts entrainment. In this panel, a pacemaker (red star) has been positioned within the slow zone of the reentrant circuit, and has been set to pace at a cycle length slightly shorter than the cycle length of the ventricular tachycardia. Each paced beat exits the zone of slow conduction at the same point at which the reentrant impulse exits, and then follows the same pathway used by the reentrant arrhythmia. As a result, each paced impulse "resets" the tachycardia at a slightly faster rate. When pacing stops, the last paced impulse simply continues cycling around the reentrant pathway, reestablishing the original tachycardia at the original cycle length. Panel C shows an ECG taken during and immediately after entrainment. Note that the cycle length during the last two paced beats (that is, during entrainment) is slightly faster than the cycle length of the reestablished tachycardia seen after pacing stops. Further, observe the long delay between the pacing spikes and the ensuing QRS complex, indicating that pacing is taking place in a zone of slow conduction (see text for details).

Because the fusion happens in the slow zone, it is "invisible" on the ECG and on most intracardiac electrograms. This kind of entrainment therefore is said to occur with "concealed fusion."

In addition to concealed fusion, pacing from the slow zone in reentrant ventricular tachycardia results in an abnormally long delay between the paced impulse and the QRS complex, since it takes more time for the impulse to exit the slow zone. This pace-to-QRS delay is illustrated in Figure 10.12, panel C.

If this kind of entrainment can be identified during reentrant ventricular tachycardia, the catheter is not only likely to be within the zone of slow conduction, but also at a potentially critical point within that zone – that is, a zone required by the reentrant circuit. Entrainment can therefore help identify areas suitable for ablation of ventricular tachycardias.

Entrainment mapping is performed by pacing at a rate 20–30 ms faster than the cycle length of the ventricular tachycardia, and at an output sufficient to capture local myocardium but not so much to capture wide areas. Usually a 5–10 mA impulse is ideal.

Two caveats to keep in mind with entrainment mapping are noncapture of the stimulus and functional delay of the pacing train. Noncapture is sometimes tricky to recognize. It is important to pace long enough to assure acceleration of the tachycardia. It is also important to recognize that the last paced beat may occur many milliseconds after the pacing stimulus, since stimulus-to-QRS times can be delayed at entrance sites. Functional delay, which results in a longer postpacing interval, can be induced if the pacing rate is much faster than the tachycardia, so entrainment should be attempted at rates only 20–30 ms faster than the tachycardia.

There are three key features to look for when doing entrainment mapping: first, determine if there is QRS fusion. If you see fusion of the QRS, you are not in the circuit, you are in an outer loop site or a site remote from the scar. In this case, the catheter should be moved to a new site. Finding concealed entrainment is critical; this means, specifically, that the tachycardia is accelerated to the pacing rate and the QRS is identical (notch for notch) to the tachycardia. Acceleration with concealed fusion is a good sign. It means you are at least close to a critical area.

The second key feature is that, once entrainment with concealed fusion has been found, the postpacing interval should be equal to (or within 10–30 ms of) the tachycardia cycle length. The postpacing interval is measured from the last pacing stimulus to the next electrogram seen on the ablation catheter tip. The postpacing interval represents the conduction time from the pacing site *to* the circuit, *through* the circuit, and *back* to the pacing site. If it is longer than the tachycardia cycle length (plus 10–30 ms), you are not in the critical isthmus. You are in either an inner loop or a bystander site

(Figure 10.11). The extra time represents conduction time to the isthmus. This is not an effective area for ablation, and mapping should continue. If you have (i) a middiastolic signal on the ablation catheter, (ii) concealed entrainment, and (iii) a postpacing interval close to the tachycardia cycle length, you are *very* close to the successful site.

The third key feature has to do with local intervals, in particular the comparison between stimulus-to-QRS interval and the local electrogram-to-QRS interval. The difference between these two intervals helps determine if you are in an adjacent bystander area or the actual critical isthmus. During entrainment, the interval from the pacing stimulus to the QRS is measured. Then, during reentrant tachycardia, the electrogram-to-QRS interval is measured. If the electrogram-to-QRS is equivalent to the stimulus-to-QRS, you are very likely in a critical isthmus and ablation should be performed at that spot. If the stimulus-to-QRS is longer than then the electrogram-to-QRS, you are probably in an adjacent bystander zone (sites D and E in Figure 10.11). This region is still close to the isthmus, and ablation at that spot might still be reasonable. However, better sites are likely close by.

The exit point of the reentrant circuit (X in Figure 10.11) can be confirmed with pacing maneuvers. During sinus rhythm, pacing from sites close to the exit should approximate the QRS complex while in ventricular tachycardia. During ventricular tachycardia, pacing at exit sites within the critical isthmus should have three properties: concealed fusion, a postpacing interval equal to the tachycardia cycle length, and a short stimulus-to-QRS duration. Pacing from entrance points (Y in Figure 10.11) during ventricular tachycardia will produce concealed entrainment, a postpacing interval equal to the tachycardia cycle length, but longer stimulus-to-QRS distance. If the stimulus-to-QRS distance is very long (≥70% of the tachycardia cycle length), you are likely in an inner loop that will not be useful for ablation (B in Figure 10.11). The stimulus-to-QRS duration at an ideal site for ablation is approximately 30–50% of the tachycardia cycle length; that is consistent with a site midway into the isthmus.

When ablation terminates reentrant ventricular tachycardia, it is a good idea to ablate a few millimeters north, south, east, and west of the successful site. It is also important to attempt reinduction of VT after the ablation, as areas of scar can have multiple potential loops.

If different morphologies of VT are noted, repeat the process of steps 1–4.

Ablation of hemodynamically nontolerated ventricular tachycardia

In many cases, ventricular tachycardia is too fast and too hemodynamically compromising to allow it to continue long enough to map by such methods. Recent studies, however, suggest that a substrate- or anatomic-based ablation approach may be effective for these patients.

For unstable VTs, start with steps 1 and 2 described above. If the ECG of the ventricular tachycardia has been recorded, this will give clues about the exit site. If the tachycardia is causing implantable cardioverter-defibrillator (ICD) shocks, and has been seen only on intracardiac electrogram recordings from the ICD, it should be induced in the laboratory so that the operator can get a sense of morphology. If unstable, the ventricular tachycardia is pace-terminated or cardioverted. The rest of the ablation proceeds during sinus rhythm. But if you have recorded a 12-lead ECG of the ventricular tachycardia, you can estimate the general area of the exit point.

Similar to step 2 above, the operator forms a 3-D map of bipolar signal amplitude during sinus rhythm. Color coding can demarcate the low-voltage scar areas. Signals of less than 1.5 mA form the area of interest. Pace mapping can be done from the scar border at a cycle length within 100 ms of the induced tachycardia. When a near morphologic match is found, the operator moves the catheter closer to the scar, now looking for a good morphology match and a stimulus-to-QRS delay. A series of radiofrequency (RF) lesions can be done at these sites parallel to the scar border but not in areas of normal signals. The operator then attempts reinduction.

Some electrophysiologists advocate for an even simpler approach to scar-related VT ablation. These purely anatomic procedures use 3-D mapping to identify the scar area and border zones. Then ablation is done at all sites with late fractionated signals, as shown in Figure 10.8. Some centers ablate around the border zones, encircling the scar, while others do more of a homogenization process in which ablation is carried on over the entire area of scar. These are long, arduous procedures in which the operator tries to empirically eliminate all potential channels from within the scar border. Sometimes it helps to switch operators after an hour or so. Great patience and a systemized approach are critical to this methodology. Ideally, at the end of the procedure, the VT should be either noninducible or much less easily induced. While this technique seems radical, keep in mind that it is being applied only to patients who are having recurrent, rapid VT, which is usually causing ICD shocks despite aggressive medical therapy. Further, ablation within noncontractile scar is unlikely to substantially worsen contractile function.

VT ablation in nonischemic cardiomyopathy

Similar to ischemic disease, scar zones in nonischemic disease create the milieu for reentry. However, the scar seen in patients with non-ischemic disease is less predictable, often patchy, and not transmural. Typical areas for scar zones in nonischemic disease tend to occur in the base of the heart, adjacent to the mitral annulus and in the intraventricular septum.

Multiple morphologies of VT are common in these patients, making ablation generally more challenging. But the principles of mapping spelled out in the previous section still apply. One important caveat in patients with nonischemic and dilated cardiomyopathy is the possibility of bundle branch reentry tachycardia, as described above. Be suspicious of this arrhythmia, especially in the presence of prolongation of the His–Purkinje interval, and typical bundle branch morphology tachycardia.

Epicardial mapping

Another caveat when ablating in nonischemic disease is the increased likelihood of an epicardial source of the ventricular tachycardia. Estimates vary but approximately 10–20% of ventricular tachycardias in nonischemic disease require ablation at an epicardial source.

Micropuncture needles have made epicardial access less risky. Obviously, patients who have had prior heart surgery have significant pericardial adhesions and epicardial mapping is virtually impossible in these patients.

Once in the pericardial space, mapping is performed similarly to endocardial mapping. Techniques include activation mapping (early sites and exit points), entrainment mapping, and pace mapping. Epicardial fat can mimic low-voltage signals, which falsely suggest scar. It is best to pay attention to double potentials and fragmented signals.

Recently, newer mapping catheters have aided our ability to identify areas of slow conduction in the epicardial space. One such catheter is called the "grid" catheter, shown in Figure 10.13. It is a soft, flat,

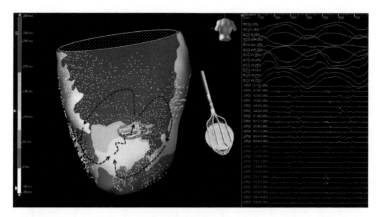

Figure 10.13 Use of a "grid" catheter in ablating ventricular tachycardia. The location of the grid is superimposed on the color-coded activation map. Electrograms from the grid catheter are shown in the right panel. As shown, the grid has been located at a critical location in the figure-of-eight tachycardia, and ablation at this site eliminated the VT. See text. Source: Courtesy of Rod Tung, MD, University of Arizona.

multielectrode catheter that covers an area slightly larger than that of a dime. This can identify areas of middiastolic potentials as shown in the right portion of the figure. Each one of the color-coded electrograms corresponds to a spline on the grid. The image on the left color codes the activation. In this case, ablation at the site covered by the grid eliminated the figure-of-eight VT.

Epicardial mapping can be done with other multielectrode catheters as well. Figure 10.14 depicts a 10-pole catheter placed in the epicardial space of a patient with nonischemic VT. The arrows depict the areas of slow conduction in middiastole. Ablation at that site terminated the VT. Interestingly, this patient had previously had endocardial mapping and no areas of abnormal conduction or scar were found. The substrate for VT in this case was isolated in the epicardium.

Multiple factors complicate ablation in the pericardial space. On one hand, lack of the cooling effect of the blood pool means temperatures can rise quickly with application of RF energy but on the other hand, sometimes pericardial fat limits lesion creation. Careful titration of power from lower to higher power is preferred. If saline-irrigated catheters are used in the pericardium, drainage of fluid is necessary every 15–20 minutes.

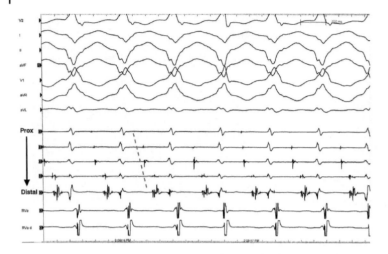

Figure 10.14 A 10-pole catheter recording from the epicardial space of a patient with nonischemic VT, in whom endocardial mapping revealed no areas of abnormal conduction or scar. The five bipolar electrograms recorded from this catheter (labelled "Prox" to "Distal"), show middiastolic potentials indicating areas of slow conduction. Ablation at this epicardial site terminated the VT.

Two particular concerns that limit the safe delivery of epicardial energy are proximity to the left phrenic nerve (noted by diaphragm capture with pacing) and the proximity to the coronary arteries. Most operators perform a coronary angiogram before delivering energy in the epicardial space. Some have also proposed novel ways of moving the phrenic nerve from the ablation window, when the focus is close to the phrenic nerve.

Although any disease of cardiac muscle can lead to an epicardial source of VT, nonischemic cardiomyopathy, ARVC, and cardiac sarcoidosis are three conditions in which the operator should be particularly suspicious of an epicardial focus.

Complications of ventricular tachycardia ablation

We feel conflicted about making this the last section of the chapter. Both the ventricular tachycardia itself and the ablation procedure carry substantial risk of harm. Ventricular tachycardia ablation is a serious procedure that is often done in ill patients with little organ reserve.

First, do no harm is the guiding principle of medical practice, and this rule takes on special importance in the current era of electrophysiology – one in which technologic advances allow us to offer ablation earlier in the course of heart disease. The skilled electrophysiologist balances the risks of the disease and its treatment, and then frames the options for the patient so that a shared decision can be made.

The risk of complications depends on the substrate. Obviously, patients with normal ventricles who have VT originating in the RVOT have a lower probability of procedural harm than a patient with advanced heart failure and incessant, scar-related VT.

The three most common major complications of VT ablation are vascular injury, thromboembolism, and cardiac perforation. In patients with scar-related VT, clinical trials have generally reported complication rates from centers of excellence that range from 6% to 13%. Death can and does occur during the procedure. A clinical trial of VT ablation versus acceleration of medical therapy, called the VANISH Trial (Sapp et al., N Engl J Med 2016;375:111), reported nine procedure-related adverse events in 132 patients (7%) in the ablation arm. A database survey study looking at more than 4600 patients who underwent ablation for ischemic VT over a 10-year period reported a major complication rate of 11.2% and in-hospital mortality of 1.6%. Interestingly, the complication rate and death rate did not decrease over the decade-long period (Harikrishnan P et al., JACC 2014;63:12-S).

11

Ablation of Atrial Fibrillation

Ablation of atrial fibrillation (AF ablation) is different from all other ablation procedures. When we use a catheter to ablate arrhythmias other than atrial fibrillation (AF), we target a focal source. For nonatrial fibrillation arrhythmias, such as accessory pathways, atrioventricular (AV) nodal reentry atrial tachycardia, atrial flutter and outflow tract ventricular tachycardia, ablation success rates are superb. These are focal diseases targeted by a focal treatment.

Atrial fibrillation is rarely a focal disease. Simply stated, we do not fully understand the mechanisms of atrial fibrillation. That is what makes it so hard to ablate. Despite many technology improvements in catheter design and mapping techniques, single-procedure long-term (5-year) success rates for AF ablation hover around 50–60%, and up to one in 10 patients requires multiple ablation procedures. Furthermore, the definition of a "successful" ablation has been controversial, and is in the process of being redefined.

Since we do not know the mechanisms for atrial fibrillation, we likewise do not really know the best target. Is atrial fibrillation due to focal drivers within the pulmonary veins? Is it due to multiple wavelets within the atria? Is it due to high-frequency sources or rotors? Or some combination of all these? We do know that atrial fibrillation is a heterogeneous arrhythmia, and very likely has variable mechanisms among and perhaps within patients.

History of atrial fibrillation ablation

In the late 1990s, a group of heart rhythm doctors from Bordeaux, France, first described a special sort of atrial fibrillation that seemed

Fogoros' Electrophysiologic Testing, Seventh Edition. Richard N. Fogoros and John M. Mandrola.
© 2023 John Wiley & Sons Ltd. Published 2023 by John Wiley & Sons Ltd.

to be occurring from within a pulmonary vein. Until this seminal discovery, most people thought of the pulmonary veins as simple pipes that carried oxygenated blood from the lungs to the heart, and not as a potential source of arrhythmias.

The French group showed that these veins could harbor a focus of a rapid irregular rhythm that looked like AF. The discovery that this single focus from within the vein could be ablated with a catheter ignited the practice of AF ablation. The French researchers combined their electrical observations with previous anatomic observations showing that the pulmonary veins are actually wrapped in heart muscle cells. This led to the concept that the pulmonary veins harbored the cause, or at least the triggers, of atrial fibrillation.

Within a few years, the typical AF ablation procedure morphed into one which uses multiple ablation lesions to build wide circles of electrical blockage around the orifices of all four pulmonary veins. The best way to think about pulmonary vein isolation (PVI) is to consider what it is meant to accomplish. Made from single point-to-point burns or circular freezes, the ablation line acts as an electric fence. Even though AF can occur from within the vein, the "fence" prevents it from getting out to the atrium.

Multiple trials have confirmed PVI as the best ablation approach, even for patients with advanced forms of AF. However, experts in electrophysiology (EP) debate almost every other aspect of AF ablation.

For instance, the debate regarding success has been rekindled. The standard now is that even 30 seconds of asymptomatic AF is considered a procedure failure. Some experts advocate getting rid of this "30-second" rule. Newer monitoring devices, such as implantable loop recorders, have allowed the measurement of "AF burden" – the percentage of time a person is in AF. Some have therefore proposed that a substantial reduction of AF burden should be used as a marker of success, though what is meant by a "substantial reduction" here is also a point of contention.

Another debate considers what it even means to have AF. Emerging research raises the provocative thought that AF episodes may simply be a marker of stroke risk rather than a direct cause.

It is still not established that successful ablation reduces the risk of stroke. Studies meant to look at this question have been hampered by enrollment difficulties, and even by disagreements over how to define successful ablation. For now, most experts believe that patients who had an indication for anticoagulation prior to ablation still have that same indication after ablation. But there are ongoing trials looking at removal of anticoagulation after successful ablation.

Experts also debate whether ablation is best used earlier or later in the course of treating AF, and whether add-on ablation in areas outside the pulmonary veins is useful or potentially proarrhythmic.

Pulmonary vein isolation with RF ablation

Preparation

PVI is an anatomic procedure. The target is not a focal source of arrhythmia but the muscle bundles surrounding the pulmonary veins. Because the procedure entails making multiple lesions in the left atrium, most doctors use anticoagulant therapy before and after the procedure. Choices for anticoagulation include warfarin (adjusted to an INR >2) or any of the new oral anticoagulant (NOACs) drugs, such as dabigatran, rivaroxaban, and apixaban. Anticoagulation is continued both before and after the procedure. During the procedure, heparin is given to keep the activated clotting time greater than 300 seconds.

Little agreement exists on the use of transesophageal echocardiography (TEE) before the procedure. The idea of TEE is to look into the left atrial appendage for a blood clot. Some operators do TEE on every case, while others do it in selected cases. Proponents of TEE say it is important to exclude clots in the appendage, while others cite studies showing that, with modern anticoagulation protocols, identifying the presence or absence of a clot is unnecessary. While a TEE is low risk, it adds expense and logistical challenges to the ablation, and complications, while rare, include damage to the esophagus.

Even less agreement exists on the use of preablation imaging. In the early years of AF ablation, most centers performed a CT scan or MRI of the heart before the procedure. These images provided details on left atrial geometry and the variable pulmonary veins. Radiation exposure, costs, difficulty registering the images with the 3-D maps, and advances in 3-D mapping have led many centers to stop doing preprocedural imaging.

In the EP laboratory

Most electrophysiologists in the United States use general anesthesia when they do AF ablations. Anesthesia allows controlled respiration, which reduces thoracic movement during ablation. It also limits movement of the 3-D map, and helps patients tolerate the procedure.

Vascular access during PVI can be somewhat challenging because it is done during full anticoagulation. Many operators use ultrasound guidance and/or micropuncture technique to visualize the vessels to be accessed.

Many vascular approaches are used for PVI. A typical approach is to place two vascular access points in the left femoral vein, which are used for a multipole coronary sinus catheter and right atrial catheter. Some operators use the internal jugular vein for these catheters. The transseptal sheaths are placed into the right femoral vein.

Intracardiac echocardiography

In recent years, catheters that have an ultrasound probe at the tip have become available. These deflectable catheters allow the operator to see most of the structures in the heart. For instance, the left atrium, including the fossa ovalis region, can be seen with the intracardiac echocardiography (ICE) catheter tip in the right atrium. Advantages of ICE during AF ablation include guiding of the transseptal puncture, seeing thrombus build-up on the catheters, visualizing the catheter position in the left atrium, and enabling real-time monitoring for pericardial effusion. ICE is widely used in the United States, but the catheters are expensive and are not routinely used in most European centers. The use of ICE has not been studied in a randomized clinical trial, so their use is guided by expert opinion only. In addition to cost, an ICE catheter requires an extra vascular access.

3-D mapping systems

We know of no laboratory performing AF ablation today without the use of 3-D mapping systems. The electrical and anatomic information from these systems has transformed AF ablation. 3-D mapping allows virtual maps of anatomic landmarks like the pulmonary vein orifices, left atrial posterior wall, anterior ridges, left atrial appendage, mitral annulus, coronary sinus, and even the esophagus. In the recent past, creation of the virtual left atrial map required point-to-point movement of the catheter, registering of the map with a CT or MRI scan, or tracing of the left atrial wall from the ICE catheter. With newer technology, the electrophysiologist makes a virtual map in a matter of seconds to minutes simply by moving the catheter around in the left atrium – a so-called "fast anatomic map."

These advanced imaging systems combined with ICE have allowed many operators to perform AF ablation with either zero (or minimal) X-ray exposure.

Transseptal puncture

To perform point-to-point radiofrequency (RF) ablation, some operators make two transseptal punctures. A long sheath and low-profile dilator are advanced from the inferior vena cava into the superior vena cava. A preformed needle is placed inside the dilator. This assembly is pulled slowly down into the right atrium until it "drops" into the region of the fossa ovalis. If ICE is used, the operator sees tenting of the septum at this point. The dilator/needle is advanced into the fossa until the operator feels it "pop" across the septum. When the operator is certain the tip of the dilator is in the left atrium, the sheath is advanced over the dilator and into the left atrium. Through one of the transseptal sheaths, a circular mapping catheter is placed into each of the pulmonary veins. The ablation catheter is placed through the second transseptal sheath. Some operators use long deflectable sheaths, which have the advantages of increasing catheter stability and making it easier to reach the inferior aspects of the left atrium. (The authors note that there are many variations on the mechanics of PV isolation – many operators use one transseptal puncture.)

One of the "tricks" that makes PVI much easier is a good transseptal puncture. For point-to-point RF, it is best to perform the transseptal inferiorly and posteriorly in the fossa. Access to the left atrium that is superior and anterior makes it extremely difficult to get adequate contact in the right inferior pulmonary vein region.

Pulmonary vein isolation – general

The key to durable PVI is to make every RF lesion as effective as possible. This is no small feat since PVI usually requires many point lesions. This requires a lot of focus on the part of the operator. Signs of an effective RF lesion include diminution of the local electrogram, a drop in impedance and, if a force-sensing catheter is used, an adequate force-time interval. Some of the newer 3-D software automatically marks lesions that have these characteristics. (However, electrophysiologists need to be wary of automated programs, because they are only as good as the humans programming them. Automated mapping systems can be easily manipulated to show operators pretty maps, whether or not they represent effective ablations.)

The first step of PVI is to generate the virtual 3-D map of the left atrium. This map does not have to be overly detailed but should include the pulmonary veins, the posterior wall, and the anterior ridges of the veins. Once these structures are identified, the map is adequate.

There are many ways to do PVI. Generally, lesions are delivered in a circular fashion around the pulmonary veins. Most experts believe the posterior wall of the left atrium is continuous with the pulmonary vein myocardium, thus most believe the circles formed from the RF lesions should encompass wide areas of isolation. A presumed added benefit of wide area isolation is that "areas of interest" (sites with high-frequency electrograms or rotors) are more likely to fall within these wider circles. (The use of the phrase "more likely to" highlights our deficit of knowledge regarding atrial fibrillation.)

An anatomic safety lesson that early atrial fibrillation ablators relearned the hard way is that the esophagus lies immediately behind the posterior left atrial wall. Early in the AF ablation experience, case reports of death from atrial–esophageal fistulas taught electrophysiologists to avoid thermal injury to the esophagus. Avoidance of esophageal damage is crucial because patients with AF are usually relatively healthy people who are in no danger of death from their rhythm – only (potentially) from the procedure. Today, several techniques are available for preventing thermal injury. These include using short-duration (4–8 seconds) burns on the posterior wall, and, using esophageal temperature probes, coming off RF power immediately with any significant rises in esophageal temperature. Some operators begin the circular lesion set with ablations on the anterior ridges, believing this approach may minimize the burden of posterior wall lesions.

Left-sided pulmonary vein isolation

Isolation of the left superior and left inferior pulmonary veins requires special attention, because of the thickness of the PV-left atrial appendage (LAA) anterior ridge – a ridge of tissue that divides the smooth-surfaced posterior left atrium (where the pulmonary veins are located), from the more anterior, more muscular left atrial appendage.

Once again, there are many techniques for successful left-sided PV isolation. This operator (JMM) uses the Hamburg, Germany, approach. RF energy begins in the left superior pulmonary vein area at about the 12 o'clock area. Ablation there is continued until separation is noted of the left atrial and pulmonary vein electrograms. This separation allows for an electrogram-guided ablation of the anterior ridge. The ablation catheter is then placed into the left superior pulmonary vein, and is gradually withdrawn with counterclockwise torque on the long sheath. Eventually, it falls into the appendage. This marks the area of the ridge, which can be noted on the virtual map. The operator then goes back into the vein and withdraws with counterclockwise torque, right to the ridge. The electrogram at that point shows a large pulmonary vein potential. Ablation is performed in a point-to-point manner, moving down the ridge from superior to inferior, to the 6 o'clock area of the left inferior pulmonary vein. RF ablation then proceeds from south to north along the posterior wall, from left inferior to left superior pulmonary vein. Care is taken in this area to avoid thermal injury to the esophagus. The resulting wide, circular ring of RF lesions is depicted in Figure 11.1. Figure 11.2 shows some of the changes in the pulmonary vein electrograms commonly seen during RF ablation.

If a circular catheter is used to record electrical activity within the pulmonary veins during RF delivery, one can see change of the pulmonary vein activation as the lesion set progresses and the vein becomes electrically isolated. Ideally, if the circular set of lesions is done carefully, total electrical isolation of the veins should occur when the set is completed (see Figure 11.2). When this occurs, we say there is *entrance block* of conduction into the pulmonary vein. At this point, the operator should also confirm exit block by pacing from one of the electrodes within the pulmonary veins. If local capture of the pulmonary vein myocardium is seen without changing left atrial activation, then there is exit block. At this point, the operator moves

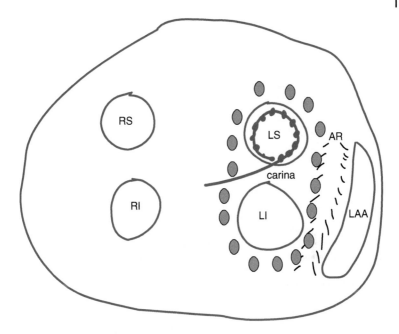

Figure 11.1 PVI of the left pulmonary veins. This figure depicts the left atrium during an RF procedure to electrically isolate the left pulmonary veins from the rest of the left atrium. A loop catheter has been placed into the left superior pulmonary vein to monitor electrical activity there during the ablation. The gray dots surrounding the two left pulmonary veins represent the developing wide circle of ablation lesions currently being created, that will isolate the left-sided veins. Once ablations are completed, there will no longer be any gaps between the points of ablation, and a complete line of block will be formed. A similar procedure will be conducted to isolate the right-sided pulmonary veins. AR, the anterior ridge that lies between the left-sided veins and the left atrial appendage; carina, the space between adjacent pulmonary veins; LAA, opening of the left atrial appendage; LI, left inferior pulmonary vein; LS, left superior pulmonary vein; RI, right inferior pulmonary vein; RS, right superior pulmonary vein. See text for details.

along to the remaining pulmonary veins and begins a waiting period to assess for reconnection in the veins just isolated (see below).

Right-sided pulmonary vein isolation

The right-sided pulmonary veins harbor some particularly tricky areas. This operator begins isolation in the area of the right inferior pulmonary vein. It is usually possible to see separation of the

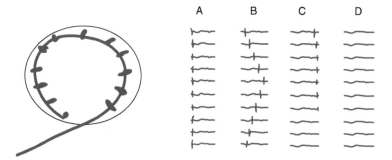

Figure 11.2 Pulmonary vein electrograms during RF ablation. This figure depicts electrograms obtained from a circular (loop) catheter within a pulmonary vein while RF ablation is being performed to isolate the vein. Prior to ablation (panel A), distinct atrial activity is recorded from all points within the vein. As ablation progresses (panels B and C), the electrical activity within the vein becomes progressively delayed and less distinct. With complete electrical isolation of the vein (panel D), electrograms from atrial depolarization are no longer distinguishable. See text.

electrograms at this area during ablation. (Note: this area is much easier to ablate with a low and posterior transseptal puncture. Using a deflectable sheath may make it easier to reach this far southerly area.)

Ablation is then carried along the anterior ridge of the right inferior vein northward to the right superior vein. The superior aspect of the right superior vein can be challenging because it is easy to lose catheter contact. Care and patience are required with this maneuver. Sometimes it is helpful to have the anesthesiologist transiently hold the patient's breath during RF delivery at this location. Once at the top of the right superior pulmonary vein, ablation then proceeds down the posterior wall from north to south. The posterior superior aspect of the right superior vein is an area that frequently reconnects (i.e., regains its ability to conduct electrical impulses). This is another region that requires care, making sure all electrograms are eliminated from ablated tissue. Once the circle is completed, entrance block should be present. Again, exit block should be confirmed by pacing from within the veins.

Ablation in the PV carina region

Pulmonary vein anatomy varies a lot from person to person. Sometimes people have common orifices of the veins. Other times, there are clearly demarcated spaces between the veins. These spaces, essentially an isthmus between pulmonary veins, are called the carina. (A carina is illustrated in Figure 11.1.) Most pulmonary veins can be isolated *en bloc*, that is, without having to create lesions within the wide circle of ablation. However, sometimes it is necessary to ablate within the carina, because triggers for AF often originate from these areas. If a large electrogram is identified in the carina region, ablation of that area can complete the isolation of the pulmonary vein.

Waiting period, and confirmation of durable PV isolation

Once PV entrance and exit block have been shown, most operators wait for a period of time, usually 15–45 minutes, to look for any pulmonary vein reconnection. During this time, a cavo-tricuspid isthmus (CTI) ablation can be done if the patient has had atrial flutter (see Chapter 12). This "waiting period" is also a good time to do a basic EP study, assessing the integrity of the conduction system and looking for inducible supraventricular tachycardias.

Isolation of the PV is confirmed by recording from within the isolated vein with a loop catheter, and demonstrating that the vein is electrically isolated from the rest of the left atrium. Figure 11.3 illustrates findings from a patient in whom the initial ablation proved to be incomplete. In this patient, a gap was identified that was treated by making further ablation lesions at the area of "leakage."

Confusing post-PVI electrograms

Care must be taken not to mistake far-field atrial signals for PV potentials. In the left pulmonary veins, far-field electrograms from the LAA can mimic pulmonary vein potentials. To sort this out, pacing from the LAA or distal coronary sinus will "bring in" the far-field potential close to the pacing stimulus (Figure 11.4). Similarly, in the right superior pulmonary vein, far-field atrial signals from the right atrium/superior vena cava region can be confusing. Clues that a right superior pulmonary vein signal is actually a far-field signal from the right atrium are that it occurs very early in the p wave; the ring electrode that shows the questionable signal is located anteriorly in the pulmonary vein (close proximity to the right atrium); and pacing from the right atrium brings the signal closer to the pacing spike.

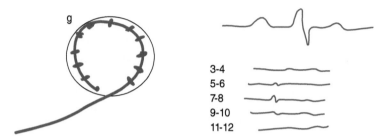

Figure 11.3 Identification of incomplete PVI. This figure shows a case in which reconnection of the pulmonary vein was identified after a 30–60-minute waiting period following the ablation. The figure depicts a loop catheter within the pulmonary vein, as well as recordings made from a surface electrocardiogram (ECG) lead and several leads taken from the loop catheter. Note that in the signal recorded from electrodes 7 and 8, atrial activity is seen within the pulmonary vein, corresponding with the P wave on the surface ECG. This indicates that electrical activity from the atrium is still making its way into the vein, at the area marked by a "g" (for gap) on the diagram. Further ablations in this area will be required to complete the isolation of this vein.

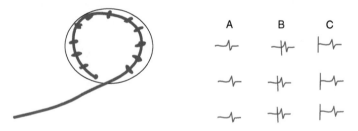

Figure 11.4 Identifying far-field potentials within a pulmonary vein. A loop catheter is depicted within a pulmonary vein after ablation. As shown in panel A, electrical potentials are seen within the pulmonary vein corresponding with atrial activity. Pacing from the left atrial appendage is then performed. In panel B, the atrial potentials move close to the pacing spike, indicating that the potentials represent far-field sensing of atrial activity and do not represent reconnection. In panel C, the atrial potentials are separated away from the left atrial pacing spikes. This indicates that the potentials are local, from within the pulmonary vein, and are not far-field potentials. Thus, panel C represents a case in which reconnection has occurred. See text.

Drug testing post PVI

Drugs are sometimes administered after ablation to help determine whether isolation of the pulmonary veins is complete. The two drugs most commonly used for this purpose are isoproterenol and adenosine. Experts differ on the usefulness of these drugs. Isoproterenol is used to increase adrenergic stimulation, which can unmask a dormant pulmonary vein connection, induce nonpulmonary vein triggers (such as from the coronary sinus, LAA, or right atrial crista), and promote induction of reentrant arrhythmias. Some operators use isoproterenol only when they are suspicious that another arrhythmia may be present, for example, in the presence of discontinuous AV nodal conduction or AV nodal echo beats (see Chapter 6). The problem with isoproterenol when used in patients who are under general anesthesia is hypotension.

Adenosine causes hyperpolarization of ablated myocardium at the pulmonary vein–left atrial junction, and can unmask a dormant pulmonary vein connection. If reconnection of a pulmonary vein is seen during the few seconds of the adenosine effect, the location of the reconnection is noted and further ablation is performed at that area. Studies looking at the utility of administering adenosine have revealed conflicting results. Some show improved procedural success but others do not. Both adenosine and isoproterenol are expensive drugs.

Ablation beyond PVI

Recent data from clinical trials show that PVI alone is sufficient treatment for patients with paroxysmal atrial fibrillation. That is, of course, if there are no other inducible or clinical arrhythmias. Surprisingly, a large contemporary clinical trial showed that PVI alone proved to be equivalent to more extensive left atrial ablation strategies, even in patients with persistent or long-standing persistent AF. Linear lesions across the left atrial roof, mitral isthmus, or anterior wall can be used to treat left atrial flutter, but consensus opinion now is that these lines should be avoided during the initial AF ablation procedure. Arrhythmias are like bears – angrier when injured.

Some have recently advocated searching for "areas of interest" outside the veins, in particular, for areas showing complex fractionated atrial electrograms (CFAE). Presumably, such areas may be triggers for atrial fibrillation. However, it has not been demonstrated that ablation at these sites improves procedural success and, further, the "extra" ablations performed in going after CFAE can often lead to postablation organized atrial flutters. Even more recently, proprietary software programs have shown some promise in locating rotors or areas of focal impulses that could sustain AF. But early studies show conflicting results, and larger trials employing this technology are ongoing.

Re-do AF ablation

If it becomes necessary to repeat an ablation for AF, the second procedure is different from the initial procedure. Atrial arrhythmias after initial PVI procedure are common and come in the form of recurrent AF, atrial flutter, and focal atrial tachycardia. The therapy of these postablation arrhythmias depends on when they occur and how much they bother the patient.

Blanking period

In the days to weeks following the index procedure, ablation lesions cause inflammation in the heart and sometimes pericardium. Electrophysiologists call this 4–6-week period after ablation the "blanking period." The term "blanking" is used because electrophysiologists try not to pay attention to them. Arrhythmias occurring in this early phase may be due to inflammation and, given time, the rhythm may normalize. Therefore, these early arrhythmias are generally ignored. Although studies that look at predictors of recurrences after ablation show that blanking-period arrhythmia is in fact a predictor for future AF, a significant number of people enjoy long-term success despite having transient arrhythmia in the blanking period. The take-home message is to give these arrhythmias time to resolve, if possible.

Left atrial flutter occurring in the blanking period can make it hard to wait. These tachycardias are often organized and, as such, are associated with a rapid ventricular rate and troublesome symptoms. (Remember the principle of AV nodal function in which slower atrial rates lead to faster nodal conduction because of less concealed conduction.) In highly symptomatic patients with organized atrial flutter, cardioversion can sometimes buy some time but often, early repeat ablation may be necessary.

The incidence of post-AF ablation flutter has declined as electrophysiologists have reduced the amount of left atrium (LA) ablations they routinely perform outside the areas of the pulmonary veins. The approach to ablating these "atypical" flutters is discussed in Chapter 12.

Repeat PVI with reconnected pulmonary veins

The best-case scenario during a repeat ablation procedure occurs when the operator finds obvious gaps in the PVI lines and the reconnected vein is actively driving AF (Figure 11.5).

When this situation is identified, the operator places a circular catheter in the vein and the gap is noted by the earliest pulmonary vein signal. The ablation lesions are targeted to that area. If a second gap is present in the same vein, the ablation lesion changes activation and a new area of early activation is observed. Reisolation of each of the pulmonary veins can proceed in similar fashion. In patients with paroxysmal AF, reisolation of the pulmonary veins is usually sufficient and is the preferred strategy. It is not uncommon for a re-do ablation to be a focal procedure with only one or two gaps to ablate. You can think of this procedure as a "spot-welding" maneuver.

If gaps are identified in PV isolation in patients without AF, most experts feel the best strategy is to use the circular catheter to guide reisolation of the reconnected veins. After reisolation of all reconnected veins, some operators will also perform an empiric cavo-tricuspid ablation line during the re-do procedure. CTI ablation (described in Chapter 12) is usually quite easy, and would prevent the necessity of a third ablation procedure for right atrial flutter.

It is also generally a good idea during a re-do procedure to repeat programmed stimulation to look for a reentrant supraventricular tachycardia (SVT) or atrial tachycardia. These arrhythmias can be fickle. If a stable atrial flutter is induced, it can then be mapped and ablated. However, adding linear lesions of any sort in patients with paroxysmal AF should be done only if necessary. Partial lines or recurrent conduction across lines can set the stage for iatrogenic macroreentrant flutters.

Repeat PVI with isolated pulmonary veins

The good news about finding isolated veins in a re-do procedure is that the first PVI was effective – the operator did a good job. The bad

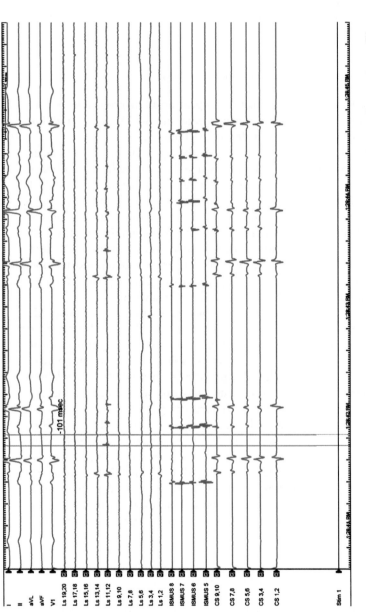

Figure 11.5 Reconstruction of a pulmonary vein. This tracing shows ECGs leads (I, II, aVL, aVF, V₁), electrograms from a LS Lasso™ catheter which is placed in the right inferior pulmonary vein, Ismus™ catheter in the right atrium, and coronary sinus catheter (CS 9–10 to1–2 is proximal to distal). Note the spontaneous electrical activity (focal atrial fibrillation) coming from within the pulmonary vein (seen earliest in Ls 11–12). This spontaneous activity propagates to the rest of the atrium with a delay of 101 ms. The earliest activation at Ls 11–12 indicates that a gap is present at this location. Ablation adjacent to that area isolated the vein.

news, and make no mistake, it is mostly bad news, is that AF is not coming from the veins, and there is no reliable way to find the triggers or drivers – if there are indeed triggers or drivers. Remember, we do not know the exact mechanisms of atrial fibrillation.

The first practical step in this situation is to make sure the veins are actually isolated. Sometimes during AF, the pulmonary vein signals can be small. A cardioversion to restore sinus rhythm makes it easier to confirm complete isolation. If it is determined that the veins are truly isolated, there exists no general agreement on the most effective approach to take.

Some experts in this situation advocate giving high doses of isoproterenol to look for nonpulmonary vein triggers for recurrent arrhythmias. If seen, these premature atrial beats can be ablated. Figure 11.6 shows such a case in which the AF-initiating premature atrial contractions (PACs) originate from the midcoronary sinus.

When no obvious triggers are found, some authors would not ablate further. (See the section below on atrial substrate modification.) Other experts would induce AF and perform linear ablations in the left atrial roof, mitral isthmus, anterior wall, and coronary sinus, hoping to organize AF into atrial tachycardia that could then be mapped. This stepwise approach invariably leads to intraatrial conduction delay and likely to reduced atrial contractile function. Still others would induce AF and look for "areas of interest," that is, areas displaying abnormal or unusual electrical activity that might be serving as triggers for AF. Multiple centers are studying different proprietary mapping systems, both intracardiac (basket catheters) and extracardiac (multielectrode vests), to try to identify the "best" ablation sites for patients with persistent AF despite PVI.

There remains no consensus on what to do next. In this situation, there are almost as many approaches as there are electrophysiologists, further highlighting the knowledge gap of AF.

Cryoballoon AF ablation

Another way to form encircling lesions around pulmonary veins is to use cryothermal energy delivered by a cryoballoon catheter positioned in the ostia of each pulmonary vein (Figure 11.7).

The cryoballoon catheter consists of a noncompliant outer balloon and a second inner balloon. Refrigerant nitrous oxide is injected into the inner balloon. Temperature is recorded from the proximal end of

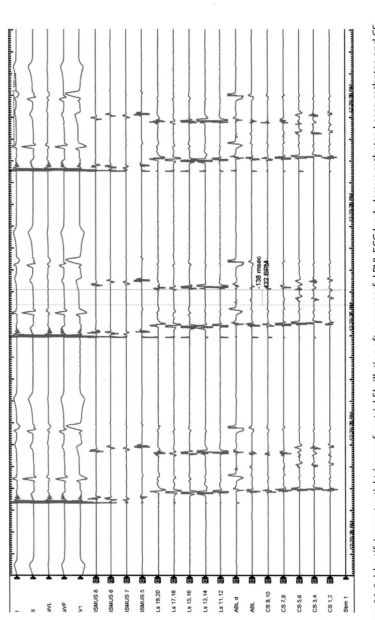

Figure 11.6 Identifying potential triggers for atrial fibrillation after successful PVI. ECG leads, Ismus catheter, Lasso catheter, and CS catheter are shown, as in Figure 11.5. In this case, the Lasso catheter has been placed in the left atrial appendage, as all pulmonary veins were successfully isolated. Two electrograms from a roaming ablation catheter are also shown (ABL and ABL d). Following an atrial paced beat, a PAC is seen to arise from the midportion of the coronary sinus 138 ms before the surface p wave. A single RF lesion in the CS eliminated the PAC and recurrent atrial fibrillation.

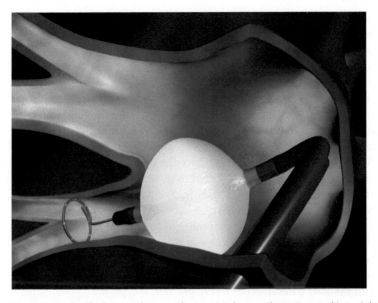

Figure 11.7 Cryoballoon catheter with mapping loop catheter inserted into right inferior pulmonary vein. Source: Image of the Arctic Front Advance Cryoballoon, and Achieve® Mapping Catheter, reproduced with permission from Medtronic, Inc.

the balloon and is dependent on blood flow from the targeted vein. The better the occlusion of the vein, the lower the temperature achieved.

In the EP lab, there are important technical differences with cryoballoon PV isolation. The balloon catheter goes through a larger, more rigid left atrial sheath. This sheath has to be placed over a guidewire through a typical low-profile sheath that has been inserted transseptally. Appropriate transseptal placement is key to successful cryoballoon ablation. Whereas a posteriorly directed septal puncture is best for point-to-point RF ablation, a low and anteriorly directed puncture works best for the cryoballoon. An anterior approach allows more room to direct the stiff sheath and balloon to the right inferior vein.

Another crucial aspect of the cryoballoon technique is avoiding phrenic nerve injury (and diaphragm paralysis) when freezing the right-sided pulmonary veins. The phrenic nerve runs just inside the ostia of the right upper and sometimes right lower pulmonary veins. Two specific maneuvers are used to avoid phrenic nerve injury. One is to place a catheter high in the superior vena cava to pace the phrenic nerve during the freeze. Diaphragm stimulation can be easily felt by placing a hand on the chest. Any diminution or loss of diaphragm contraction warrants immediate termination and deflation of the balloon. The second maneuver to avoid phrenic injury is to avoid deep-seating the balloon in the vein. This is most often a problem with large right superior pulmonary veins.

The current generation of the cryoballoon comes with a multipole spiral catheter that is used both as a guidewire to push the balloon into the ostium of the vein and as a recording catheter to show loss of PV potentials during the freeze. Once the operator places the balloon into the ostium, contrast is injected to show that the vein is occluded. Some operators use color Doppler from intracardiac echo to confirm balloon occlusion. When the freeze begins, the console shows the rate of temperature drop and the minimum temperature. These parameters correlate with adequate and durable PV isolation, as does the time to PV isolation – shorter is better. Different operators use different protocols regarding the time of the freeze and number of freezes for each vein. Roughly 3 minutes per freeze per vein is typical.

The potential advantages of cryoballoon isolation include:

- ability to employ a "single shot" for PVI
- need for only one transseptal puncture
- less need for manual dexterity leads to a shorter learning curve
- low rate of pulmonary vein stenosis
- shorter procedure time
- histologic studies suggest a more uniform lesion.

The drawbacks of cryoballoon isolation include:

- cannot be used for other arrhythmias, such as CTI-dependent flutter or SVT
- phrenic nerve injury is more common
- requires use of contrast
- anatomic variants (common veins) are more difficult.

How Do RF and cryoballoon ablation compare?

In the cleverly named Fire and Ice trial, European investigators compared RF ablation and cryoballoon ablation. They enrolled 762 patients with paroxysmal AF from 16 highly experienced centers in eight European countries. The results of this randomized comparison were nearly identical: 34.6% of patients in the cryoballoon arm experienced atrial fibrillation vs 35.9% in the RF arm. Complications also did not differ statistically: 10.2% with cryoballoon ablation vs 12.8% for RF. Cryoballoon ablation resulted in shorter procedure times (124 vs 141 minutes on average) but longer average fluoroscopy times (17 vs 22 minutes on average). Multiple large studies, including a metaanalysis and a German registry, have also shown comparable outcomes with the two techniques (Kuck KH et al., N Engl J Med 2016;374:2235).

It is widely believed (with some supportive evidence) that cryoballoon-based AF ablation may be most beneficial in the hands of operators with less experience, since RF ablation for AF requires a steeper learning curve.

Pulsed field ablation

As we mentioned in the introductory chapters on ablation, pulsed field ablation (PFA) is a promising strategy for ablating atrial myocardium. The major advantages of PFA are its speed and selectivity for myocardial cells. Multipolar ablation catheters can be used to isolate pulmonary veins, create lines of block, and modify atrial substrate.

This technology is being used in Europe but at the time of this writing is not yet approved for use in the US. The promise of not causing extracardiac damage (esophageal or phrenic injury) is highly appealing, but many questions remain to be answered in ongoing trials.

Atrial substrate modification

In recent years, Australian investigators have shown the importance of cardiometabolic risk factor management for AF. Through a novel approach using a physician-led risk factor management clinic in which overweight or obese patients with AF are encouraged to lose weight, gain fitness, reduce alcohol intake, control blood pressure, and treat any sleep apnea, these investigators have demonstrated reduced AF symptoms and AF episodes without drugs or ablation.

In animal models and in preliminary data from humans, they have also observed resolution of interstitial atrial fibrosis, and improved atrial conduction velocity and voltage. The ability to improve atrial structural and electrical health with risk factor treatment has important mechanistic and therapeutic implications for future AF research. In a large observational cohort study from this group, overweight patients who successfully lost 10% of their body weight enjoyed nearly fivefold greater success rates after ablation. Gains in physical fitness added to the benefit of weight loss (Pathak RK et al., J Am Coll Cardiol 2014;64:2222–2231).

This data has direct implications for AF ablation. For instance, in overweight patients with AF, a reasonable approach could be to isolate the pulmonary veins, which eliminates triggers, while aggressive treatment of risk factors acts to improve atrial structural disease. That brings us back to the original problem of AF ablation: the lack of understanding of the mechanisms of atrial fibrillation.

If you use the analogy of the approach to SVT ablation, PVI is akin to ablating the PACs that induce SVT. Success is high for SVT ablation, not because we ablate the PACs but because we ablate the cause – the abnormal pathway (the slow pathway in AV node reentract tachycardia or the accessory pathway in Wolff–Parkinson–White). To increase the success rate of AF ablation, we need to move past the equivalence of merely ablating the PACs and find the underlying cause. But the work on reversal of AF by risk factor management raises a provocative possibility: the best treatment of many forms of AF may not be with a catheter.

12

Ablation of Atrial Flutter

The technique for catheter ablation of atrial flutter depends on the type of atrial flutter being treated. Atrial flutter is a macroreentrant arrhythmia, that is, the reentrant circuit is large. As with every reentrant circuit, those that cause atrial flutter include a barrier (either anatomic or functional) that creates unidirectional block, as well as an area of slowed conduction so that tissue can recover and become excitable again. Successfully ablating atrial flutter requires identifying the anatomic pathway of the reentrant circuit and, in particular, understanding the nature of the barrier that allows the arrhythmia to become established. With this understanding, ablation lesions can usually be created in a critical area of the reentrant pathway, to create a conduction block that then prevents the atrial flutter from becoming established.

Several types of atrial flutter can be seen and identified. The increased use of catheter-based atrial fibrillation (AF) ablation, surgical ablation, and cardiac surgery that create scars (and thus potential barriers) in the atrial tissue has increased the prevalence of various "nontypical," iatrogenic atrial flutters.

"Typical" atrial flutter: CTI-dependent flutter

The most common form of atrial flutter involves macroreentry of the electrical impulse around the right atrium (RA) – so-called "typical" flutter. In this typical flutter, the crista terminalis acts as the anatomic barrier. Slowed conduction, usually in the area of the isthmus between the inferior vena cava orifice and the tricuspid valve annulus, allows for a large reentrant circuit within the right atrium.

Fogoros' Electrophysiologic Testing, Seventh Edition. Richard N. Fogoros and John M. Mandrola.
© 2023 John Wiley & Sons Ltd. Published 2023 by John Wiley & Sons Ltd.

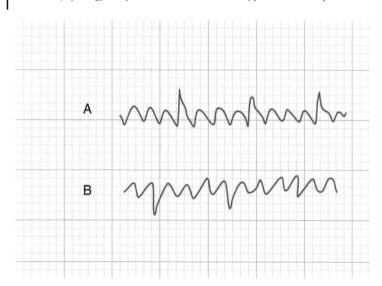

Figure 12.1 Electrocardiographic differences in CTI-dependent right atrial flutter. Leads AVF are shown from two different patients with CTI-dependent right atrial flutter ("typical" atrial flutter). In patient A, the reentrant impulse is traveling counterclockwise through the reentrant circuit within the right atrium (see text). A sawtooth pattern of atrial activity can be seen, with predominantly negative deflections. In patient B, the flutter is traveling clockwise. Here, the flutter waves are predominantly positive. Because a sawtooth-like pattern is seen in both patients, the difference is somewhat subtle.

The new name for typical atrial flutter is cavo-tricuspid isthmus (CTI)-dependent flutter. The rotation of the electrical impulse within the right atrial circuit can be either counterclockwise (negative flutter waves or sawtooth pattern in leads II, III, AVF) or clockwise (positive flutter waves in leads II, III, AVF) (Figure 12.1).

Figure 12.2 depicts the typical reentrant pathway in CTI-dependent atrial flutter. This schematic depicts the interior right atrium, demonstrating the important anatomic features that determine the reentrant pathway for atrial flutter. Two key features should be noted. First, it is the crista terminalis (a ridge of tissue running roughly from the superior to the inferior vena cava) which presents the electrical barrier that defines the reentrant circuit and allows atrial flutter to develop. Second, in typical atrial flutter, the flutter wave must pass through a narrow isthmus defined by the inferior vena cava and the tricuspid annulus.

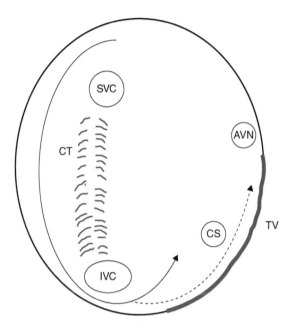

Figure 12.2 Reentrant pathway for CTI-dependent atrial flutter. The right atrium is depicted, including the inferior vena cava (IVC), superior vena cava (SVC), tricuspid annulus (TV), AV node (AVN), os of the coronary sinus (CS), and crista terminalis (CT). The CT is a ridge of tissue roughly connecting the SVC and the IVC. In most patients with atrial flutter, the CT functionally divides the right atrium into two sections. The flutter circuit (indicated by the arrows) must pass through the narrow isthmus between the IVC and the tricuspid annulus. This isthmus thus presents a favorable target for ablation. Note that this figure depicts a counterclockwise movement of the electrical impulse through the reentrant circuit – the more common type of CTI-dependent flutter. However, a clockwise rotation can also be seen, and in some patients successive episodes of flutter can rotate in opposite directions. See text for details.

It is this latter feature that makes radiofrequency (RF) ablation a viable option for many patients with atrial flutter. If a linear lesion can be made, extending from the tricuspid annulus to the opening of the inferior vena cava, then electrical blockade of the necessary isthmus can be created (Figure 12.3).

If CTI-dependent atrial flutter is suspected, it is vital to first confirm the correct diagnosis. This can be done in three ways. First, during the atrial flutter, the activation of the coronary sinus should occur proximally to distally. Activation in the coronary sinus that is not

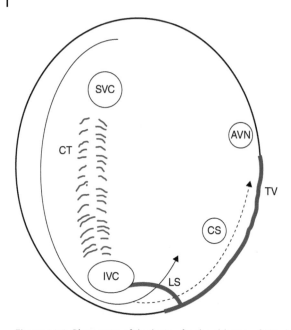

Figure 12.3 Placement of the lesion for the ablation of CTI-dependent atrial flutter. The anatomic features shown here are the same as in Figure 12.2. The ablation lesion (the thick red line indicated by LS) is depicted. This lesion transects the isthmus between the IVC and the tricuspid annulus, blocking the pathway necessary for typical atrial flutter. See text for details.

clearly proximal to distal should suggest a flutter of left atrial origin. Second, during CTI flutter, pacing from the isthmus 20–30 ms faster than the tachycardia cycle length should entrain the flutter with concealed entrainment *and* the postpacing interval (PPI) should equal the tachycardia cycle length. (See Chapter 10 for a discussion of entrainment.) Third, 3-D electrical-anatomic mapping should show rotation around the right atrium. For instance, in counterclockwise flutter, 3-D electroanatomic activation appears as a broad wavefront exiting from the medial CTI isthmus, proceeding from south to north up the septum and then down the lateral right atrial wall. Early breakthrough of the flutter from the intraatrial septum suggests a left atrial origin.

Ablating CTI-dependent flutter

The essence of ablation of CTI flutter is to establish conduction block across the CTI, as in Figure 12.3. The ablation catheter is advanced into the right atrium and deflected down to the tricuspid valve isthmus. Many operators use a long sheath to stabilize the catheter tip. The linear lesion in the isthmus is best performed at or slightly lateral to 6 o'clock in the left anterior oblique (LAO) view. More septal lesions risk injury to the circumflex or right coronary artery. Because the CTI area can be thick and sometimes longer than the "typical" 20 mm described in anatomy books, persistence is important. Catheter choices include an 8 mm tip catheter or a saline-irrigated catheter. Force-sensing catheters are increasingly common and provide feedback on the number of grams of contact force at the catheter tip. RF lesions with less than 5 g of contact force are unlikely to be effective.

Ablation of the isthmus can be performed during atrial flutter or during sinus rhythm. If the patient is in sinus rhythm, most operators perform ablation with coronary sinus pacing.

Ablation begins on the tricuspid annulus. The "ideal" catheter position on the annulus is confirmed by demonstrating a small atrial deflection and large ventricular deflection. It is tempting to move inferiorly quickly but that urge should be resisted. The area where the linear block is most likely to be incomplete is in the region of the tricuspid valve, because making good catheter contact on the annulus can be challenging. Force-sensing catheters may help with this problem.

Once adequate ablation of the valve annulus is assured, the catheter is "dragged" inferiorly toward the inferior vena cava orifice, moving it a few millimeters every 30 seconds or so. Adequate ablation at a particular atrial site can be confirmed by observing a flattening or elimination of the local atrial electrogram. The area of the Eustachian ridge, at the junction of the right atrium and inferior vena cava, is often another tricky area. Sometimes moving slightly lateral or slightly septal at this area can help stabilize the catheter and allow adequate contact. Since the catheter wants to "fall" into the inferior vena cava from the Eustachian ridge, the operator must take care to maintain good contact, as the inferior vena cava junction is another common area of reconnection.

The linear lesion thus created must produce complete electrical blockade between the inferior vena cava and the tricuspid annulus. It is wise to wait 20–30 minutes after CTI block has been noted to assess for recurrent conduction. During that period, "insurance burns" can be applied. An electrical impulse can pass through even a minute discontinuity in the line of block, and atrial flutter will continue.

Confirming conduction block at the CTI

Whenever ablation is used to make lines of block (anywhere in the heart), it is critical to confirm that complete block has been achieved. Catheter ablation, like antiarrhythmic drugs, can be proarrhythmic. Partial block causes delayed conduction, and delay sets the stage for reentry.

Confirming complete block across the CTI is usually straight-forward. Operators differ on how they assess for complete block. Some use two multipole catheters, one in the coronary sinus and one along the lateral right atrium (Figure 12.4). With this method, complete block is confirmed during coronary sinus pacing, when lateral right atrial activation proceeds from proximal to distal. The last pole activated should be closest to the line of block. Merely delayed conduction through the isthmus – indicating incomplete block – is noted when the distal RA electrodes are not the last ones activated. It is important to pace from both sides of the isthmus as block must be bidirectional. The time from lateral right atrium to the coronary sinus should be the same as coronary sinus pacing to the right atrium. Use of multipole catheters makes CTI block easier to see, especially during ablation, as activation changes as the isthmus is ablated.

Multipole catheters make it easier to see CTI block, but they are not necessary. 3-D mapping systems can be used to confirm conduction block. During coronary sinus pacing, the mapping catheter is moved across the isthmus. In the presence of complete block, the latest point of activation should be immediately lateral to the line of block. (Be mindful of 3-D mapping because the color-coded map depends on where the human operator marks the timing of an electrogram.)

Yet another way to assess for complete block is to pace at varying distances from the line of block while recording from the other side of block. This is typically done while pacing on the lateral right atrial wall. As the pacing site on the lateral right atrial wall is moved from superior to inferior (closer to the line of block), the time to the recording in the

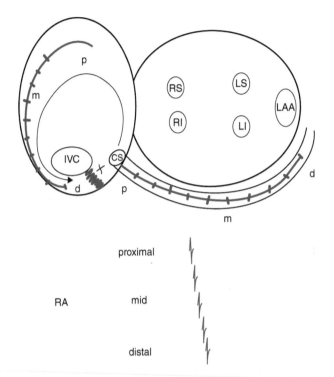

Figure 12.4 Confirming complete block of the CTI. Both right and left atria are depicted. After ablation of the cavo-tricuspid isthmus (CTI), pacing from the coronary sinus (CS) is performed. The paced impulse is blocked at the line of ablation (dense squiggly line marked with an "x"), and must travel counterclockwise through the right atrium. Also shown are the signals recorded from a multielectrode catheter placed in the right atrium (RA). This reveals a proximal-to-distal pattern, confirming that the last part of the right atrium to be depolarized is immediately adjacent to the line of block. Thus, the block is complete. See text for details. Right atrial and CS electrode catheters are depicted as heavy lines with cross-hatching. IVC, inferior vena cava; LAA, left atrial appendage; LI, left inferior pulmonary vein; LS, left superior pulmonary vein; RI, right inferior pulmonary vein; RS, right superior pulmonary vein.

coronary sinus should get longer. Finally, double potentials recorded from the isthmus should be greater than or equal to 110 ms apart. If less than 90 ms apart, incomplete block across the isthmus is likely.

Another trick to assess for complete block across the isthmus is to pace at very slow cycle lengths. Rate-dependent isthmus block (partial block at slow cycle lengths and complete block at faster cycle lengths) indicates the need for more ablation along the isthmus.

One pitfall to guard against is placement of the recording catheter posterior to the Eustachian ridge. Since the coronary sinus is also a posterior structure, recording from a posteriorly placed catheter can give the false appearance of partial isthmus block. 3-D mapping systems help identify location of catheters.

Ablation of atypical or non-CTI-dependent atrial flutter

Some forms of atrial flutter are atypical; while they are still macroreentrant in nature, their reentrant circuits follow pathways other than the CTI as depicted in Figure 12.2.

The three most common reasons why patients have non-CTI flutters are previous atrial fibrillation ablation, previous heart surgery (especially congenital repair or valve surgery), and intraatrial scar tissue.

Non-CTI-dependent flutters are harder to target with catheter ablation because they use highly variable pathways for reentry. Successful ablation of these flutters depends on the underlying substrate, the ability to identify the involved circuit, and the feasibility of creating conduction block between discrete landmarks.

Non-CTI-dependent atrial flutters can occur in either the right or left atrium. With atrial flutters of all types, the patterns of activation during flutter as recorded in the right atrium, and especially in the left atrium (reflected by the coronary sinus electrograms), are of critical importance in making the correct diagnosis. Electrophysiologists rely on these electrograms as the very first step in performing ablation procedures for any atrial flutter. Figure 12.5 depicts the typical patterns of activation recorded from right atrial and coronary sinus catheters with the major types of atrial flutter.

Non-CTI-dependent right atrial flutter

Most right atrial flutter(s) that do not use the CTI as a critical part of the reentrant circuit occur in patients who have had previous heart surgery. The suture line in the right atrium can create barriers that may lead to reentry, as can scar tissue from atrial dilation. In rare cases,

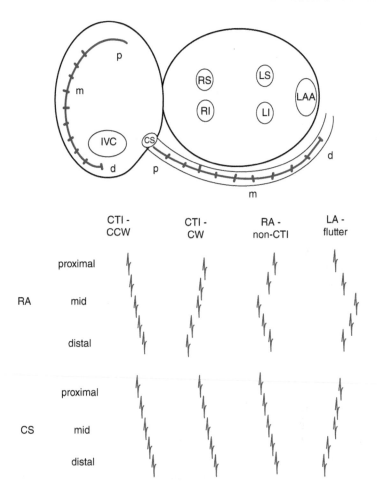

Figure 12.5 Patterns of atrial activation with the major types of atrial flutter. Labels are the same as in Figure 12.4. During atrial flutter, the activation patterns obtained from multielectrode catheters placed in the right atrium (RA) and coronary sinus (CS) often reveal which type of atrial flutter is present. In this schematic, electrograms from RA and CS catheters are depicted for four major types of atrial flutter. With *CTI-dependent, counterclockwise right atrial flutter* (CTI-CCW), the activation pattern in both catheters is proximal to distal. With *CTI-dependent clockwise right atrial flutter* (CTI-CW), the activation pattern from the RA catheter is distal to proximal. With *non-CTI right atrial flutter* (RA-non-CTI), the midportion of the RA lateral wall is activated early. Note that with all three types of right atrial flutter, activation of the CS proceeds from proximal to distal. With *left atrial flutter* (LA-flutter), the lateral right atrial wall is activated late. CS activation with LA flutter in this diagram is shown as going distal to proximal, but CS activation varies depending on the type of left atrial flutter (see Figure 12.6).

atrial cardiomyopathy may set the stage for macroreentry in the right atrium.

Two electrocardiogram (ECG) features suggestive but not diagnostic of non-CTI-dependent right atrial flutter are a completely negative flutter wave in lead V_1 (anterior to posterior forces) and isoelectric periods between flutter waves. With intracardiac electrodes, right atrial flutter should have proximal-to-distal activation of the coronary sinus. A multipole right atrial catheter (isthmus catheter) usually shows early activation from the lateral wall, that proceeds superiorly and inferiorly (Figure 12.5).

When ablating non-CTI-dependent right atrial flutter, it is important to anticipate the most likely pathways for reentry. Usually, the location of the flutter circuit depends on the location of a scar. The two most common sites of scar (and thus of critical isthmuses that can serve as targets for ablation) are found along the right atrial free wall or around a central obstacle involving the superior vena cava.

Mapping the arrhythmia first requires a stable electrode to use as a reference. This is typically provided by one of the leads in the coronary sinus catheter, ideally a lead with a large-amplitude atrial signal.

A 3-D electroanatomic map is often done; this allows both electrical (early vs late) and anatomic mapping. If the flutter is 300 ms, one sets the window of mapping for 150 ms before and 150 ms after the reference catheter. Then the ablation catheter can be used to record points in the right atrium. Newer multipolar recording catheters represent a significant advance because an operator can now take hundreds of points during tachycardia in a matter of minutes. These catheters can quickly show the arrhythmia circuit. However, it is essential to point out once again that with these newer mapping systems, it is essential to take great care in recording these points. Color-coded 3-D maps are only as good as the data that goes into building them.

If the macroreentrant tachycardia is located within the right atrium, the 3-D map should include more than 90% of the cycle length. In post-surgical right atrial flutters, low-voltage areas are usually recorded in the area of the lateral or posterolateral right atrium. On the 3-D map, these areas are typically in regions where early activation and late activation are in close proximity – where "early meets late."

At these sites, low-voltage fractionated electrograms can often be observed from the catheter tip. These are areas of interest for ablation. It is useful to attempt entrainment from these sites. If the catheter is in a critical isthmus, pacing 20–30 ms faster than the cycle length will entrain the tachycardia with concealed fusion *and* the PPI should be equal to the tachycardia cycle length. If there is not fusion or if the PPI is more than the tachycardia cycle length, the catheter is not in a critical isthmus and mapping should continue.

Before ablating in the lateral right atrial wall, especially in the superior right atrium, high-output pacing should be performed (10 mA or greater) to check for phrenic nerve stimulation. Phrenic capture results in obvious diaphragm stimulation. Ablations should be strictly avoided at these sites because injury to the phrenic nerve could result in paralysis of the diaphragm. Some operators will place anatomic markers on the 3-D map at sites that have shown phrenic nerve capture.

If there are areas of right atrial scar, a critical isthmus is often identified between the scar and a nearby anatomic boundary, such as the tricuspid annulus, crista terminalis, or superior vena cava. Creating a complete linear lesion across that isthmus most often eliminates the atrial flutter.

When ablation at a critical isthmus in the right atrium terminates the atrial flutter, it is useful to perform "insurance" ablation in the same general vicinity. Ablation of macroreentry flutter in the right atrium slows conduction and creates boundaries, and thus creates a favorable milieu for CTI-dependent flutter. It is best therefore to add CTI ablation if it has not yet been done. After completion of ablation, it is important to attempt reinduction of atrial flutter with programmed stimulation and burst pacing. If linear ablation lesions were performed, one should confirm complete block across the line. Widely spaced double potentials and differential pacing (and recording) from either side of the line confirm complete block.

Left atrial flutter ablation

Left atrial flutter (and left atrial tachycardia) have become much more common in the era of ablation of atrial fibrillation. In any patient presenting with new atrial flutter after an ablation procedure, left atrial flutter should be strongly suspected. Left atrial flutter occurring in this setting, especially in the few weeks to months after the index procedure, is often incessant and poorly tolerated.

While the ECG is not diagnostic of left atrial flutter, positive flutter waves in leads V_1 (posterior to anterior forces), negative flutter waves in leads 1, AVL and V_6 (left to right forces) and isoelectric periods between flutter waves suggest a left atrial origin. It is not merely of academic importance to suspect left atrial flutter before beginning the electrophysiology (EP) study. Because ablation in the left atrium requires transseptal catheterization and, usually, more extensive ablation, it carries a higher risk. This higher risk should be conveyed to the patient, and the balance of potential benefits to potential harms should be thoroughly discussed. During placement of intracardiac catheters, the pattern of coronary sinus activation is *the* key observation. As the coronary sinus wraps posteriorly around the mitral annulus, its activation provides the electrophysiologist with a window to left atrial activation. Examining this activation pattern should be the first step.

During atrial flutter, activation of the coronary sinus that is simultaneous (e.g., proximal coronary sinus is activated at the same time as the distal coronary sinus), or activation that occurs distally to proximally, confirms a left atrial flutter. However, documenting proximal-to-distal coronary sinus activation does not definitely indicate right atrial flutter. Perimitral flutter in the counterclockwise direction can also display proximal-to-distal coronary sinus activation. In this case, pacing maneuvers from the CTI and right atrium show entrainment with fusion, and very long PPIs.

Once coronary sinus activation patterns have been evaluated, the next step is to exclude pulmonary vein-dependent atrial tachycardia or flutter. As discussed in Chapter 11, pulmonary vein reconnection (i.e., failure of pulmonary vein block) after ablation of atrial fibrillation is common. These gaps in conduction can allow pulmonary vein tachycardia to exit into the left atrium; the gaps can also form an anchor point for microreentry. In the presence of left atrial tachycardia or left atrial flutter and pulmonary vein reconnection, performing a reisolation of the pulmonary veins is usually the first step. If this procedure terminates the tachycardia, the problem is solved. It should be noted that in any re-do procedure following AF ablation, reisolation of the pulmonary veins will be required in any case.

If the pulmonary veins are reisolated and the tachycardia continues, the next step is looking for variability in the atrial tachycardia cycle length. This assessment requires a stable catheter position, usually with a multipole coronary sinus catheter or a circular catheter placed in the left atrial appendage. If the variability in cycle length is greater than 15%, or in rare cases if the tachycardia displays a start/stop pattern, a focal atrial tachycardia is highly likely. The focal source may be an area of either enhanced automaticity or microreentry. In either case, mapping can be directed toward identifying the earliest site of the atrial activation.

On the other hand, if the pulmonary veins are isolated and the tachycardia displays a stable cycle length, the diagnosis is likely macroreentry, i.e., flutter. As with the ablation of non-CTI-dependent right atrial flutter, the search for the ablation target begins with knowledge of the possibilities of the potential circuits.

The most common left atrial macroreentrant flutter circuits include perimitral (clockwise or counterclockwise), in which the reentrant circuit courses around the mitral annulus; roof-dependent flutter, in which the reentrant circuit courses up the anterior left atrial wall and down the posterior wall (or vice versa); a combination of both of these; anterior wall reentry through areas of scar; and, less commonly, intraseptal reentry or atrial appendage reentry. To distinguish among all these various possibilities, it is particularly important to assess coronary sinus activation during the arrhythmia.

Perimitral flutter

Coronary sinus activation patterns are important in making the diagnosis of perimitral flutter. If the activation of the coronary sinus is either purely distal to proximal (clockwise) or purely proximal to distal (counterclockwise), perimitral reentry is possible. Note, however, that coronary sinus activation represents only posterior wall activation. Activation of the anterior left atrium can be assessed by recording from sites on the left atrial anterior septum and lateral wall. These additional recordings can confirm perimitral rotation. For instance, in clockwise (distal to proximal in the coronary sinus) perimitral flutter, the anterior septal signal should precede the anterior lateral signal (Figure 12.6).

When the pattern of activation is consistent with perimitral reentry, the next step is to perform pacing maneuvers to look for concealed entrainment. Pacing at a rate 20–30 ms faster than the cycle length in the mitral isthmus or the distal coronary sinus should entrain the tachycardia with concealed fusion, and the PPI should be equal to or within 10–20 ms of the tachycardia cycle length. The same entrainment maneuvers can also be performed from anterior septal sites along the mitral annulus.

Once the diagnosis is established, an appropriate linear ablation lesion can interrupt the circuit. Most operators create a line of block

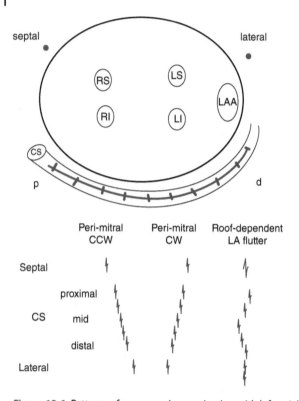

Figure 12.6 Patterns of coronary sinus activation with left atrial flutters. Labels are the same as in Figure 12.4. Activation patterns are shown for the three common types of left atrial flutter, recorded from a multielectrode CS catheter, as well as from electrodes placed near the anterior septum (septal) and lateral wall (lateral). With *perimitral atrial flutter rotating in the counterclockwise direction* (perimitral CCW), CS activation proceeds from proximal to distal, with septal activation preceding proximal CS activation and lateral atrial activation following distal CS activation. With *perimitral atrial flutter rotating in the clockwise direction* (peri-mitral CW), CS activation proceeds from distal to proximal, with lateral atrial activation preceding distal CS activation and septal activation following proximal CS activation. With *roof-dependent left atrial flutter* (roof-dependent LA flutter), the activation of the proximal and distal CS is simultaneous (see text).

in the isthmus defined by the left inferior pulmonary vein and the mitral annulus. This can be a difficult ablation, which often takes persistence. It is usually helpful to employ a long sheath, often a deflectable sheath, to improve catheter stability. A little clockwise torque on the sheath helps stabilize the catheter.

The operator "drags" the catheter inferiorly and slightly anteriorly from the pulmonary vein down to the mitral annulus, targeting large-amplitude atrial signals. Slowing of the tachycardia cycle length can be observed during the ablation but the operator should also be alert for changes in tachycardia activation. It is not uncommon to see perimitral tachycardia change to roof-dependent tachycardia (see below) during RF delivery.

Sometimes mitral isthmus fibers course in the epicardium, in which case ablation in the coronary sinus may be necessary to achieve complete block. Experts debate how often ablation in the coronary sinus is necessary, but it appears to be required in more than a third of cases. The far distal coronary sinus comes around anteriorly along the mitral isthmus. When ablating in the coronary sinus in this region, one should begin with low power, and use high levels of saline irrigation, to minimize the risk of complications.

Some authors have proposed another approach to perimitral flutter. With this alternative approach, a linear ablation is made from the mitral annulus, across the anterior wall (anterior to the left atrial appendage) to the right superior pulmonary vein and a previously formed roof line. This so-called "anterior line" lessens the chance of causing tamponade, but increases the odds of creating electrical isolation of the left atrial appendage (which increases the risk of thrombus), as well as creating the substrate for a gap-related left atrial flutter in the anterior wall.

It is a good sign when perimitral flutter terminates during the ablation procedure but this should not be the endpoint of ablation. As with CTI-dependent flutter, it is crucial to confirm mitral isthmus block when ablating perimitral flutter. One way to do this is to pace from the left atrial appendage, which should show complete reversal of coronary sinus activation – proximal-to-distal activation. Also, successive pacing can be performed from the middle to the distal coronary sinus. As the site of pacing moves closer to the distal coronary sinus and the line of block, activation time to the left atrial appendage should get longer.

Vein of Marshall Alcohol Ablation

Another recent development in aiding the elimination of conduction in the mitral isthmus is ablating the vein of Marshall using alcohol (Figure 12.7). The vein of Marshall is an embryological remnant of the left superior vena cava. It runs northward from the coronary sinus in

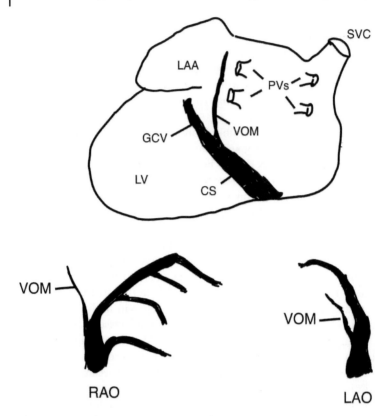

Figure 12.7 A schematic representation of the vein of Marshall. The top panel shows the posterior aspect of the heart. The vein of Marshall arises near the junction of the coronary sinus and the great cardiac vein, and courses superiorly between the left-sided pulmonary veins and the left atrial appendage. Alcohol ablation of this vein can produce block in the mitral isthmus, and can also eliminate epicardial fibers that have been implicated in atrial arrhythmias (see text). The two bottom panels illustrate the position of the vein of Marshall as typically seen during angiography in the RAO and LAO projections. CS, coronary sinus; GCV, great cardiac vein; LAA, left atrial appendage; LV, left ventricle; PVs, pulmonary veins; SVC, superior vena cava; VOM, vein of Marshall.

the area of the mitral isthmus between the left-sided veins and atrial appendage (or so-called ridge) (see Figure 12.7).

The vein of Marshall has been implicated as a cause of AF as it can be a source of triggering beats as well as a tract for neural innervation. A recent trial, called VENUS, found that the addition of vein of Marshall ethanol infusion to catheter ablation, compared with catheter ablation alone, increased the likelihood of remaining free of AF or atrial tachycardia at 6 and 12 months in patients with persistent AF (Valderrábano M et al., JAMA 2020;324(16):1620).

The main reason, however, why retrograde infusion of alcohol and ablation of the vein of Marshall has gained popularity lately is that it aids in creating mitral isthmus block for the elimination of perimitral flutter.

As we wrote previously, the mitral isthmus often includes epicardial fibers, which can be impossible to reach with ablation from the endocardium. The vein of Marshall runs in the epicardium and ablation there has been shown to aid in the creation of mitral isthmus block.

The technique for ablation of this vein is depicted in Figure 12.7. The first requirement is to identify the vein of Marshall, which arises near the junction of the great cardiac vein; then a guiding catheter is placed and contrast injected. The next step is to place a small over-the-wire angioplasty balloon to occlude the vein. Once occlusion is confirmed (Figure 12.8), small doses of pure alcohol are injected slowly. This creates a blushing and ablates epicardial tissue in the mitral isthmus inferior to the left inferior pulmonary vein.

The authors want to emphasize that this technique is promising but more studies are needed with regard to long-term efficacy. It is not without potential complications, which can include pericardial effusion and tamponade and AV block (from injecting the wrong vein).

Roof-dependent LA flutter

Flutter involving the left atrial roof is also a common type of atrial flutter seen after AF ablation. The key diagnostic sign is simultaneous coronary sinus activation (see Figure 12.6), in which neither proximal-to-distal nor distal-to-proximal activation is seen. While other arrhythmias can give the pattern of simultaneous coronary sinus activation, roof-dependent macroreentry is the most common.

Simple mapping maneuvers can confirm this tachycardia. By recording from the ablation catheter low in the anterior wall near the mitral annulus, and then near the anterior roof, the direction of activation is determined relative to a reference channel. This same maneuver is then repeated on the posterior wall. The pattern of activation should proceed in opposite directions on the anterior and posterior wall. For example, if the impulse goes south to north on the anterior wall, it should travel north to south on the posterior wall. If

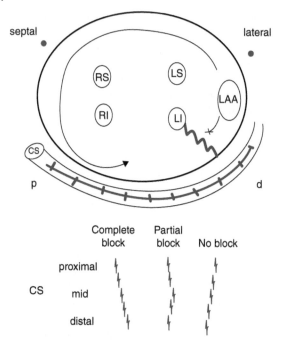

Figure 12.8 Confirming block after ablation of the mitral isthmus for perimitral atrial flutter. Labels are the same as in Figure 12.4. A linear ablation has been performed across the isthmus between the LI and mitral valve annulus (red squiggly line). To confirm that complete block has been accomplished, pacing is performed from the LAA, and the resultant electrograms are recorded from the CS catheter. With complete block, the electrical impulse from the LAA must travel counterclockwise around the pulmonary veins in order to reach the region of the distal CS. Consequently, with complete block the CS activation pattern is proximal to distal. If the block has failed, the activation pattern is distal to proximal. With partial block, the impulse crosses the line of block but only slowly – so CS activation proceeds from both directions. See text for details.

the direction of activation is similar on both the anterior and posterior walls, then the roof is a bystander and not part of the reentrant circuit. 3-D mapping systems are useful but not necessary to confirm this activation pattern. Younger operators often rely on computerized mapping systems with multipole catheters to do this automatically. We believe, however, that it is important to confirm this activation and, more importantly, understand how the computer maps are generated.

Pacing maneuvers using entrainment will confirm roof-dependent flutter. Again, with the ablation catheter in the circuit, usually on the roof, pacing 20–30 ms faster than the tachycardia cycle length will entrain the tachycardia with concealed fusion and the PPI will be equal to the tachycardia cycle length.

With the aid of the 3-D mapping system, ablation of the roof is straightforward. The catheter is positioned at either the right upper or left upper pulmonary vein, and ablation is performed by moving the catheter across the superior aspect of the roof by a few millimeters every 30 seconds. Diminution of atrial electrograms, confirming that electrical block is being created, is easy to observe on the roof. Termination of the flutter (or a change in flutter morphology) often occurs before the roof block is complete. It is important to finish creating the linear block even after the arrhythmia terminates, and then confirm that the block is complete by pacing on either side of the line. An easy way to confirm block across the roof is to pace from the left atrial appendage and record from the posterior wall. The latest electrogram should be closest to the line in the superior posterior left atrium. That is because when the roof is blocked, activation proceeds down the anterior wall, around the floor and up the posterior wall.

Ablating the left atrial roof requires special precautions. The roof can be a thin-walled structure, and the superior posterior aspects of the left atrium can be close to the esophagus. It is not necessary to use high-wattage outputs during the ablation. Some experts advocate for the use of esophageal temperature monitoring during the ablation, to help avoid a serious complication.

Left atrial anterior wall flutter

The left atrial anterior wall is not usually targeted during procedures for atrial fibrillation. However, this area can harbor areas of low voltage and fibrosis, which can serve as barriers for macro- or microreentry. Patients susceptible to this pathology, and thus to left anterior wall flutter, tend to be older, female and more often have persistent or long-standing persistent AF. Although these anterior circuits can occur spontaneously, they usually are seen in patients who have had previous linear ablation along the left atrial roof and mitral isthmus.

3-D electroanatomic mapping is useful but not necessary for ablation of these circuits. The characteristic features of these arrhythmias include low-voltage, fractionated potentials in the anterior wall. Sometimes the entire tachycardia circuit localizes to the anterior wall. Pacing maneuvers confirm concealed entrainment and the PPI is equal to the tachycardia cycle length from these areas of abnormal substrate.

Experts do not agree on the best approach for ablating these arrhythmias. Some recommend focal ablation in the critical isthmus, and others suggest that an anterior line be created from the mitral isthmus to the right superior pulmonary vein. Either approach can create problems, hence the controversy.

The problem with focal ablation is that it creates an opportunity for recurrent flutter rotating around a new barrier of anterior scar. (In this light, the lack of reinduction of flutter after ablation may not be predictive of success.) The problem with creating anterior lines of block is that, in the presence of new or preexisting roof and mitral isthmus lines of block, left atrial appendage isolation may result, or left atrial contractility can be compromised, or both – again, creating a substrate for thrombus. Ablation in the anterior wall often leads to activation of the appendage *after* the QRS, and hence after ventricular systole. With such an extreme delay in left atrial activation, the hemodynamic contribution of atrial systole to cardiac output must necessarily be compromised and, to the extent that it occurs simultaneously with ventricular syncope, atrial systole may become counterproductive.

Even worse than delaying the appendage activation is isolating the appendage. While this often prevents future flutters, it renders the appendage noncontractile and even more of a potential nidus for clot formation. Numerous studies have found that patients with an electrically isolated appendage are at very high risk of stroke with even transient interruption of oral anticoagulation.

Other left atrial flutters

Rarely, after extensive ablations in the left atrium, microreentry can occur in the intraatrial septum, left atrial appendage, and coronary sinus. The approach to these arrhythmias is similar to that for anterior wall flutter.

De Novo left atrial flutter

The heart of the electrophysiologist sinks a bit when the coronary sinus catheter shows distal-to-proximal activation in a patient who has had neither heart surgery nor previous ablation in the left atrium.

This pattern indicates the patient has a *de novo* left atrial flutter. These are very challenging arrhythmias, because almost all these patients have significant atrial substrate disease – why else would they have macroreentrant atrial flutter?

Unlike CTI-dependent flutter, left atrial flutter can use any of the macroreentrant circuits previously discussed, and in addition they may have reentry around either or both the nonisolated pulmonary veins. What is more, no atrial flutter occurs spontaneously. All atrial flutter requires triggering from premature atrial beats or, more commonly, short bursts of atrial fibrillation. Thus, when ablating these *de novo* flutters, it is usually necessary to perform pulmonary vein isolation in addition to whatever other ablation lesions may be needed. This combination can make for a long day in the laboratory, and achieving adequate control of the arrhythmia is substantially less likely than it is with most other forms of atrial flutter.

Indeed, the ablation of these *de novo* flutters should only be undertaken after much circumspect thought. Given the underlying atrial structural disease that is virtually always present, the need for extensive ablation, and the high recurrence rates, more conservative management of the arrhythmia – possibly including atrioventricular node ablation with pacemaker placement – is very often a more reasonable alternative.

13

Conduction System Pacing

Cardiac pacing is one of the purest forms of medical practice: patients with symptomatic bradycardia need our help, and pacing provides it. A properly placed pacemaker resolves the problem, whether it was due to sinus nodal, AV nodal or His–Purkinje disease. Patients who had been suffering often feel better immediately after a pacemaker is implanted.

Still, since the invention and refinement of catheter ablation, cardiac pacing hasn't generated much intellectual enthusiasm amongst electrophysiologists. That is, not until the advent of conduction system pacing. The ability to place pacing leads in the region of the His bundle or left bundle branch (LBB) has reignited excitement in pacing. Conduction system pacing as a field is rapidly evolving. In this chapter, we will provide an overview of the basics, what is known currently, and some educated guesses on what the future holds.

Standard RV pacing

For decades, electrophysiologists have placed pacing leads into the right ventricular muscle. This can be done with an active fixation (screw in) or passive fixation (tined) lead. The electrode at the distal tip of the pacing lead senses cardiac activity, and if it does not "see" a native beat within the programmed time (e.g., 1 second for a lower rate of 60 beats per minute), the pacemaker delivers a stimulus down the lead that then captures the local myocardium at the tip.

Once the local myocardium is activated (or captured), the wave of depolarization propagates by muscle-to-muscle conduction to the RV and LV (Figure 13.1). Because the right ventricle is depolarized first, and because the wave of conduction bypasses the rapidly conducting

Fogoros' Electrophysiologic Testing, Seventh Edition. Richard N. Fogoros and John M. Mandrola.
© 2023 John Wiley & Sons Ltd. Published 2023 by John Wiley & Sons Ltd.

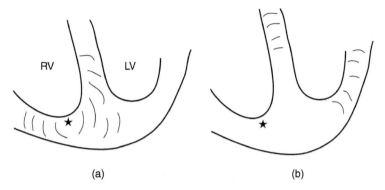

Figure 13.1 Asynchronous ventricular depolarization with right ventricular pacing. (a) The wave of depolarization during the first 50–100 ms following delivery of a pacing impulse to the right ventricular apex (denoted by the star). Note the depolarization wave traveling across the right ventricular and septal myocardium, well before reaching the bulk of the left ventricle. (b) The wave of depolarization 125–150 ms after the paced impulse. The bulk of the left ventricle and the rest of the ventricular septum are finally being depolarized. Because the right ventricle is stimulated first, and because the depolarization wave is propagated muscle-to-muscle and not via the Purkinje system, ventricular depolarization takes a relatively long time, and is asynchronous.

His–Purkinje system, left ventricular depolarization is relatively late. This results in a very wide QRS complex with a left bundle branch block (LBBB) morphology.

The problem with RV pacing

Because standard RV pacing depolarizes the heart from right to left via muscle-to-muscle conduction, a dyssynchronous ventricular activation pattern occurs. Simply speaking, this means that the two ventricles contract sequentially, first the right ventricle, then the left. This is in contrast to the normal condition, in which rapid conduction through the His–Purkinje system activates the right and left ventricles nearly simultaneously. The ventricular dyssynchrony induced by RV pacing causes ventricular systole to become less efficient than normal.

In fact, while we don't fully understand the mechanism, numerous studies have found that dyssynchronous activation of the heart through standard RV pacing can cause left ventricular dysfunction. Estimates of RV pacing-induced cardiomyopathy range from 12% to

20%. As a result, cardiac resynchronization therapy (CRT) is often used to correct pacing-induced cardiomyopathy, just as it is for other kinds of heart failure characterized by ventricular dyssynchrony. (CRT is discussed in detail in Chapter 14.)

The promise of conduction system pacing

The major advantage of conduction system pacing is that it avoids the dyssynchrony problem. It does this by activating the right and left ventricles simultaneously, via the rapidly conducting His–Purkinje system.

Until recently, conduction system pacing would have meant His bundle pacing. Now, however, most electrophysiologists perform conduction system pacing by pacing the left bundle branch area (LBBA) on the left side of the septum.

His bundle pacing

During normal cardiac activation, as described in Chapter 4, the cardiac impulse first travels through atrium to the compact AV node, which is on the atrial aspect of the tricuspid annulus. The His bundle starts just after the AV node, still on the atrial aspect, and is contained within the central fibrous body. See Figure 1.1.

The anatomy varies a lot, with some His bundles quite superficial and others deeper within fibrous tissue. The varied anatomy explains the ease or difficulty in placing pacing leads in this area. Obviously, a relatively superficial His bundle is easier to capture.

The His bundle then traverses the membranous septum on the right side of heart. After a few millimeters, it penetrates the septum at the top of the muscular septum and then breaks into RBB and LBB. The LBB stays in the subendocardium and then undergoes extensive arborization.

His bundle pacing involves placing a specialized (usually, but not exclusively) thin lumenless lead on either the atrial or ventricular side of the tricuspid valve. It is a challenging area in which to place leads, and often requires specialized sheaths that direct the lead toward the septum.

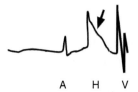

A   H   V

Figure 13.2 Current of His bundle injury with His bundle pacing lead. A His bundle electrogram is shown as recorded from a His bundle pacing lead. Note the current of injury (arrow) following the His spike on this electrogram. This injury current is a good sign that the lead is well placed for reliable His bundle pacing.

The operator aims to record a small atrial deflection, a visible His deflection and ideally a large ventricular deflection. The lead is then rotated to actively fixate it in that position. A good sign is a current of injury after the His deflection, indicating firm fixation. Pacing and sensing thresholds are then obtained (Figure 13.2).

The operator then observes the paced QRS. The ideal outcomes are shown in Figure 13.3. A nonselective response, in which the pacemaker captures a small amount of septal myocardium as well as the His bundle, results in a QRS akin to preexcitation over an accessory pathway. The initial QRS has a slight slur in the upstroke, representing capture of the peri-His septal myocardium, then becomes sharp and narrow as the His bundle itself is depolarized.

A selective response occurs when the His bundle itself is directly captured. The electrogram shows a pacing spike, then a very brief

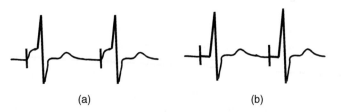

(a)   (b)

Figure 13.3 Nonselective and selective capture with His bundle pacing. Lead V6 is depicted in both panels. (a) Nonselective pacing, in which the pacing lead is in the near vicinity of the His bundle. Note the delta wave-like slurring of the upstroke of the QRS complex, immediately following the pacing spike. This early electrical activity represents capture of the septal myocardium near the His bundle. (b) Selective His bundle pacing, in which no septal myocardium is captured directly by the pacing lead. Both selective and nonselective capture are considered acceptable for chronic His bundle pacing.

isoelectric phase (of a duration equal to the HV interval, usually 30–50 ms), followed by a narrow QRS. The tip of the electrode is fixated in the His bundle and captures only the specialized conduction system, without any direct capture of ventricular myocardium.

Studies looking at left ventricular function and clinical outcomes suggest that both selective and nonselective His bundle pacing perform similarly in terms of preventing dyssynchronous contraction of the two ventricles.

A fascinating discovery from His bundle pacing has been its ability to correct LBBB. This seems counterintuitive because the His bundle is "north" of the left bundle. You would expect that capture of the His would still run into the block in the more distal left bundle. But the situation turns out to be more complex than we have traditionally envisioned. His bundle pacing has led to the discovery that there are protected fibers that traverse the conduction system. Conducting fibers within the His bundle that are destined for the left and right bundles become segregated from one another, within the His bundle itself. So LBBB may occur at any level once segregation of these protected fibers occurs, even before the His splits into its two main bundle branches. So His bundle pacing may actually capture distal to the level of LBBB or it may capture local fibers that bypass the block (Figure 13.4).

His bundle pacing is effective, but it is associated with several limitations. His bundle pacing can be hard to perform. The anatomy of the His region varies a lot, and successfully pacing the His bundle requires a long learning curve. In addition, His bundle pacing often results in higher pacing thresholds, which can increase further over time. This leads to lower battery life of the pacemaker and the need for more generator change surgeries, which then expose the patient to added risk.

Another problem with His bundle pacing is with sensing – both oversensing of the atrial or His signal (leading to inhibition of pacing) and undersensing of the ventricular signal. Sensing issues arise because the area around the tricuspid annulus often has large atrial signals and small ventricular signals.

Finally, while His bundle pacing can overcome a LBBB, this often requires a high-voltage pacing stimulus to capture the committed fibers within the fibrotic tissue. This too can cause premature battery depletion.

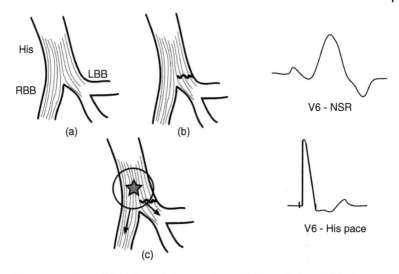

Figure 13.4 How His bundle pacing can overcome left bundle branch block (LBBB). (a) The His bundle is composed of individual protected Purkinje fibers that eventually divide into the left and right bundle branches. (b) In many cases of LBBB, the site of block is actually located in the distal His bundle. This panel shows such a case. Here, a block in the distal His bundle interrupts the left-sided His fibers, producing LBBB proximal to the LBB itself. (c) How His bundle pacing may overcome this type of LBBB. The site of pacing is depicted by the star, and the area captured by the pacing impulse is shown by the circle surrounding the star. In this example, left-sided His fibers distal to the site of block are captured by the pacing impulse, and as a result there is no LBBB in the paced beat. The electrograms to the right of (a), (b) and (c) show lead V6 during normal sinus rhythm (NSR), demonstrating LBBB, and with His bundle pacing, showing resolution of the LBBB.

Left bundle area pacing

While His bundle pacing has become a useful way of achieving effective conduction system pacing, because of its several limitations it has now largely been supplanted by a different technique – LBBA pacing. With LBBA pacing, the pacing lead is placed distally to the His bundle, in the region where the LBB branches into its major components (Figure 13.5).

Figure 13.5 shows the basic anatomy of the LBB relative to the septum. The idea behind pacing the left bundle area stems from both

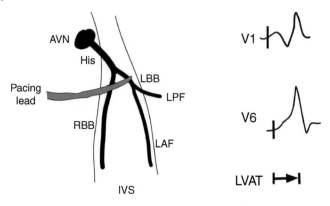

Figure 13.5 Left bundle branch area pacing. The diagram on the left shows the optimal positioning of the pacing lead to achieve left bundle branch area pacing (LBBAP). The tip of the pacing lead penetrates the intraventricular septum (IVS), and is directed to an area distal to the division of the His bundle into the right and left bundle branches (RBB and LBB), close to the point where the LBB divides into its anterior (LAF) and posterior fascicles (LPF). Pacing from this area will achieve immediate capture of the LBB, along with adjacent septal myocardium. The electrograms on the right of this figure confirm LBBAP. Leads V1 and V6 are depicted. LBBAP is confirmed during pacing by demonstrating a qR or rsR' configuration in lead V1, and rapid left ventricular capture, as demonstrated by a short left ventricular activation time (LVAT) of less than 80 ms. The LVAT is measured from the pacing spike to the peak of the R-wave in lead V6.

geography and physiology. Geographically, if you successfully pace the left bundle, you are distal to the level of the block. Physiologically, pacing the left bundle preserves the normal left-to-right septal activation and prevents the delayed left ventricular activation seen in LBBB or standard right ventricular pacing.

Mechanistic studies confirm that pacing in the area of or directly on the left bundle provides the same synchrony of contraction that is seen in His bundle pacing. This, of course, would be exactly what one would expect given that pacing in the left bundle prevents delayed LV activation.

Figure 13.5 also shows the typical pattern of LBB activation. Lead VI shows a pattern seen in RBBB and lead V6 shows that the time from stimulus to peak of the R wave is short (less than 80 ms is felt to be enough to avoid LV delay and dyssynchrony). The time from stimulus to peak of the R wave in V6 indicates the initial forces of depolarization that are traveling to the LV lateral wall.

Operators accomplish left bundle area pacing by placing a lead about 1–2 cm past the His bundle area on the septum and then actively fixating the lead deep into the septum. This usually requires a sheath and a fair amount of active fixation force. You can see the tip of the lead develop a bit of a "beak-like" appearance on X-ray.

There are many advantages of left bundle area pacing. These include a technically easier implant. There is minimal to no mapping for signals. We use anatomy to guide placement of the sheath. Differently shaped sheaths are now available to accommodate varied anatomy. Another major advantage of left bundle area pacing is the robust pacing parameters that are usually achieved. Because the lead is in the septum, there are no atrial signals to oversense and there are large ventricular signals. Pacing thresholds in this area are low, which translates to less battery drain and longer times between generator changes.

While there is great excitement surrounding left bundle area pacing, there remain uncertainties. We do not know whether leads placed in the septum will have the same longevity as standard leads. Some experts worry about the hinge-like effect of the tip of the lead over the course of decades. Will this cause early lead failure?

While left bundle branch area pacing leads to pleasingly narrow QRS complexes, and early studies suggest synchronization is similar to His bundle pacing, there are minimal data on clinical outcomes.

Cardiac resynchronization therapy (see Chapter 14) with biventricular pacing has been thoroughly studied in blinded trials that have delivered impressive clinical benefits. We do not have these sorts of studies for conduction system pacing. At the time of writing, exciting news has come that the US government has funded a large multicenter outcomes trial of conduction system pacing vs CRT in patients eligible for CRT. In the years to come, we will learn whether clinical results with this technique compare favorably to the standard of CRT with biventricular pacing.

14

Cardiac Resynchronization: Pacing Therapy for Heart Failure

Electrophysiologists have always been intrigued with the notion that, somehow, pacemakers can improve the function of the failing heart. When permanent pacemakers were first developed, many thought that they would be able to improve cardiac function in patients with heart failure simply by increasing the heart rate. Since cardiac output equals stroke volume times heart rate, they reasoned that pacing the heart a little faster ought to increase cardiac output. What they failed to realize (hemodynamics never being the strong suit of most electrophysiologists) was that the heart does not determine the cardiac output; the body does. The heart merely responds to the metabolic demands of the body. So, unless a patient is in overt low-output failure at rest, increasing the resting heart rate does not appreciably increase cardiac output. Instead, since the heart can only pump whatever volume of blood the body returns to it, the stroke volume falls; the cardiac output remains the same, only now at the cost of an increased heart rate and higher cardiac workload. If anything, patients with heart failure feel worse with pacemaker-induced rapid heart rates.

Then, a few years later, when dual-chambered pacemakers became available, many electrophysiologists decided to goose the other determinant of cardiac output – the stroke volume – by figuring out how to optimize the AV delay. This goal proved elusive. Attempts at optimizing the AV delay generated a confusion of literature – some experts proposing shorter AV delays, others proposing longer ones – that successfully boosted a few academic careers but not in any reliable way the cardiac function of patients with heart failure.

So, we can readily understand why, when yet another attempt at improving heart failure with pacing therapy was proposed in the

Fogoros' Electrophysiologic Testing, Seventh Edition. Richard N. Fogoros and John M. Mandrola.
© 2023 John Wiley & Sons Ltd. Published 2023 by John Wiley & Sons Ltd.

mid-1990s, it was initially viewed with great skepticism. This time, however, the pacing therapy worked.

Cardiac resynchronization therapy

How it works

Cardiac resynchronization therapy (CRT) is aimed at improving the disordered patterns of ventricular contraction – referred to as ventricular dyssynchrony – seen in some patients with heart failure. CRT is accomplished by pacing both ventricles simultaneously, or the left ventricle alone, in order to improve the coordination and efficiency of ventricular contraction.

CRT pacemakers have three pacing leads instead of two: a right atrial lead, a right ventricular lead, and a left ventricular lead. They work similarly to DDD pacemakers except for two things. First, with CRT pacing, in most cases *both* ventricles are paced instead of just the right ventricle. Second, biventricular pacing itself, rather than rate support, is the primary desired therapy – CRT pacemakers are thus programmed to pace virtually 100% of the time, under all conditions.

CRT pacemakers are used to correct ventricular dyssynchrony. Ventricular dyssynchrony is most obviously present in patients with wide QRS complexes. Since the QRS complex reflects the activation sequence of the ventricular muscle, a wide QRS complex indicates that the ventricles are being activated abnormally. Specifically, a bundle branch block implies that one ventricle is being activated before the other – that is, the ventricles are being activated sequentially instead of simultaneously.

This sort of ventricular dyssynchrony may not produce any noticeable hemodynamic consequences in people with otherwise normal hearts. But in patients with systolic dysfunction, ventricular dyssynchrony can produce enough inefficiency in ventricular contraction to cause or worsen symptoms of heart failure and, potentially, can exacerbate ventricular remodeling and a further reduction in the ventricular ejection fraction. In these cases, by pacing both ventricles simultaneously, one can often resynchronize ventricular contraction sufficiently to improve ventricular efficiency, reduce symptoms, and improve clinical outcomes.

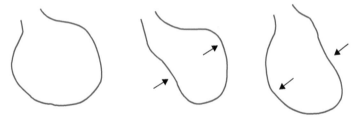

Figure 14.1 How ventricular dyssynchrony causes reduced ventricular function. The three panels in this figure illustrate left ventricular systole in a patient with cardiomyopathy and LBBB. The panel on the left shows the dilated left ventricle at end-diastole. The middle panel shows the first 60 ms of systole. Here, the left ventricular septum (which is activated along with the right ventricle) is already contracting, but the left ventricular free wall has not yet been activated. In fact, the free wall bulges outward. The panel on the right shows the last 60 ms of systole. The left ventricular free wall is now finally being activated but now the septum, which has already finished contracting, is pushed outward. As a result of this dyssynchrony, with each systole much of the energy expended by this diseased ventricle is applied toward creating a useless, swaying, "hula"-type movement, instead of toward ejecting blood into the aorta.

Figure 14.1 illustrates how left ventricular dyssynchrony caused by left bundle branch block (LBBB) can affect ventricular function in a patient with heart failure. The panel on the left shows a dilated left ventricle at end-diastole. The middle panel shows the first 60 ms of systole. Here, the septum (which is activated along with the right ventricle) is already contracting, but the left ventricular free wall has not yet been activated (due to the bundle branch block). In fact, the left free wall bulges outward. The panel on the right shows the last 60 ms of systole. The left ventricular free wall has finally been activated and is contracting but now the septum, which has already finished contracting, is pushed outward. As a result, with each systole, much of the precious energy being expended by this diseased ventricle is used to create a useless, swaying, "hula"-type movement, swishing blood around inside the cardiac chamber instead of ejecting it out into the aorta.

Figure 14.2 illustrates how CRT might benefit such a ventricle. The panel on the left again shows the same dilated left ventricle at end-diastole. The panel on the right shows what happens when biventricular pacing is activated. Here, the right and left ventricles are paced simultaneously; both the septum and the left ventricular free wall contract at the same time. The energy expended by the ventricle

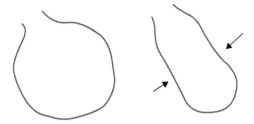

Figure 14.2 How biventricular pacing improves ventricular function. The two panels in this figure illustrate how biventricular pacing improves the function of the dyssynchronous, cardiomyopathic left ventricle illustrated in Figure 14.1. The panel on the left shows the dilated left ventricle at end-diastole. The panel on the right shows what happens when biventricular pacing is activated. Here, the right and left ventricles are paced simultaneously; both the septum and the left ventricular free wall contract at the same time. The energy expended by the ventricle now goes toward ejecting the blood, instead of merely swishing it around inside the cardiac chamber. Ventricular contraction becomes much more efficient and effective.

now goes toward ejecting blood. Ventricular contraction becomes much more efficient and effective.

Between 20% and 30% of patients with congestive heart failure have intraventricular conduction delays, and in many if not most of these, it is left ventricular activation that is delayed.

The effects of CRT

Several clinical studies have documented the benefits of CRT in appropriately selected patients.

Hemodynamic effects

CRT has consistently yielded improved hemodynamic function in patients with heart failure and LBBB, including improved cardiac output and cardiac index, increased aortic pulse pressure, and reduced pulmonary capillary wedge pressure.

Contractility

Measures of left ventricular contractility improve with CRT, including enhanced global contraction and increased left ventricular ejection fractions. In contrast to other forms of therapy that have boosted ventricular contractility in patients with heart failure (such as the inotropic agents amrinone and milrinone), CRT actually *reduces* myocardial energy expenditure. Thus, ventricular contraction is not only more effective but also more efficient.

Reverse remodeling

Remodeling of the left ventricle – manifested by ventricular dilation, increased ventricular mass, and reduced ejection fraction – is a fundamental response to reduced systolic function. In essence, the cardiac enlargement that occurs with remodeling is a compensatory mechanism which allows the ventricle to eject a near-normal stroke volume despite reduced contractility. Aside from the fact that remodeling itself is ultimately harmful, the degree of remodeling reflects the degree of systolic dysfunction.

CRT has been demonstrated to reverse left ventricular remodeling. Specifically, it has been shown to reduce the end-systolic and end-diastolic dimensions of the left ventricle, as well as the left ventricular mass. This reverse remodeling is thought to reflect a fundamental improvement in ventricular systolic function.

Clinical studies with CRT

Numerous clinical trials have now been completed to assess the benefits of CRT in patients with heart failure due to systolic dysfunction. These trials have demonstrated that patients with symptomatic heart failure due to left ventricular dysfunction and left ventricular delay benefit from CRT. That said, there are gray areas. Most of these stem from the fact that the QRS duration from an ECG is merely a surrogate for left ventricular activation. Certainly, when there is typical LBBB and a long-duration QRS ($\geq 150\,ms$), one can be reasonably assured that lateral LV wall activation is delayed and the electrical therapy from CRT will prove beneficial.

But what about cases in which LBBB is present but the QRS duration is less than 150 ms? The result of CRT here is harder to predict because, while there is some degree of delay in left ventricular activation, correcting this lesser amount of delay with an LV lead may not improve ventricular dysfunction very much.

What if there is a wide QRS but not a typical LBBB morphology? This could mean the delay is in muscle-to-muscle conduction instead of in the bundle branches, and a left ventricular lead may not substantially correct this delay. This type of conduction disturbance is often seen in patients with prior myocardial infarction. Another gray area is that most of the studies underpinning CRT were done in patients with sinus rhythm. But patients with atrial fibrillation can also have LBBB, and develop the same problems with dyssynchrony. Should these patients have the option of CRT despite the lack of supporting clinical trials? Most electrophysiologists think the data gathered in patients with sinus rhythm also apply to patients with atrial fibrillation.

When CRT is used in patients with atrial fibrillation, there is an additional challenge related to heart rate. Namely, if the heart rate increases beyond the pacing rate of the CRT, the pacemaker will be inhibited, and there will be no correction of dyssynchrony. It makes no sense for a CRT to be in place and not be pacing. So if CRT is to be used in a patient with atrial fibrillation with a frequently rapid ventricular response, every step ought to be taken to control the heart rate, including AV node ablation to create permanent AV block. This then permits 100% CRT pacing.

Implanting CRT devices

The difference between implanting a CRT device and a pacemaker (or between implanting a CRT-D device and an ICD) is the need to place an additional lead for left ventricular pacing.

Left ventricular pacing is usually accomplished by placing a pacing lead in the coronary sinus. A variety of tools are available for placement of specially designed pacing leads in the coronary venous system. These tools allow the electrophysiologist to rapidly and safely insert left ventricular pacing leads via the coronary sinus. In most cases, these leads can be placed, positioned, and tested in 30 minutes or less.

In placing left-sided leads, the os of the coronary sinus is generally first engaged with an introducer designed specifically for this purpose. Dye is injected to visualize the cardiac venous system. A "target" vein is identified. A pacing lead is chosen whose handling characteristics are likely to suit the anatomy of the target vein, and is then inserted and positioned.

It is critical that this vein go to the left ventricle, preferably to the area of the left ventricle that is activated last. Remember, CRT is essentially preexcitation of the part of the left ventricle that is activated latest.

Usually, but not always, the geographic distance between the RV lead and LV lead is a decent marker of a good target. When possible, an operator can measure the activation time from RV to LV, and then place the lead at the latest site.

Operators should always use a left anterior oblique view to assure that the vein goes to the lateral left ventricle. Unfortunately, even today it is not rare for a coronary sinus lead to be placed into an anterior vein, which essentially paces the RV and thus does not correct dyssynchrony.

Figure 14.3 shows an AP and lateral chest X-ray of a patient whose CS lead was mispositioned. This patient did not respond to CRT. In the AP projection, the leads look well separated but in the lateral projection, you can see that the CS lead overlies the right ventricle. Thus, there is no resynchronization. The lateral film – which can be approximated in the lab with a steep LAO projection – is crucial to assure LV placement of the CS lead. Anything posterior to the dotted line in this figure is usually acceptable.

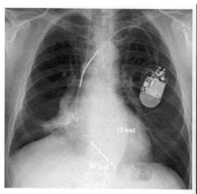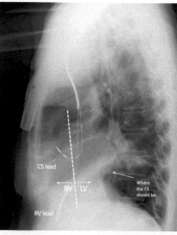

Figure 14.3 PA and lateral chest X-ray demonstrating mispositioning of a CS lead. In the PA projection (left panel), the positioning of the RV lead and CS lead appears to be adequate. However, the lateral projection (right panel) shows that the CS lead has been placed into an anterior branch of the CS, and is actually pacing the right ventricle. The dotted line in the right panel demonstrates the approximate division between the right and left ventricles. When placing a CS lead for resynchronization therapy, it is important to check the LAO projection to assure the CS lead is placed posteriorly.

When testing the left-sided lead, the operator looks for adequate R-wave voltage, pacing threshold, and impedance measurements, but also for evidence of diaphragmatic stimulation – the most common problem with pacing from the coronary veins. This problem occurs because the left phrenic nerve traverses near the lateral LV epicardium. If the pacing lead is in close proximity, the stimulus may capture the phrenic nerve, leading to uncomfortable diaphragm stimulation.

In years past, diaphragmatic stimulation meant moving the lead. That was a problem because manipulating the lead increased the risk of dislodgment. Most coronary sinus leads now have four pacing electrodes (quadripolar), and this allows the operator to "electronically reposition" by changing the vector configurations of available electrodes.

Complications from CRT

Coronary sinus perforation and subsequent pericardial tamponade is the most feared procedural complication unique to left-sided lead placement. Additional complications with CRT implantation include diaphragmatic pacing, pneumothorax, and infection.

Unresolved issues with CRT

Responders versus nonresponders

From the very earliest days of CRT therapy, doctors took note of the fact that many patients with heart failure who received these devices had very dramatic responses. These patients improved rapidly from NYHA class III to I, or from class IV to II, and were able to accomplish physical tasks they had not been able to perform for months or years. These patients were exceedingly grateful for their new lease of life and, accordingly, the doctors were exceedingly gratified. Such patients were quickly deemed to be "responders" or even "super-responders." Roughly 40–60% of patients who receive indicated CRT devices for heart failure fall into this category.

Naturally, patients who did not have such dramatic improvements in well-being began to be regarded as "nonresponders." This designation is probably unfortunate. The tendency to consider the lack of a dramatic response to CRT as equivalent to a lack of any meaningful response is shortsighted. It seems very unlikely that CRT will produce an "all-or-nothing" effect, where either patients have remarkable, raising-the-dead-style symptomatic improvement or no improvement at all. More likely, some patients are benefited by CRT in a more subtle way, such that, while they may not feel dramatically better, the "trajectory" of their illness improves, so that they have fewer hospitalizations over a given period of time or an improvement in mortality.

As it turns out, these more subtle benefits of CRT are the very benefits that the randomized trials were designed to measure. From these trials, the magnitude of overall benefit to the population probably cannot be explained by the proportion of patients who (if the "responder"/"nonresponder" parameter had been tabulated) would have been classified as "responders." For instance, in the CARE-HF study (Cleland JG et al., N Engl J Med 2005;352:15390), mortality in the CRT group was reduced by 33%, a magnitude that would be very difficult to attribute to the 50% or so who likely responded "dramatically" to the therapy. More likely, this impressive benefit in CARE-HF was distributed among both "dramatic responders" and "nondramatic responders."

How much QRS delay is needed?

While it is sometimes difficult to predict the magnitude of response from CRT, it has become clear that CRT provides no benefit to patients with a narrow QRS. A trial called EchoCRT (Ruschitzka F et al., N Engl J Med 2013;369:1395) tested CRT in patients with narrow QRS complexes but dyssynchrony detected by echocardiography. The trial was stopped early for futility and there was a trend toward higher death rates in the CRT arm.

This result makes sense because CRT is quite simply an electrical therapy. If ventricular dyssynchrony is not related to an electrical delay, then CRT cannot help.

One caveat of this trial was the fact that while the entry criteria included a QRS ≤130 ms, the mean QRS duration of the enrolled patients in the trial was substantially lower than this cutoff value – 105 ms. This sets up a gray area around 130 ms. While we can say with confidence that patients with QRS duration of 105 ms clearly do not benefit, there remains uncertainty for those with QRS durations closer to 130 ms who have left bundle branch patterns.

Right bundle branch block

As discussed earlier, a typical right bundle branch block delays activation of the right ventricle. The LV is not delayed. CRT, therefore, would be unlikely to benefit these patients.

We write "unlikely" because some wide QRS patterns can have a right bundle branch appearance but there can actually be left ventricular delay. These cases are uncommon and difficult to sort out, but in general are associated with very wide QRS complexes.

Optimization of CRT

Beyond the original notion that pacing the ventricles simultaneously will help to resynchronize dyssynchronous ventricular contraction, relatively little has been accomplished so far in systematically studying how the benefits of CRT might be optimized in each individual patient. Several methods for optimizing CRT have been proposed and, if developed sufficiently, one or more of these might improve the overall benefits of CRT.

AV interval

In general, a relatively short AV delay (between 90 and 120 ms) is used with CRT pacing, to diminish native AV conduction and maximize biventricular pacing, and some studies have correlated these short AV delays with better clinical outcomes.

Shortened AV delays may not be optimal for every patient, however. In patients with intraatrial conduction delays, for instance, a short AV interval may cause the left ventricle to contract before left atrial contraction is completed. Some clinicians conduct "AV optimization" procedures with echocardiography in an attempt to maximize LV performance with CRT therapy. Studies have not demonstrated a group benefit in doing such AV optimization, but it is possible that some individual patients might benefit from it.

VV interval

Classically, CRT is accomplished by pacing the left ventricle simultaneously with right ventricular activation (or pacing). However, it may be the case that different timing sequences between the two ventricles (the VV interval) would improve the efficacy of CRT in some patients. Data exist, for instance, suggesting that in some patients, pacing only the left ventricle (in advance of any right ventricular activation) might be better than biventricular pacing.

The VV interval ought to be viewed as a continuum of potential ventricular activation sequences, all the way from right ventricular-only pacing (i.e., the pacing mode used in all "standard" pacemakers) to left ventricular-only pacing. For all we know, the optimal VV interval may vary from patient to patient or even within the same patient.

CRT devices exist today that allow the physician to vary the VV interval. The makers of the CRT devices now provide optimization algorithms. In many cases, the algorithm appears to maximize synchrony. We caution, however, that part of good CRT management is making sure that the algorithm is indeed working. This can be accomplished in the clinic by recording 12-lead ECGs and observing QRS duration and morphology while pacing with different VV intervals.

Should CRT be the standard mode of pacing?

If spontaneous LBBB produces ventricular dyssynchrony, and is thus detrimental to patients with systolic heart failure, then would not iatrogenic LBBB created by right ventricular pacing also be detrimental to these patients? Is it really a good idea for patients who require pacing most or all of the time to have LBBB-inducing right ventricular pacing – especially patients with systolic dysfunction?

In the BLOCK HF trial (Curtis AB et al., N Engl J Med 2013;368:1585), patients with class I, II, or III heart failure and left ventricular ejection fractions of 50% or below, and who needed pacemakers for AV block, received CRT pacemakers. They were then randomized to receive biventricular or right ventricular pacing. After 3 years, the clinical outcomes (mortality, urgent heart failure therapy, or worsening ventricular function) were significantly better in the biventricular pacing group.

In summary, CRT pacing appears to be superior to right ventricular pacing in patients with moderate heart failure who are likely to be in a paced rhythm most of the time.

The notion of CRT pacing for all has great allure because it would prevent dyssynchrony and provide better cardiac contraction. The problems with this thinking are that CRT is not free. CRT adds cost, complexity, and likely lower battery life of the generator. What is more, most patients with standard RV pacing do not develop pacing-induced cardiomyopathy.

In the coming years, conduction system pacing, discussed in Chapter 13, may reduce the risk of pacing-induced cardiomyopathy, and in some cases may provide the same synchronizing effect as CRT – with one ventricular lead rather than two. The only way to sort out these questions is with trials – which are in the planning stage.

15

The Evaluation of Syncope

The evaluation of patients with syncope (sudden transient loss of consciousness and posture) has classically been difficult. This challenge stems from the very nature of syncope itself: syncope occurs most often in a sporadic and relatively unpredictable fashion, and between episodes, patients with syncope often appear to be (and frequently are) quite normal. Worse, almost no patient with syncope is wearing a heart monitor at the time!

Electrophysiologists are regularly involved in the evaluation of patients with syncope for two reasons: first, cardiac arrhythmias are often either a direct cause or a prominent feature of syncope. Second, techniques developed in the electrophysiology laboratory have often proven helpful in revealing the etiology of syncope. In this chapter, we review the causes of syncope and discuss the evaluation of syncope in light of the lessons that have been learned in the electrophysiology laboratory over the past few decades.

Causes of syncope

Table 15.1 lists the major causes of syncope, divided into five major categories. Diagnosing syncope associated with the first four categories depends on taking a careful history and performing a careful physical examination. The majority of patients with syncope, however, fall into the fifth category: syncope associated with cardiac arrhythmias. In most cases, therefore, the clinician is left with having to assess whether the patient has syncope directly caused by cardiac arrhythmias (bradyarrhythmias or tachyarrhythmias), or instead (and much more commonly), a variant of vasodepressor syncope, in

Fogoros' Electrophysiologic Testing, Seventh Edition. Richard N. Fogoros and John M. Mandrola.
© 2023 John Wiley & Sons Ltd. Published 2023 by John Wiley & Sons Ltd.

Table 15.1 Major causes of syncope.

Syncope from neurologic disorders

Vertebrobasilar transient ischemic attacks	Normal-pressure hydrocephalus
Subclavian steal syndrome	Seizure disorders

Syncope from metabolic disorders

Hypoxia	Hyperventilation
Hypoglycemia	

Syncope from psychiatric disorders

Panic disorders	Hysteria

Syncope from mechanical cardiac disease

Aortic stenosis	Obstructive cardiomyopathy
Mitral stenosis	Left atrial myxoma
Pulmonary stenosis	Prosthetic valve dysfunction
Global ischemia	Pulmonary embolus
Aortic dissection	Pulmonary hypertension

Syncope associated with cardiac arrhythmias

Bradyarrhythmias – sinus node dysfunction, AV conduction disease

Tachyarrhythmias – supraventricular and ventricular tachyarrhythmias

Vasodepressor syncope

which bradycardia is often a prominent, but usually not a causative, feature.

Bradyarrhythmias that cause syncope

Although bradyarrhythmias are often assumed to be a common cause of syncope, they actually cause less than 5% of syncopal episodes. Nonetheless, bradyarrhythmias are an important cause of syncope because they are always completely treatable. The evaluation of patients with bradyarrhythmias has been discussed in detail in Chapter 5. In this section, we review the causes and evaluation of bradyarrhythmias only briefly.

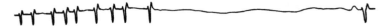

Figure 15.1 Prolonged pause following termination of atrial fibrillation. In people with both sinus nodal dysfunction and atrial fibrillation, significant overdrive suppression of the sinus node may occur during the arrhythmia. When the atrial fibrillation terminates, a prolonged asystolic period often occurs before the sinus node finally recovers, as shown in this figure. Because sinus nodal dysfunction is often associated with atrial fibrillation (so-called brady-tachy syndrome), this mechanism of syncope is much more common than usually realized.

Sinus nodal dysfunction

Abnormalities of the sinus node are common in elderly patients and are most often caused by idiopathic fibrous degeneration of the sinus node. Sinus nodal dysfunction is frequently associated with a similar fibrous degeneration of the AV conduction system, producing AV block, or of the atrial tissue, producing atrial tachyarrhythmias. Although sinus nodal disease is rarely a life-threatening disorder, the potential for serious injury or even sudden death is real in patients whose sinus nodal dysfunction is severe enough to produce syncope. When sinus node disease produces syncope, it often does so in association with a supraventricular tachycardia (as illustrated in Figure 15.1).

In most patients with syncope due to sinus nodal dysfunction, abnormalities of the sinus node are quite overt, and are usually seen during simple cardiac monitoring. In years past, electrophysiologic testing was occasionally used to investigate the sinus node. The advent of modern monitoring devices has rendered use of the invasive electrophysiologic testing mostly obsolete. Newer monitoring devices, such as patch ECG monitors, outpatient cardiac monitors, implantable loop recorders, and even smart watches, allow for the diagnosis of intermittent bradycardias.

AV block

AV nodal disease, while not uncommon, only rarely produces syncope. In contrast, block in the His–Purkinje tissue is the most common cause of syncope due to bradyarrhythmias. When syncope is due to AV block, the ECG and cardiac monitoring most often reveal clues as to the etiology of syncope. Obviously, complete heart block in a patient presenting with syncope is an indication for pacing. Second-degree AV block should also be regarded as a strong clue. Even more subtle findings that can usually be safely ignored, such as intraventricular conduction disturbances or first-degree AV block, should be regarded with a high degree of suspicion in patients presenting with syncope. In such patients, electrophysiologic testing can be strongly considered, especially if no other etiology for syncope presents itself.

Tachyarrhythmias that cause syncope

Supraventricular tachycardias

Although supraventricular tachycardias are relatively frequent arrhythmias, they only rarely cause syncope. In most cases in which syncope is associated with supraventricular tachycardia, a second condition is responsible for it. Most commonly, this second condition is sinus nodal dysfunction. In a patient with sinus nodal dysfunction, supraventricular tachycardia (usually atrial fibrillation or flutter) causes exaggerated overdrive suppression of the diseased sinus node, as described in Chapter 5. When the arrhythmia terminates, there is a prolonged sinus pause, leading to loss of consciousness (Figure 15.1).

Syncope that accompanies supraventricular tachycardias without sinus nodal dysfunction usually implies other conditions. One is the initiation of the vasodepressor reflex, in which the tachycardia itself may simply be the triggering stimulus for the vasodepressor response that produces syncope. Other possibilities include rapidly conducting tachycardia in the presence of cardiac conditions such as aortic stenosis, severe left ventricular hypertrophy or the concomitant use of blood pressure-lowering drugs, for example in patients with heart failure.

When syncope is associated with supraventricular tachycardia, loss of consciousness is frequently preceded by a prominent and unambiguous sensation of palpitations. Such a history should lead the physician immediately to suspect tachycardia as an etiology. Electrophysiologic testing should be considered early in the evaluation of such patients.

Ventricular tachyarrhythmias

Although ventricular arrhythmias were not generally recognized until the mid-1980s as a major cause of syncope, it is now apparent that these arrhythmias are frequently responsible for syncope, especially in patients with underlying cardiac disease. Ventricular tachycardia or fibrillation probably represents the cause of syncope in many patients with heart disease who present with this symptom. Because syncope due to ventricular tachyarrhythmias is a sign of impending sudden death, the new onset of syncope in patients with significant underlying heart disease should be evaluated as a medical emergency.

Syncope caused by ventricular tachyarrhythmias usually occurs suddenly and without warning, although in some patients with sustained ventricular tachycardia, the sensation of a rapid heart rate may precede loss of consciousness. The syncope can be quite fleeting, lasting only for moments, or it may present as dramatically as a self-terminating cardiac arrest. No other cause of syncope is likely to produce the type of pulseless, apneic, cyanotic patient produced by a ventricular arrhythmia. Many patients referred to electrophysiologists for syncope of unknown etiology are immediately reclassified as having had an aborted cardiac arrest after careful interrogation of witnesses.

Because most ventricular tachyarrhythmias are reentrant in nature, and because most reentrant circuits require the substrate produced by myocardial fibrosis, ventricular arrhythmias are unlikely to be the cause of syncope unless a disorder of the ventricular myocardium is present. Rarely, a normal-ventricle VT can cause syncope, such as with the long QT syndromes, Brugada syndrome, and catecholaminergic polymorphic ventricular tachycardia (see Chapter 7).

But the main point here is that when myocardial disease is present, ventricular arrhythmias must be considered as being the most likely cause of syncope until proven otherwise. In fact, the very first question a clinician must ask when evaluating a patient with syncope is whether the patient has underlying cardiac disease. If there is substantial heart disease, the focus must immediately shift away from merely preventing syncope and toward preventing sudden death.

Accordingly, if a careful history and physical examination do not yield the cause of syncope, a noninvasive cardiac workup to assess the status of the ventricular myocardium must be considered an essential part of the evaluation of the patient. If ventricular function is normal and there is no ventricular hypertrophy, ventricular arrhythmias can usually be dismissed as a cause for syncope.

If the cardiac evaluation reveals segmental wall motion abnormalities or a reduced left ventricular ejection fraction, potentially lethal ventricular arrhythmias must be strongly considered.

Ambulatory monitoring should play a relatively small role in diagnosing ventricular arrhythmias as a cause of syncope, for three reasons. First, ventricular arrhythmias producing syncope are sporadic and unpredictable. The odds of capturing a syncope-producing ventricular arrhythmia while monitoring for a few days or a few weeks are small, and in a patient with underlying cardiac disease, the absence of such arrhythmias on ambulatory monitoring should not be particularly reassuring. Second, the presence or absence of asymptomatic ventricular ectopy in such patients has extremely low specificity (so finding ectopy on ambulatory monitoring does not bring the clinician any closer to making a diagnosis). Third, once a patient with significant underlying heart disease has syncope of unclear origin, that patient must be presumed to be in imminent danger of sudden death, and the time for leisurely outpatient monitoring has passed. The patient should be evaluated as if he or she had suffered not "just" syncope, but an aborted cardiac arrest.

Once it has been determined that ventricular arrhythmias are reasonably likely to be the cause of a patient's syncope, that patient should immediately be admitted to a monitored bed until lethal ventricular tachyarrhythmias have been either definitively ruled out or adequately treated. In such patients, the electrophysiology study is often the most direct way of determining the cause of syncope and deciding on appropriate therapy.

Vasodepressor syncope

Vasodepressor syncope is by far the most common cause of syncope. The fact that vasodepressor syncope is known by so many names (including vasovagal syncope, cardioneurogenic syncope, and reflex syncope) is a reflection of the fact that its mechanism is poorly understood. To make matters worse, clinical syndromes that are almost certainly subcategories of vasodepressor syncope (Table 15.2) have often been discussed in the literature as if they were completely unique and unrelated entities. This practice has led clinicians to the widespread misconception that there must be scores of causes of syncope, and accordingly, to a widespread attitude of hopelessness when faced with a patient who has syncope. In fact, patients who

Table 15.2 Syndromes of vasodepressor syncope.

Presumed afferent pathways	Syndromes	
Gastrointestinal/ genitourinary mechanoreceptors	Micturition Defecation	Postprandial Peptic ulcer
Cerebral cortex	Panic or fright Pain	Noxious stimuli
Cranial nerves	Glossopharyngeal neuralgia	Oculovagal
Cardiopulmonary baroreceptors	Carotid sinus	Tussive
Cardiac C fibers	Valsalva Upright tilt Jacuzzi Weight lifting Trumpet playing	Postexercise Volume depletion Pacemaker syndrome Supraventricular tachycardia

are prone to vasodepressor syncope often have a history of multiple syncopal episodes, and episodes experienced by a single patient will frequently match several of the syndromes listed in Table 15.2. Recognition that these different syndromes are merely variants of the same basic mechanism leads the clinician immediately to the diagnosis in the majority of cases, and is a major step toward prescribing effective treatment.

The common denominator in all varieties of vasodepressor syncope is most likely the stimulation of the medullary vasodepressor region of the brainstem. The pathways that stimulate the vasodepressor region (afferent pathways) can arise from numerous locations – the resultant clinical syndrome has most often been named by the event that results in afferent stimulation of the medullary vasodepressor region (see Table 15.2). Once the vasodepressor region has been stimulated, that region generates efferent signals that cause both increased vagal tone (via the vagus nerve) and vasodilation (by pathways that are incompletely understood). Diminished cardiac filling and bradycardia follow, leading to syncope.

It should be recognized that although bradycardia is often a prominent feature of this type of syncope, it is only rarely as important as vasodilation in producing symptoms. This is why therapy with pacemakers is usually not of significant benefit to patients suffering from vasodepressor syncope. It is also why the authors have chosen to use the term "vasodepressor syncope" from the available plethora of names.

In many of the syndromes listed in Table 15.2, stimulation of the cardiac C fibers (mechanocardiac receptors in the left ventricle) appears to be the origin of afferent stimulation of the vasodepressor region. The C fibers are stimulated when a volume-depleted ventricle is contracting vigorously, a situation that most commonly occurs when the venous return is decreased and the sympathetic tone is high.

Vasodepressor syncope tends to have characteristic clinical features that should lead the clinician directly to the correct diagnosis. Many individuals have a predisposition to vasodepressor syncope, so episodes tend to recur periodically during a patient's lifetime. The initial episode of syncope often occurs during the patient's teen years. This history is often an important clue.

Over time, such individuals may have episodes that match several of the syndromes listed in Table 15.2. Vasodepressor syncope is most often preceded by at least a few seconds of prodromal symptoms (lightheadedness, ringing in the ears, visual disturbances, diaphoresis, and nausea are the most prominent) and almost always occurs when the patient is upright (sitting or standing). Syncope resolves almost immediately when the patient assumes the supine position (often by falling). The vasodilation tends to persist for several minutes, so that if the patient tries to get up immediately after such an episode, a second syncopal episode often occurs. A prolonged feeling of being "washed out" and unable to function is common after vasodepressor syncope and is probably related to a residual autonomic imbalance triggered by the episode; unfortunately, these postdromal symptoms may be mistaken by clinicians for a "postictal" state.

Patients who are predisposed to vasodepressor syncope will often have episodes of syncope when they are in a warm environment, when they have a viral illness, when they are dehydrated, or when they are under significant stress. The syndromes related to cardiac C fiber stimulation are relatively uncommon in patients with significant cardiac dysfunction, possibly because the C fibers are affected by myocardial disease. Not uncommonly, patients prone to vasodepressor syncope will experience a *flurry* of syncopal events over a period of days or weeks. Usually the reason for these flurries is unclear.

Obviously, given these prominent clinical features of vasodepressor syncope, taking a careful history is vitally important in making the correct diagnosis. As can be seen by studying Table 15.2, a patient's activity at the time of syncope yields strong clues as to the mechanism. Syncope that occurs while micturating, defecating, coughing, or swallowing is almost always vasodepressor in origin. The same holds for syncope associated with fright, pain, noxious stimulation, or severe emotional stress. These syncopal episodes rarely cause a diagnostic dilemma, but obtaining a history of such episodes in the past may yield clues as to the etiology of more recent and less clear-cut episodes of vasodepressor syncope. Syncope that occurs immediately after stopping prolonged or vigorous exercise is usually vasodepressor in origin (as opposed to syncope that occurs *during* vigorous exercise). In the authors' experience, syncope that occurs in a church (especially during the winter holidays, when tightly packed worshippers remain bundled in layers of cold-weather clothing) is usually due to a vasodepressor response. In a related phenomenon, syncope among members of a choir is also vasodepressor in origin in most cases. No other form of syncope is as *situational* as vasodepressor syncope.

Tilt-table testing

The upright tilt-table study can be used for determining a patient's propensity to develop vasodepressor syncope, though it is much less used in recent times. When subjected to an upright, motionless tilt, patients who have vasodepressor syncope will often develop a frank syncopal episode.

The protocol used in performing tilt-table testing varies among laboratories, but most centers tilt patients for 15–45 minutes at 60–85°. "Normal" individuals compensate for such a tilt by increasing both α- and β-adrenergic tone as a result of baroreceptor stimulation, thus compensating for the decrease in venous return. In susceptible patients, however, these compensatory mechanisms eventually collapse. In such individuals, venous return is apparently never completely compensated. Thus, sympathetic tone progressively increases until, eventually, vigorous squeezing of the relatively empty ventricles results in recruitment of the cardiac C fibers. This, in turn, causes stimulation of the medullary vasodepressor region. The result is a sudden withdrawal of sympathetic tone, a sudden increase in vagal tone, sudden vasodilation, and syncope. A positive tilt-table study therefore identifies a patient who is prone to vasodepressor syncope.

The problems with tilt-table testing are poor specificity and poor sensitivity. It can be negative in patients with vasodepressor syncope, and positive in those without vasodepressor syncope. This, and the fact that it is time-consuming and not loved by patients, are the reasons it has fallen out of favor.

Treating vasodepressor syncope

The most effective form of therapy for vasodepressor syncope is educating the patient. The patient who has had one or more vasodepressor episodes should be advised as to the types of situations that predispose to vasodepressor syncope. Aggressive hydration should be advised when the patient is exercising, suffering from a viral illness or other infectious condition, or working in a hot environment. The symptoms experienced by the patient before losing consciousness – the prodrome of vasodepressor syncope – should be stressed as a warning that syncope is imminent. The patient should be advised to immediately assume the supine position under such circumstances until the symptoms pass, in order to avoid losing consciousness. Physical counterpressure – isometric actions such as tensing the arms, strongly gripping a tennis ball or other object, or crossing the legs and tensing the abdominal muscles – can abort or delay vasodepressor syncope. If prodromal symptoms are recognized, physical counterpressure techniques can be used to prevent syncope, or at least to delay loss of consciousness long enough to assume a supine position.

With such measures, especially in patients who have infrequent episodes, often no other therapy is necessary.

Pharmacologic therapy for vasodepressor syncope is not often effective, but may be employed if education and lifestyle modifications have not worked. In fact, the authors know of no drug that has proven effective for this condition when tested against placebo control.

Because bradycardia alone is only rarely the proximate cause of syncope in the vasodepressor syndromes, pacemaker therapy prevents these episodes only rarely and is generally reserved for patients who have profound and prolonged bradycardia accompanying their episodes. These patients are usually older and often have concomitant conduction system disease. If pacemaker therapy is to be used, a dual-chamber pacemaker should be implanted to maintain AV coordination during pacing.

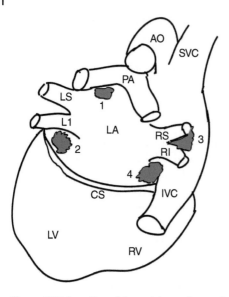

Figure 15.2 Location of the atrial ganglionated plexi. The posterior aspect of the heart is depicted, with the relative locations of the four atrial ganglionated plexi represented by the shaded areas. Shaded area one shows the superior left ganglionated plexus; shaded area two shows the inferior left ganglionated plexus; shaded area three shows the anterior right ganglionated plexus (so named because it is located anterior to the pulmonary veins); shaded area four shows the inferior right ganglionated plexus. The aorta (AO), superior vena cava (SVC), pulmonary artery (PA), left atrium (LA), left superior and left inferior pulmonary veins (LS and LI), right superior and right inferior pulmonary veins (RS and RI), inferior vena cava (IVC), left ventricle (LV), and right ventricle (RV) are also labeled.

At the time of this writing, a new but quite promising technique for using the electrophysiology laboratory is being developed for the treatment of patients with vasodepressor syndromes. The technique is called catheter ablation of the ganglionated plexi (GP), which can be considered as relay stations for neural input and output to the heart (Figure 15.2). GPs reside in the epicardial space, coincidentally in many of the same areas (pulmonary vein–left atrial junctions) that electrophysiologists ablate during atrial fibrillation ablation (see Chapter 11). The GPs contain both sympathetic and parasympathetic fibers, which influence electrical, vascular, and contractile functions of the heart.

Through a series of investigations and observations (notably, that patients who have pulmonary vein isolation for atrial fibrillation often report a slightly higher resting heart rate), various investigators have discovered that the GPs can be located and ablated. These same reports have described dramatic decreases in the frequency of vasodepressor episodes.

Because so many previously promising therapies for vasodepressor syncope have failed to pass muster when tested in placebo-controlled trials, the next step in studying this technique is comparison against a sham control. These trials are in the planning stages.

Evaluation of the patient with syncope

In the past, the evaluation of syncope centered on searching for neurologic etiologies. We cannot emphasize enough how uncommon it is for a syncope to be caused by a pure neurologic condition. This is an important notion because there is still tremendous waste of resources (and time) looking for neurologic causes of syncope. Nearly all syncopal episodes have cardiovascular causes. The physician evaluating a patient with syncope should understand this as his/her pretest prior idea.

Table 15.3 outlines a three-step approach for evaluating the patient with syncope. The most important step is to obtain a careful history and perform a physical examination. Although this step is important in the evaluation of any medical condition, it is particularly important in the patient with syncope. The history yields important clues relating to the presence of neurologic conditions, underlying cardiac conditions, and vasodepressor syncope. The authors advocate learning the exact specifics of what happened with each syncopal episode. It may seem mundane or banal to focus on historical aspects of the syncope, but the specifics are vital.

The physical examination is important in uncovering the presence of occult neurologic lesions and cardiac disorders. When you approach the patient with syncope, your attitude must be that you will not leave the bedside until a presumptive diagnosis is clear; for, once you decide that laboratory studies must be relied upon to make the diagnosis, you have got a very difficult task ahead.

The ECG is important in the patient with syncope. The presence of Q-waves, an intraventricular conduction abnormality, or ventricular arrhythmias should alert the physician to the presence of underlying cardiac disease that may predispose to lethal ventricular arrhythmias. Heart block or the presence of sinus bradycardia or sinus pauses points

Table 15.3 Evaluation of the patient with syncope.

Step 1

History and physical examination, ECG, serum electrolytes.

Step 2

If neurologic problem suspected after step 1, consider an electroencephalography (EEG), brain scan, or angiography.

If vasodepressor syncope suspected, consider further workup as necessary to rule out reversible lesions (e.g., gastrointestinal or genitourinary disease), and initiate therapy. Tilt-table testing is almost never needed.

If cardiac disease is suspected or if cause remains unclear, do noninvasive cardiac workup to assess ventricular function (echocardiogram). Where appropriate, consider treadmill testing or cardiac catheterization.

Step 3

If the cause of syncope remains unclear after step 2:

- if structural heart disease is present, do a full cardiac evaluation, then electrophysiologic testing.

- if structural heart disease is absent, consider ambulatory monitoring, treadmill testing, and observation. If syncope recurs, consider tilt-table testing and electrophysiologic testing.

---

to bradycardias as a potential etiology. A short PR interval or preexcitation indicates a bypass tract, which may be the cause of syncope. The ECG should also be examined for signs of left ventricular hypertrophy, Brugada syndrome, or a prolonged QT interval, which might indicate a propensity for torsades de pointes.

The routine performance of brain scanning or electroencephalography (EEG) has not been helpful, and these tests should not be ordered unless the history or physical examination suggests a neurologic lesion or seizures. In cases in which a seizure has occurred but the EEG is negative, tilt-table testing could be considered, because seizure-like activity can be reproduced by inducing vasodepressor syncope in some patients (thus sparing the patient the inappropriate diagnosis of epilepsy).

Tilt-table testing is not necessary in patients with a classic history for vasodepressor syncope. In these patients, therapy for vasodepressor syncope is indicated even if the tilt-table study is negative.

Exercise-related syncope is usually vasodepressor in origin in younger patients, but in older patients is more likely to be related to ventricular arrhythmias, especially if underlying cardiac disease is present. Even younger patients with exercise-related syncope should have treadmill testing, however, to look for exercise-induced arrhythmias, and echocardiograms to look for structural abnormalities that might produce syncope (especially hypertrophic cardiomyopathy).

The most important, and the most neglected, part of the evaluation of syncope is to rule out underlying cardiac disease. In middle-aged and elderly patients with syncope, especially if syncope is of recent onset, a noninvasive evaluation of ventricular function is essential. An echocardiogram is probably the most useful means of assessing cardiac function, because it also yields information relative to potential aortic outflow lesions.

Ambulatory monitoring has historically been disappointing as a means of diagnosing arrhythmic syncope. More modern recording devices are better. For instance, an implantable cardiac loop recorder (event recorder) can be helpful when transient and intermittent arrhythmias are suspected. Loop recorders are not helpful when vasodepressor syndromes are felt likely, because they invariably show profound bradycardia, and this tempts clinicians to recommend pacing. When malignant ventricular arrhythmias are suspected as the cause of syncope, however, ambulatory monitoring is inappropriate.

Electrophysiologic testing is indicated in patients with syncope of unknown origin who are found to have had a previous myocardial infarction, a depressed left ventricular ejection fraction, or nonsustained ventricular tachycardia. These patients should be presumed to be at high risk for sudden death from ventricular arrhythmias until proven otherwise, and should be hospitalized and monitored until ventricular arrhythmias are either ruled out or controlled.

The evaluation of patients with syncope has often been regarded as difficult and frustrating. However, by employing the principles outlined in this chapter, a diagnosis can be made relatively quickly in the vast majority of patients presenting with syncope.

16

Electrophysiologic Testing in Perspective: The Evaluation and Treatment of Cardiac Arrhythmias

In this final chapter, we will attempt to synthesize the information presented in the first 15 chapters into a general approach to the evaluation and treatment of cardiac arrhythmias, with emphasis on the appropriate use of the electrophysiology study.

The approach outlined in this chapter is an elementary and, indeed, almost a trivial one. Quite simply, the basic principle of our approach is to tailor the aggressiveness of the therapy to the severity of the arrhythmia being treated. Many of the serious mistakes that are made in the management of cardiac rhythm disturbances can be traced to a violation of this modest principle.

The three steps in evaluating and treating cardiac arrhythmias

The appropriate management of cardiac arrhythmias involves following a predetermined plan of therapy aimed at achieving specific goals. Those goals, in turn, are determined by the severity of the arrhythmia being treated. Thus, in evaluating and treating cardiac arrhythmias, three discrete steps are implicit.

Step 1. Assess the severity of the arrhythmia to be treated. This involves consideration of both the arrhythmia itself and the company it keeps – in terms of structural heart disease.

Step 2. Decide on the therapeutic endpoint. The physician decides whether the primary goal of treatment is to prevent death, to minimize harm, or to relieve symptoms.

Fogoros' Electrophysiologic Testing, Seventh Edition. Richard N. Fogoros and John M. Mandrola.
© 2023 John Wiley & Sons Ltd. Published 2023 by John Wiley & Sons Ltd.

Step 3. Design the treatment plan. The physician devises a treatment plan that is directly aimed at achieving the primary therapeutic endpoint.

The crucial step tying these steps together is education of the patient. The modern-day electrophysiologist must be a teacher and partner. In the early days of catheter ablation, the electrophysiology lab was primarily used to cure. The ablation of SVT, for instance, was akin to surgery. One procedure, one follow-up visit and that was it.

Electrophysiology, however, has now taken a larger role in management of chronic conditions. Atrial fibrillation is rarely cured; it requires ongoing management of comorbid conditions, such as the treatment of obesity, diabetes, and hypertension. Cardiac devices, such as ICDs, CRTs, and now conduction system pacing, require careful follow-up and partnership with patients, general cardiologists, and heart failure doctors.

Step 1. Assess the severity of the arrhythmia to be treated

As already stated, the most common and most serious mistake made in the management of cardiac arrhythmias is to institute therapy that is inappropriate for the arrhythmia being treated. This error most often results from the propensity of physicians to assign specific treatments to specific arrhythmias, without considering the setting in which the arrhythmia occurs.

The first step is obviously to diagnose the arrhythmia. In recent times, this rarely requires an invasive electrophysiology study.

The standard ECG, with its 12 looks (leads) at the heart's activation, is often the best clue. Skilled clinicians can sort out a right vs left atrial tachycardia, right vs left accessory pathways, and even the exit site of most ventricular tachycardias. But there is even more information to be gained from the lowly ECG: once the arrhythmia ceases, the baseline ECG offers clues regarding the underlying heart disease. A person who presents with wide-complex tachycardia whose baseline ECG has large q-waves and terminal delay in the QRS is likely to have scar-related VT. A person who presents with transient dizziness and near syncope who has right bundle branch block, left anterior fascicular block, and first-degree AV block may have transient complete heart block. And a patient with an atrial flutter with a slow atrial rate and long isoelectric periods between flutter waves who has had previous AF ablation likely has a left atrial flutter.

Modern-day monitoring has transformed the diagnosis of intermittent arrhythmia. From 24-hour monitors, to 2-week patch ECGs, to implantable loop recorders, the electrophysiologist has many tools with which to diagnosis an arrhythmia.

On rare occasions, the electrophysiology study can be used to sort out a diagnosis. More often than not, though, in this era, the EP study may find arrhythmias that were not previously known to exist. Examples include the induction of SVT during an AF ablation. This is an important finding as the SVT may have been a trigger for the AF. Another example is the diagnosis of a focal atrial tachycardia after ablation of an SVT.

The next step is to assess what symptoms are associated with the arrhythmia. Arrhythmias generally cause only a few types of symptoms: palpitations, lightheadedness or dizziness, loss of consciousness and sometimes fatigue and dyspnea. Palpitations are the most common symptom and are commonly associated with ectopic beats. Most patients can tolerate palpitations if this is the only symptom they experience, especially if they can be reassured that their arrhythmia is benign. Lightheadedness and dizziness, which occur with various levels of severity, tend to be associated either with bradyarrhythmias or with tachyarrhythmias that consist of more than isolated extra beats. Although many patients can tolerate occasional mild episodes of lightheadedness, others find these symptoms to be extremely disturbing.

Loss of consciousness from an arrhythmia indicates extreme hemodynamic compromise, and any bradyarrhythmia or tachyarrhythmia that produces this symptom should be considered to imply an elevated risk. An important exception to this rule is that syncope accompanied by bradycardias is most often vasoactive in nature. In such cases, the bradycardia itself is usually *not* the cause of syncope (instead, vasodilation is the cause) and should not be considered a lethal arrhythmia.

Some arrhythmias cause symptoms by producing or worsening symptoms of congestive heart failure. Any form of tachycardia that persists for weeks or months (such as persistent reentrant supraventricular tachycardia, or atrial fibrillation with a rapid ventricular response) can ultimately produce ventricular remodeling and dilation and thus congestive heart failure. In patients with diastolic dysfunction, whose noncompliant ventricles are dependent on atrial contraction to achieve a high end-diastolic pressure while maintaining a relatively normal mean atrial pressure, loss of that atrial contraction with the onset of atrial fibrillation can produce pulmonary congestion quite acutely.

When a patient has symptoms compatible with an arrhythmia, determining whether those symptoms are actually due to an arrhythmia is not always straightforward. Quite often, an ambulatory monitoring study will show arrhythmias and symptoms but will fail to show a correlation between the two. In these instances, the arrhythmia should not be construed as the cause of the symptoms. Because the appropriate treatment of many nonlethal arrhythmias depends on the symptoms they produce, every attempt should be made to document a correlation between the arrhythmia and the symptoms before any potentially toxic therapy is initiated. Further, several symptoms are often attributed to arrhythmias but in fact are only rarely due to arrhythmias. These symptoms include dyspnea, nonspecific fatigue, and seizures or localizing neurologic symptoms. Any of these symptoms, even if accompanied by cardiac arrhythmias, should prompt a thorough search for other causes.

Once it is determined that symptoms are due to the arrhythmia in question, those symptoms should be categorized in terms of their severity.

Equally important in this first step of assessing the severity of an arrhythmia is the presence or absence of structural heart disease. In the absence of structural disease, most (but not all) arrhythmias are benign.

An electrophysiologist makes this assessment with four main tools: the history (e.g., can a patient can exercise without limits?), exam, (e.g., are there murmurs of valvular disease or a third heart sound?), ECG, (as we discussed above), and noninvasive assessment. The latter includes an echocardiogram and stress testing to assess for ischemia.

The state of the heart is a huge factor in triaging and planning treatment. Keep in mind that many patients who first present with arrhythmia are fearful. When there is no structural heart disease, and you have a clear diagnosis, the patient can be reassured – which can be highly therapeutic in and of itself (Table 16.1).

Step 2. Decide on the therapeutic endpoint

Cardiac arrhythmias are treated because they produce symptoms, pose a threat to health, or have the potential to cause sudden death. Thus, there are three general therapeutic endpoints in treating cardiac

Table 16.1 Classification of the risk for sudden death imposed by arrhythmias.

High risk	Moderate risk	Low risk
Ventricular tachycardia	Complex ventricular ectopy with underlying heart disease	Premature atrial complexes
Ventricular fibrillation	Second-degree AV block	Premature ventricular complexes
Third-degree AV block with an inadequate escape	Third-degree AV block with adequate escape	Sinus node dysfunction
Wolff–Parkinson–White syndrome with rapid antegrade conduction in atrial fibrillation	Atrial fibrillation	Supraventricular tachycardias
		Complex ventricular ectopy with no underlying heart disease
		First-degree AV block

arrhythmias: to relieve symptoms, to maintain health, or to prevent sudden death. Before a treatment plan can be devised, it is vital to decide which of these goals is to be pursued and to keep that goal clearly in mind.

The appropriate goal of therapy should be chosen based on the severity of the arrhythmia and state of the underlying heart condition, as determined in step 1. The following generalizations can be made. Low-risk arrhythmias, because they do not have the potential to produce death, should be treated only if they are producing symptoms that are disruptive to the patient's life, in which case the goal of therapy is merely to reduce symptoms. High-risk arrhythmias, on the other hand, should always be treated, and the goal of therapy with these arrhythmias is to prevent sudden death.

Moderate-risk arrhythmias are the most problematic. Two arrhythmias tend to fall into this category: atrial fibrillation and complex ventricular ectopy in the setting of significant underlying cardiac disease.

Atrial fibrillation presents a problem (aside from the symptoms caused by the arrhythmia itself) because it poses a long-term risk of embolic stroke, and in some patients it can produce or exacerbate heart failure. Further, as we have discussed, "getting rid" of atrial fibrillation (with either antiarrhythmic drugs or ablation) can be extremely difficult and risky. So, in treating this arrhythmia the clinician must decide whether to use a "conservative" approach (controlling the rate response and anticoagulating) or an "aggressive" approach (trying to restore and maintain sinus rhythm). Neither of these approaches is easy or straightforward, and both may require escalating attempts at achieving the therapeutic goal (for instance, advancing from drug-based therapy to ablation-based therapy).

Complex ventricular ectopy, in the setting of significant underlying cardiac disease, is associated with an increased risk of sudden death. However, trying to abolish these arrhythmias with most antiarrhythmic drugs merely increases the risk, and treating the ectopy with amiodarone or ablation has not been shown to reduce risk. Instead, lowering the risk of sudden death in these patients usually comes down to aggressively optimizing their medical care, and deciding whether they are candidates for an implantable defibrillator.

Step 3. Design the treatment plan

The final step in the management of cardiac arrhythmias is to decide on a therapeutic plan aimed at achieving the chosen goal of therapy. Keeping the goal of therapy clearly in mind is vitally important because treatments for similar arrhythmias may vary markedly from patient to patient, depending on whether the aim of therapy is to prevent sudden death or merely to relieve symptoms. (It should be noted that in managing bradyarrhythmias, the basic therapy for both relieving symptoms and preventing sudden death is essentially the same – a permanent pacemaker. The following discussion thus pertains mainly to ectopic beats and tachyarrhythmias.)

Treating to Relieve Symptoms

When the primary goal of therapy is to relieve symptoms, the physician must determine what steps are necessary to achieve that goal. For most patients in whom symptom relief is the therapeutic endpoint, the arrhythmia being treated is benign. Thus, therapy aimed at relieving symptoms is often (and appropriately) less aggressive than therapy aimed at preventing sudden death.

The first and, in our opinion, most underrated step is education and perhaps teaching patients how to manage the arrhythmia themselves.

For instance, benign premature beats, short runs of SVT or even AF in a low-risk patient may be best approached by ignoring the symptoms or resting transiently. This strategy often works well because it is often the anxiety of an arrhythmia that causes the most distress. A calm and reassuring clinician who is knowledgeable in arrhythmia management may be able to relieve as much suffering with words as with a prescription pad or catheter.

Empiric trial-and-error therapeutic attempts are often appropriate and are frequently performed on an outpatient basis. Generally, milder therapies are tried first, moving progressively and as necessary to more aggressive treatments. Before each escalation of therapy, careful consideration is given as to whether the symptom being treated warrants yet more aggressive therapy. The use of as-needed medications has increased in favor. A patient with intermittent infrequent tachycardias not associated with heart disease may benefit from use of short-acting medications such as β-blockers or IC antiarrhythmic drugs. This pill-in-the-pocket approach avoids the use of daily medications for arrhythmias that occur much less frequently.

However, a patient may have an arrhythmia that is itself non-life-threatening but that produces severely disabling symptoms. In such instances, it may be entirely appropriate to attempt very aggressive therapy. As an example, consider a patient with severe cardiomyopathy who has chronic atrial fibrillation with a rapid ventricular response, resulting in moderate decompensation of the patient's congestive heart failure. With such a patient, one might begin with attempts to control the ventricular response pharmacologically. But if this is unsuccessful, it would be entirely appropriate to move on to more radical measures, such as His bundle ablation and insertion of a permanent pacemaker. Therefore, one may arrive at aggressive therapy in relieving the symptoms of an arrhythmia, but in general only after less aggressive measures have failed.

The electrophysiology study has only a moderate role in managing arrhythmias when the suppression of symptoms is the primary goal. Although the electrophysiology can help in assessing the presence of various nonlethal arrhythmias (such as sinus node or AV node dysfunction), this study cannot supply much information on the symptoms caused by these arrhythmias.

For several types of arrhythmia, however, the electrophysiology study can be helpful in abolishing symptoms. This is especially true for most reentrant supraventricular tachycardias, which usually can be cured with transcatheter ablation.

Treating to Prevent Sudden Death

Once the physician decides that the primary goal of therapy is to prevent the patient's sudden death, a treatment plan should be devised that reflects the urgency of the therapeutic endpoint. By its nature, sudden death occurs instantaneously and unexpectedly. Thus, when a patient is judged to be a candidate for sudden death, immediate and aggressive efforts should be made to prevent this event. Ideally, these efforts should include placing the patient in the hospital and on a monitor until adequate therapy is derived. Trial-and-error (empiric) methods of treatment are inappropriate. When the goal of therapy is to prevent sudden death, the initial therapy must be effective because the physician is unlikely to have a second chance should the initial therapy prove ineffective.

With regard to patients who are at high risk for sudden death from ventricular arrhythmias, the treatment "plan" has been greatly simplified over the past few years. In contrast to the days when the electrophysiology study was used as the cornerstone of a complex therapy selection strategy, today the "baseline" treatment strategy is almost always the same: to insert an implantable defibrillator. The electrophysiology study, when done at all, is generally used to help determine how to optimally program the implantable defibrillator, for instance in optimizing antitachycardia pacing.

For the other major variety of arrhythmia that poses an increased risk of sudden death – a bypass tract with rapid antegrade conduction – the electrophysiology study with ablation remains the mainstay of effective treatment.

Conclusion

This final chapter outlines a general approach to, and a perspective on, the use of the electrophysiology study in the management of cardiac arrhythmias. Devising a reasonable treatment plan depends on defining the goals of therapy. Those goals, in turn, depend on the severity of the arrhythmia and of the symptoms caused by the arrhythmia. The electrophysiology study can be of moderate help in assessing the severity of cardiac arrhythmias and can be extremely helpful in abolishing both the symptoms and the risk caused by several cardiac arrhythmias.

Most serious mistakes in treating cardiac arrhythmias stem from failing to match the aggressiveness of therapy to the severity of the arrhythmia being treated. Using a logical, stepwise approach to the evaluation and treatment of cardiac arrhythmias allows one to avoid this critical error.

Index

Fogoros' Electrophysiologic Testing, Seventh Edition. Richard N. Fogoros and John M. Mandrola.
© 2023 John Wiley & Sons Ltd. Published 2023 by John Wiley & Sons Ltd.

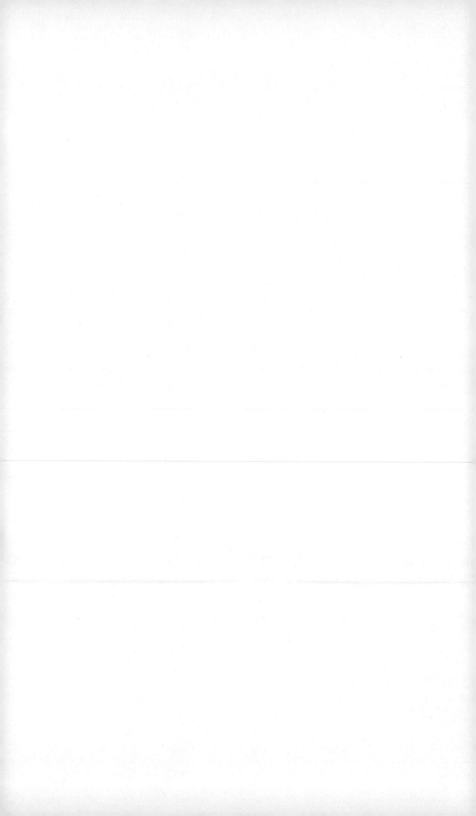